Medical Parasitology

The Practical Approach Series

SERIES EDITORS

D. RICKWOOD
Department of Biology, University of Essex
Wivenhoe Park, Colchester, Essex CO4 3SQ, UK

B. D. HAMES
Department of Biochemistry and Molecular Biology
University of Leeds, Leeds LS2 9JT, UK

★ indicates new and forthcoming titles

Affinity Chromatography
Anaerobic Microbiology
Animal Cell Culture (2nd Edition)
Animal Virus Pathogenesis
Antibodies I and II
★ Basic Cell Culture
Behavioural Neuroscience
Biochemical Toxicology
★ Bioenergetics
Biological Data Analysis
Biological Membranes
Biomechanics—Materials
Biomechanics—Structures and Systems
Biosensors
★ Carbohydrate Analysis (2nd Edition)
Cell–Cell Interactions
★ The Cell Cycle
★ Cell Growth and Apoptosis
Cellular Calcium
Cellular Interactions in Development
Cellular Neurobiology
Clinical Immunology
Crystallization of Nucleic Acids and Proteins
★ Cytokines (2nd Edition)
The Cytoskeleton
Diagnostic Molecular Pathology I and II
Directed Mutagenesis
★ DNA Cloning 1: Core Techniques (2nd Edition)
★ DNA Cloning 2: Expression Systems (2nd Edition)
★ DNA Cloning 3: Complex Genomes (2nd Edition)
★ DNA Cloning 4: Mammalian Systems (2nd Edition)
Electron Microscopy in Biology
Electron Microscopy in Molecular Biology
Electrophysiology

Enzyme Assays
Essential Developmental Biology
Essential Molecular Biology I and II
Experimental Neuroanatomy
★ Extracellular Matrix
★ Flow Cytometry (2nd Edition)
Gas Chromatography
Gel Electrophoresis of Nucleic Acids (2nd Edition)
Gel Electrophoresis of Proteins (2nd Edition)
★ Gene Probes 1 and 2
Gene Targeting
Gene Transcription
Glycobiology
Growth Factors
Haemopoiesis
Histocompatibility Testing
★ HIV Volumes 1 and 2
Human Cytogenetics I and II (2nd Edition)
Human Genetic Disease Analysis
Immunocytochemistry
In Situ Hybridization
Iodinated Density Gradient Media
★ Ion Channels
Lipid Analysis
Lipid Modification of Proteins
Lipoprotein Analysis
Liposomes
Mammalian Cell Biotechnology
Medical Bacteriology
Medical Mycology
★ Medical Parasitology
★ Medical Virology
Microcomputers in Biology
Molecular Genetic Analysis of Populations
★ Molecular Genetics of Yeast
Molecular Imaging in Neuroscience
Molecular Neurobiology
Molecular Plant Pathology I and II
Molecular Virology
Monitoring Neuronal Activity
Mutagenicity Testing
★ Neural Cell Culture
Neural Transplantation
Neurochemistry
Neuronal Cell Lines
NMR of Biological Macromolecules
★ Non-isotopic Methods in Molecular Biology
Nucleic Acid Hybridization
Nucleic Acid and Protein Sequence Analysis
Oligonucleotides and Analogues
Oligonucleotide Synthesis
PCR 1
★ PCR 2
★ Peptide Antigens
Photosynthesis: Energy Transduction
★ Plant Cell Biology
★ Plant Cell Culture (2nd Edition)
Plant Molecular Biology

★ Plasmids (2nd Edition)
Pollination Ecology
Postimplantation Mammalian Embryos
Preparative Centrifugation
Prostaglandins and Related Substances
★ Protein Blotting
Protein Engineering
Protein Function
Protein Phosphorylation
Protein Purification Applications
Protein Purification Methods
Protein Sequencing
Protein Structure
Protein Targeting
Proteolytic Enzymes
★ Pulsed Field Gel Electrophoresis
Radioisotopes in Biology
Receptor Biochemistry
Receptor–Effector Coupling
Receptor–Ligand Interactions
RNA Processing I and II
Signal Transduction
Solid Phase Peptide Synthesis
Transcription Factors
Transcription and Translation
Tumour Immunobiology
Virology
Yeast

Medical Parasitology

A Practical Approach

Edited by

S. H. GILLESPIE

Department of Medical Microbiology,
Royal Free Hospital,
Pond Street, London NW3 2QG, UK

and

P. M. HAWKEY

Department of Microbiology,
University of Leeds,
Leeds LS2 9JT, UK

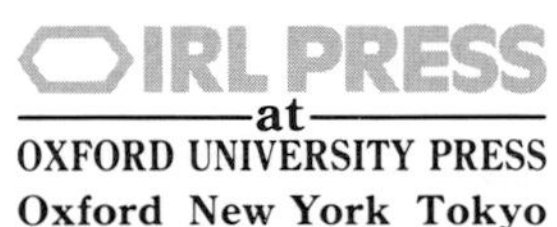

Oxford University Press, Walton Street, Oxford OX2 6DP
Oxford New York
Athens Auckland Bangkok Bombay
Calcutta Cape Town Dar es Salaam Delhi
Florence Hong Kong Istanbul Karachi
Kuala Lumpur Madras Madrid Melbourne
Mexico City Nairobi Paris Singapore
Taipei Tokyo Toronto
and associated companies in
Berlin Ibadan

Oxford is a trade mark of Oxford University Press

Published in the United States
by Oxford University Press Inc., New York

A catalogue record for this book is available from the British Library

Library of Congress Cataloging in Publication Data
Medical parasitology : a practical approach / edited by S.H. Gillespie, P.M. Hawkey.–1st ed.
(The Practical approach series ; ISSN v. 152)
Includes bibliographical references and index.
1. Medical parasitology–Laboratory manuals. I. Gillespie, S. H. II. Hawkey, P. M. (Peter M.) III. Series.
[DNLM: 1. Parasitic Diseases–diagnosis–laboratory manuals. 2. Parasitology–laboratory manuals. QX 25 M489 1995]
QR251.M43 1995 616.9'6075–dc20 94 47178

ISBN 0 19 963301 0 (Hbk)
ISBN 0 19 963300 2 (Pbk)

Typeset by Footnote Graphics, Warminster, Wilts
Printed in Great Britain by Information Press Ltd, Eynsham, Oxon.

Preface

The nature of parasitology has been changed in recent years by the development in mass foreign travel and the onset of the HIV epidemic. Parasitology is no longer the province of specialist laboratories diagnosing tropical exotica but has entered the mainstream of clinical microbiology. This book has been written to reflect this fact.

The introduction provides an overview of the main diagnostic approaches and tables of differential diagnoses. There is a chapter for each of the main species or groups of parasites written by a specialist in the field. These chapters have been particularly prepared to allow the non-specialist microbiologist to diagnose parasitological infections which are presenting in patients that are not resident in endemic areas. The book provides detailed practical protocols for diagnosis for both temperate and tropical zone parasites. We hope you find this book is a useful adjunct in your daily diagnostic work.

London S.H.G.
Leeds P.M.H.
August 1994

Contents

The colour plates referred to in the text fall between pp. xviii and 1.

Contributors

J. P. ACKERS
The London School of Hygiene and Tropical Medicine, Keppel Street, London WC1E 7HT, UK.

JAMES C. ALLAN
Department of Biological Sciences, University of Salford, Salford M5 4WT, UK.

PETER L. CHIODINI
Department of Clinical Parasitology, The Hospital for Tropical Diseases, 4 St. Pancras Way, London NW1 0PE, UK.

SHEILA CLARK
Department of Clinical Parasitology, The Hospital for Tropical Diseases, 4 St. Pancras Way, London NW1 0PE, UK.

PHILIP S. CRAIG
Department of Biological Sciences, University of Salford, Salford M5 4WT, UK.

ALASTAIR DEERY
Department of Cytopathology, Royal Free Hospital, Rowland Hill Street, London NW3 2QG, UK.

D. A. DENHAM
The London School of Hygiene and Tropical Medicine, Keppel Street, London WC1E 7HT, UK.

N. FRANCIS
Department of Histopathology, Charing Cross and Westminster Medical School, Charing Cross Hospital, Fulham Palace Road, London W6 8RF, UK.

S. H. GILLESPIE
Department of Medical Microbiology, Royal Free Hospital, Pond Street, London NW3 2QG, UK.

P. M. HAWKEY
Department of Microbiology, University of Leeds, Leeds LS2 9JT, UK.

RICHARD E. HOLLIMAN
Public Health Laboratory, Department of Medical Microbiology, St. George's Hospital, London SW17 0QT, UK.

JULIE D. JOHNSON
Public Health Laboratory, Department of Medical Microbiology, St. George's Hospital, London SW17 0QT, UK.

IAN MARSHALL
Department of Parasitology, School of Tropical Medicine, Pembroke Place, Liverpool L3 5QA, UK.

MICHAEL T. ROGAN
Department of Biological Sciences, University of Salford, Salford M5 4WT, UK.

H. V. SMITH
Scottish Parasite Reference Laboratory, Department of Parasitology, Stobhill NHS Trust, Glasgow G21 3UW, UK.

R. R. SUSWILLO
The London School of Hygiene and Tropical Medicine, Keppel Street, London WC1E 7HT, UK.

D. C. WARHURST
The London School of Hygiene and Tropical Medicine, Keppel Street, London WC1E 7HT, UK.

J. E. WILLIAMS
The London School of Hygiene and Tropical Medicine, Keppel Street, London WC1E 7HT, UK.

Plates

Plate 1

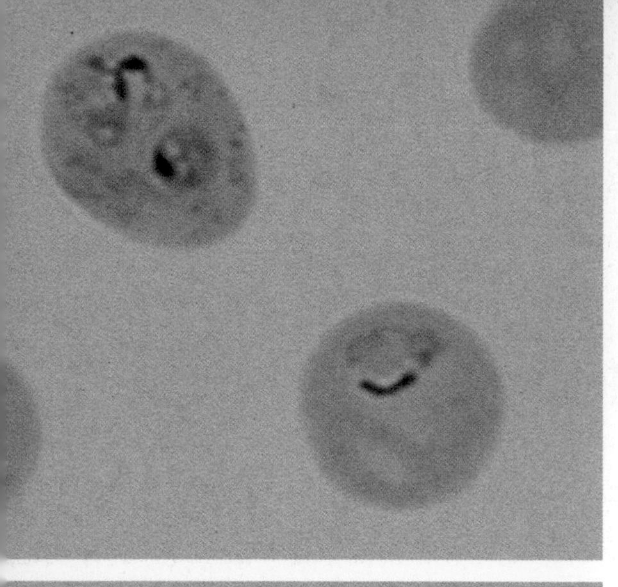

(a) *P. falciparum* early ring form and doubly infected red cell.

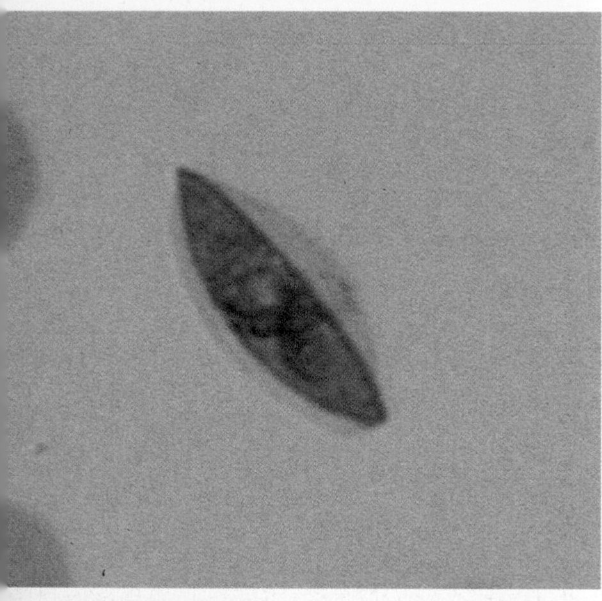

(b) *P. falciparum* gametocyte.

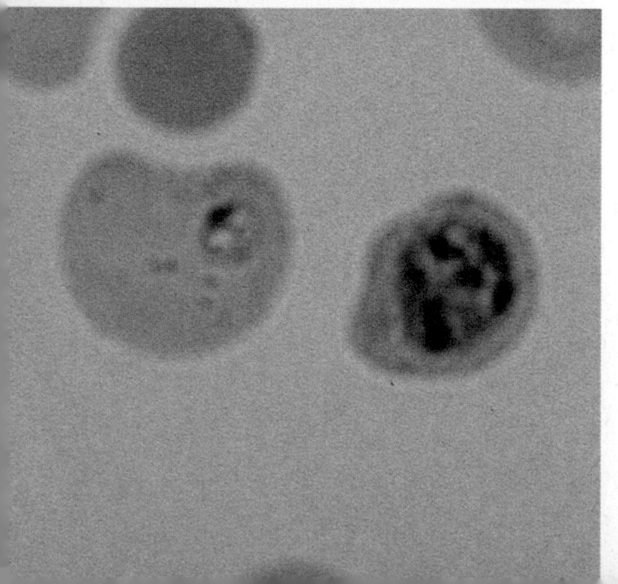

(c) *P. falciparum* early ring and pre-schizont.

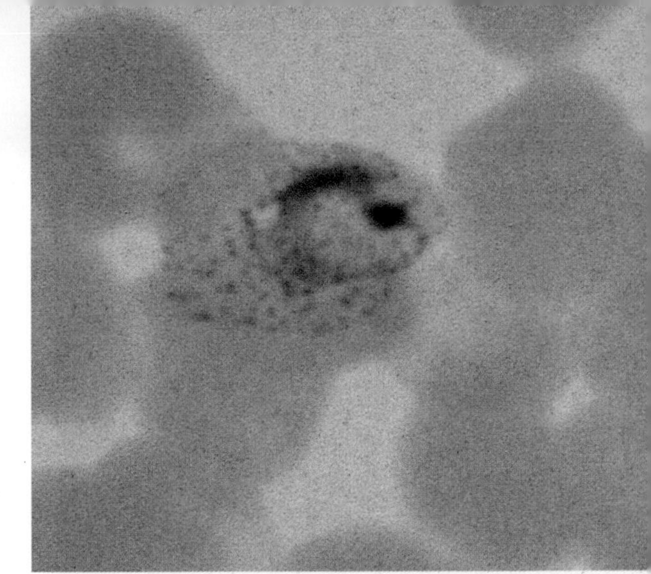

(d) *P. vivax* trophozoite with typical amoeboid morphology and Schuffner's dots.

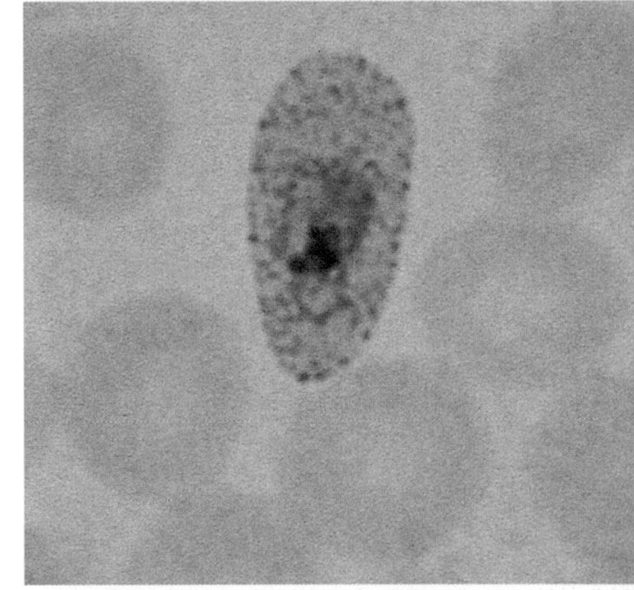

(e) *P. ovale* trophozoite with oval morphology and Jame's dots.

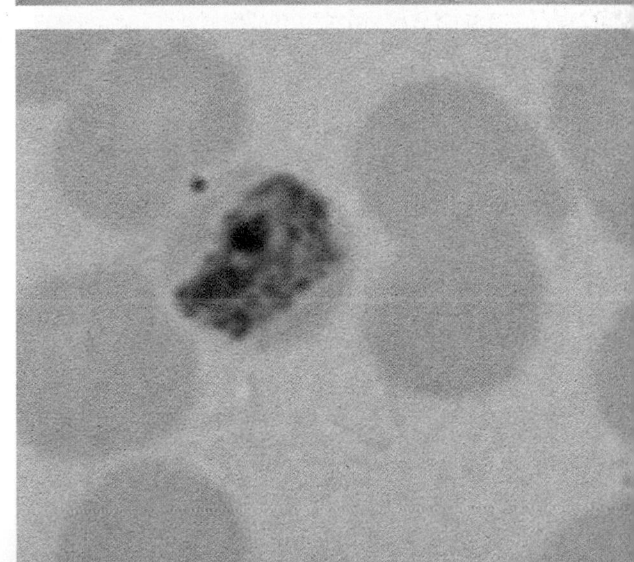

(f) *P. malariae* band form.

Plate 2

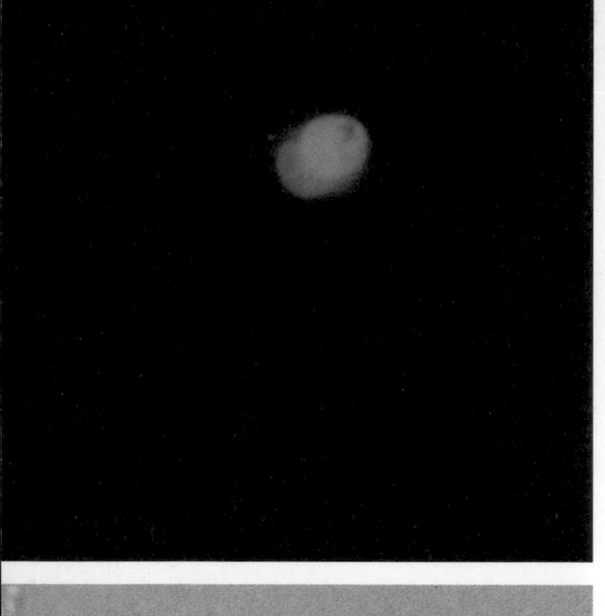

(a) *Pneumocystic carinii* identified by immunofluorescence.

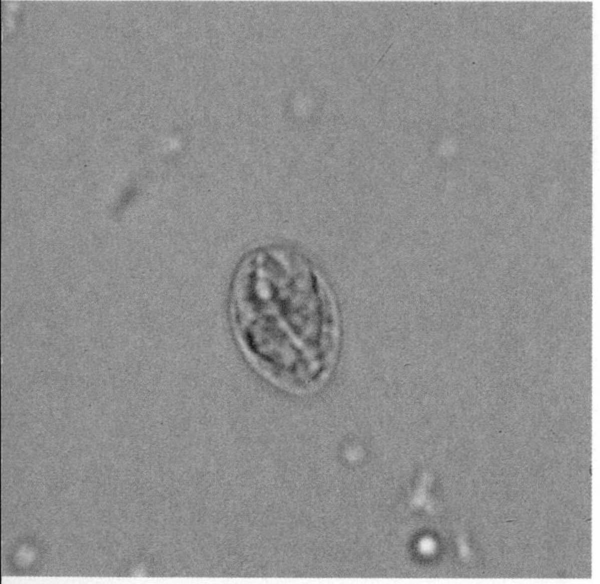

(b) *G. lamblia* cyst 9–13 μm.

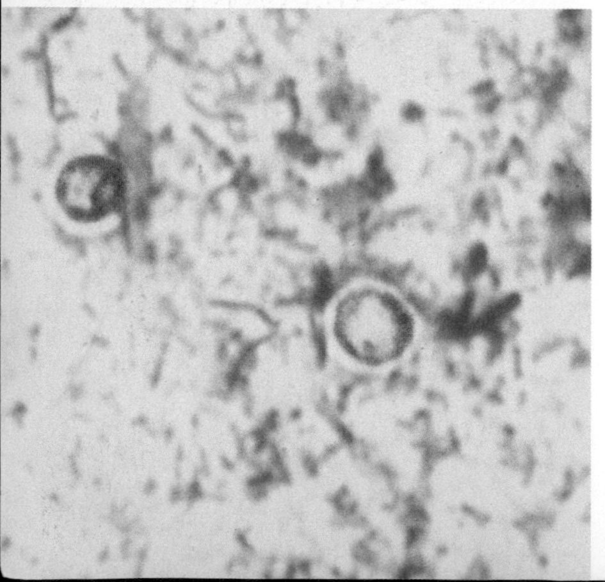

(c) Ziehl–Neelsen stained *Cryptosporidium* cysts 4–6 μm.

(d) Ziehl-Neelsen stained *Isospora belli* cysts 25–30 μm.

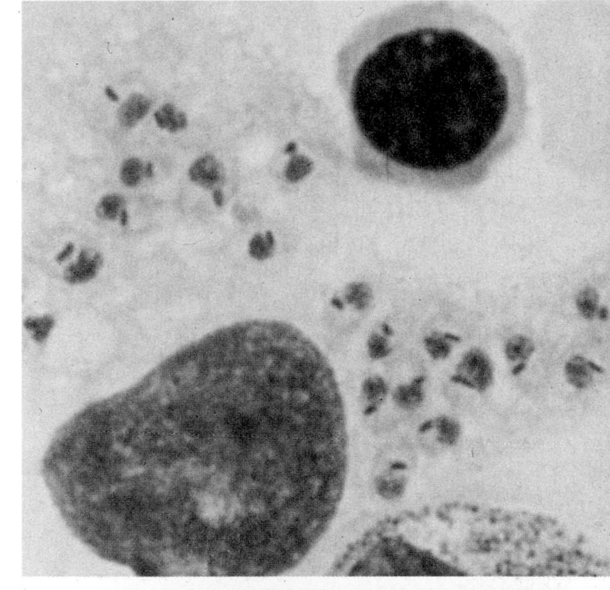

(e) Amastigote of *L. donovani* in a bone marrow smear (Giemsa).

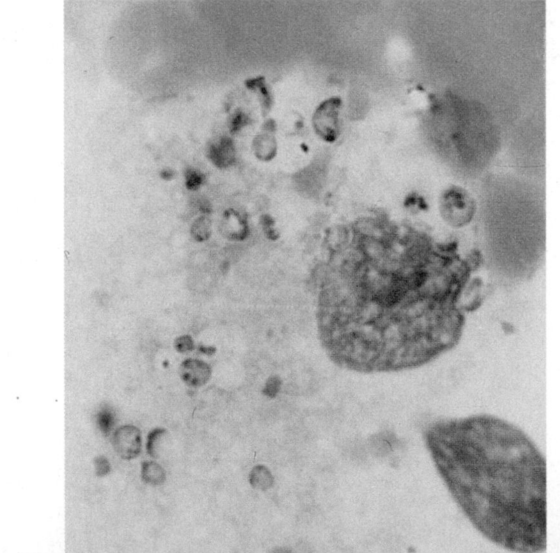

(f) *Histoplasma capsulatum* in a bone marrow smear from an AIDS patient (Giemsa).

Plate 3

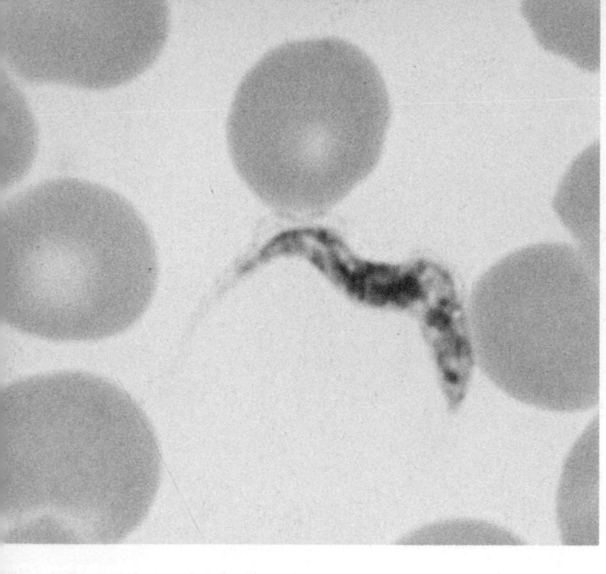

(a) Trypomastigote of *Trypanosoma brucei* var *rhodesiense* (Giemsa).

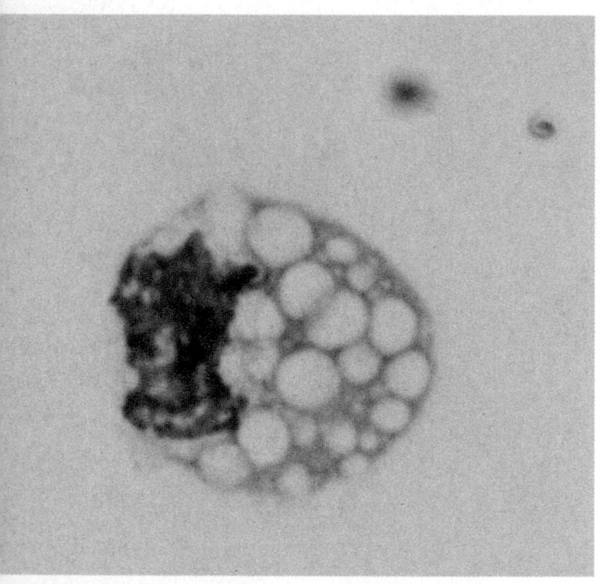

(b) Morula cell in CSF from a case of Gambian sleeping sickness (Giemsa).

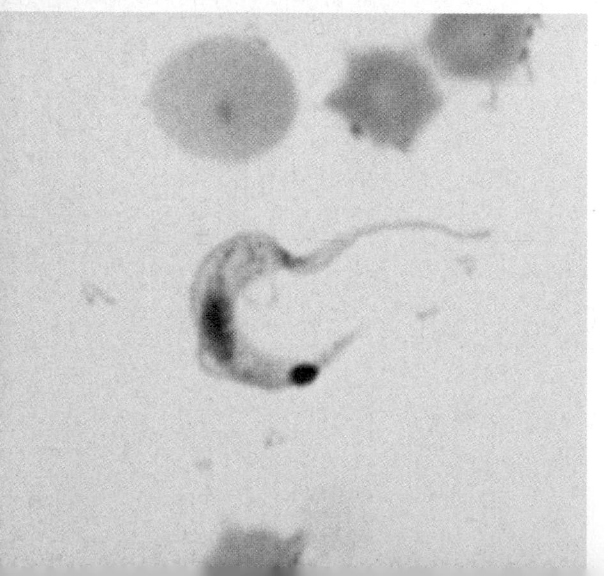

(c) Trypomastigote of *T. cruzi* (Giemsa).

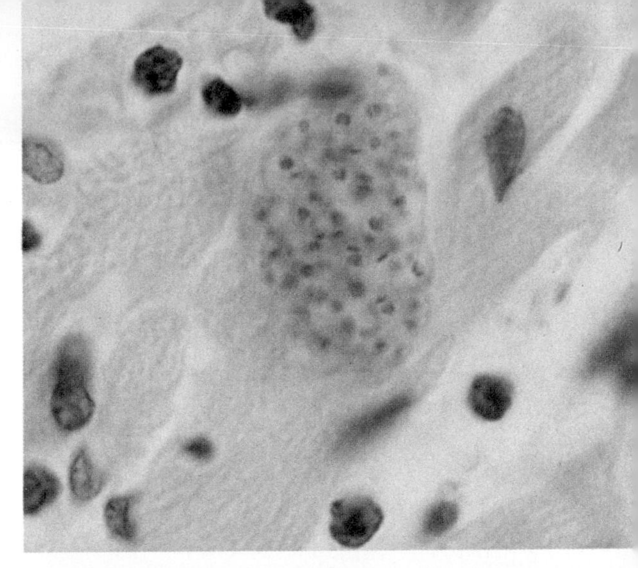

(d) Pseudocyst of *T. cruzi* in human heart muscle (H&E).

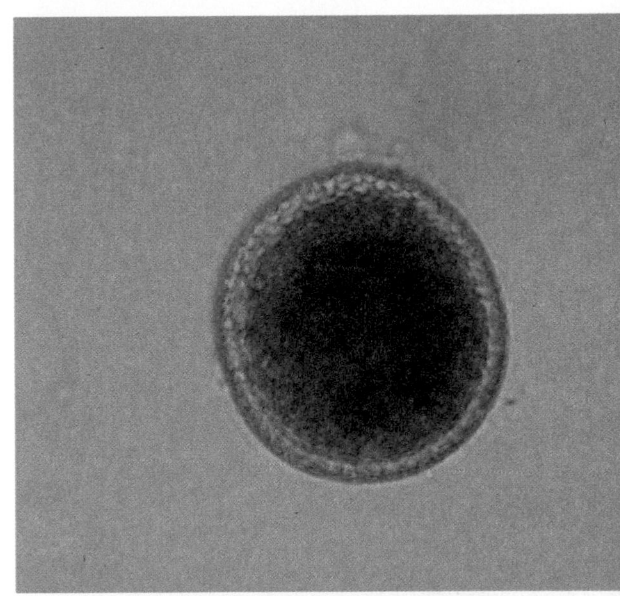

(e) *Toxocara canis* Un-embroyonated egg.

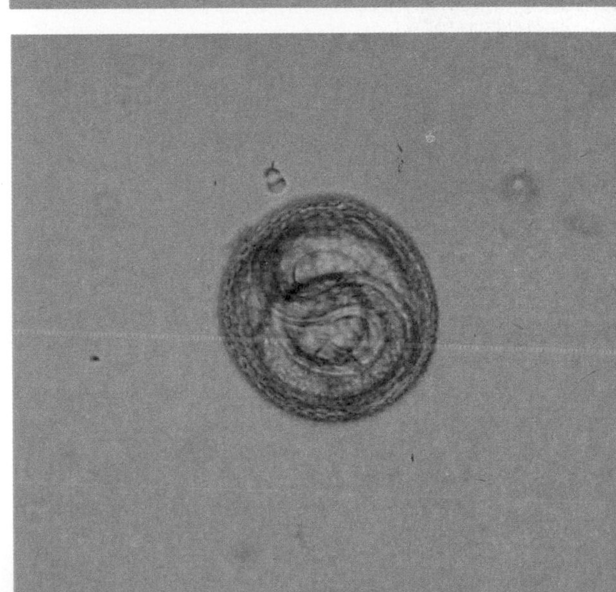

(f) *Toxocara canis* egg with developing larva.

Plate 4

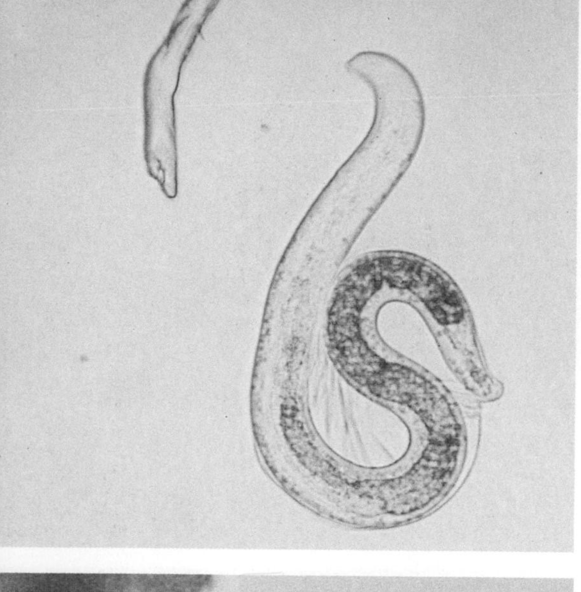

(a) *Toxocara canis* hatched larva.

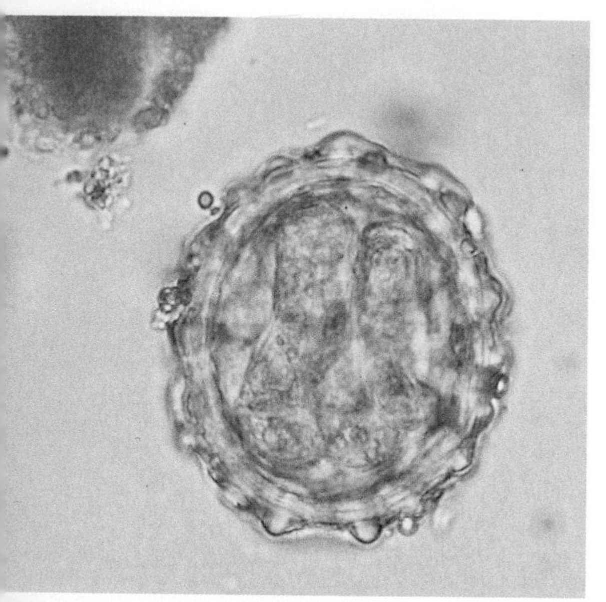

(b) *Ascaris lumbricoides* fertile ovum $40 \times 60\ \mu m$.

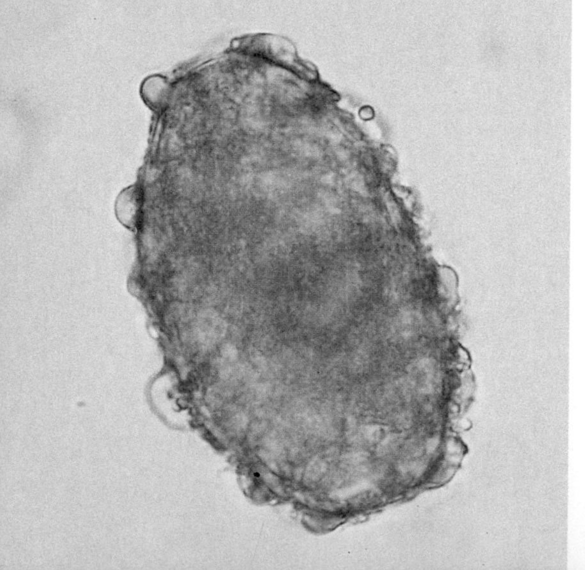

(c) *A. lumbricoides* infertile ovum $45 \times 90\ \mu m$.

(d) *Trichuris trichiura* ovum 22 × 50 μm.

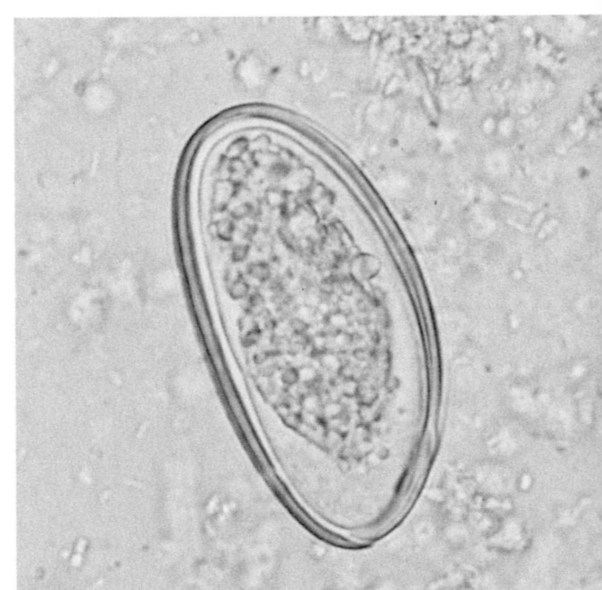

(e) *Enterobius vermicularis* ovum 30 × 55 μm.

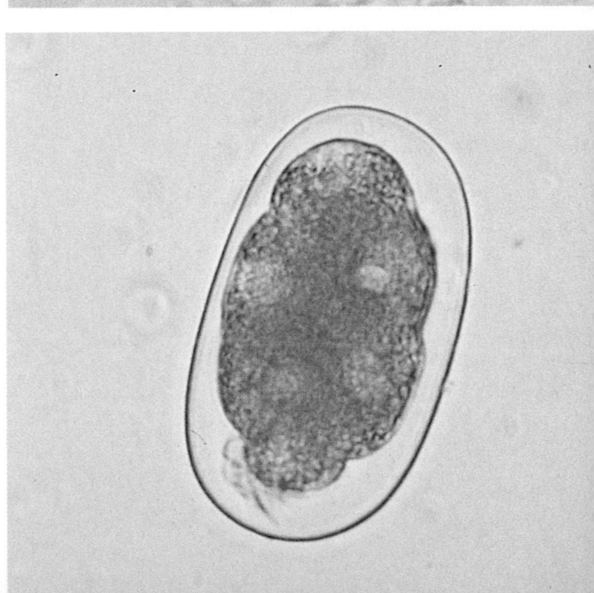

(f) Hookworm ovum 40 × 65 μm.

Plate 5

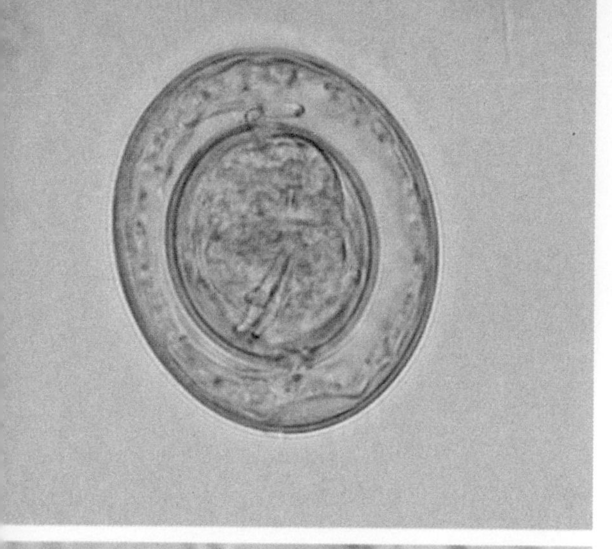

(a) *Hymenolepis nana* ovum
30×45 μm.

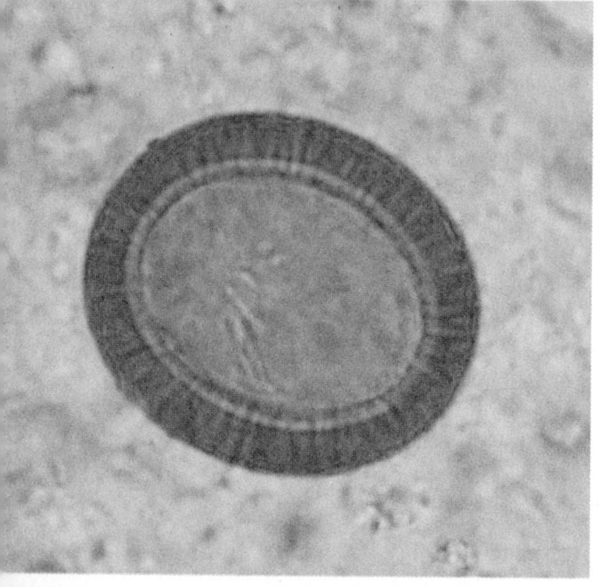

(b) *Taenia* spp. ovum 33×43 μm.

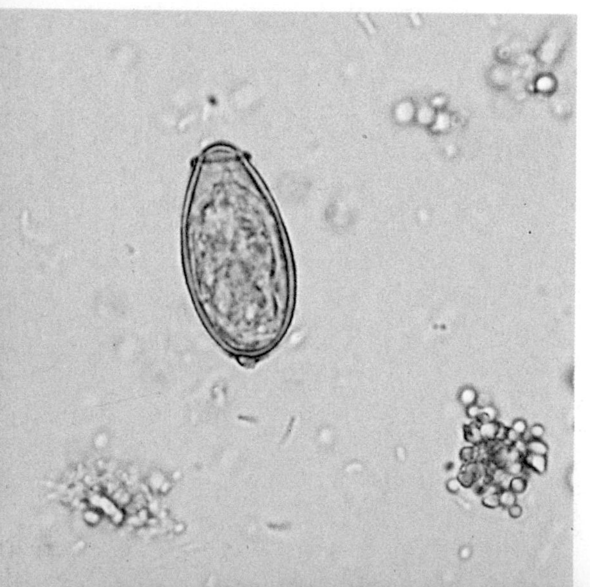

(c) *Opisthorchis sinensis* ovum
16×30 μm.

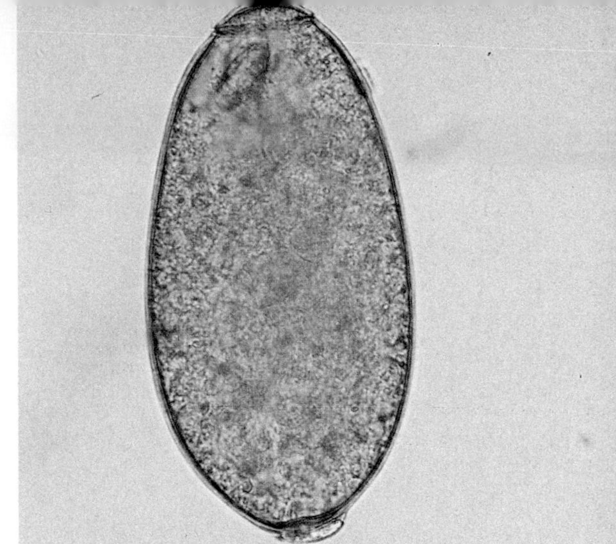

(d) *Paragonimus westermanni* ovum 50–65 × 70–100 μm.

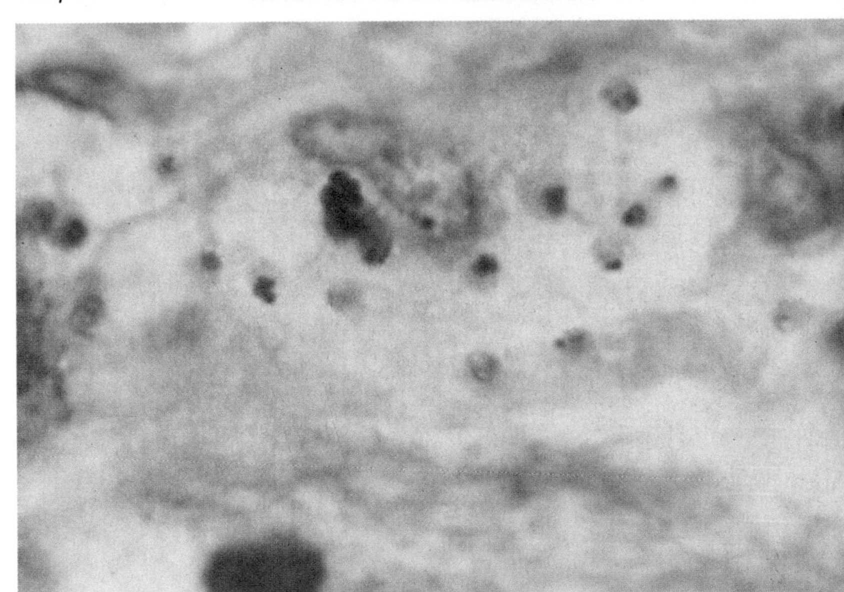

(e) *P. falciparum* parasitized red cells adhering to a brain capillary.

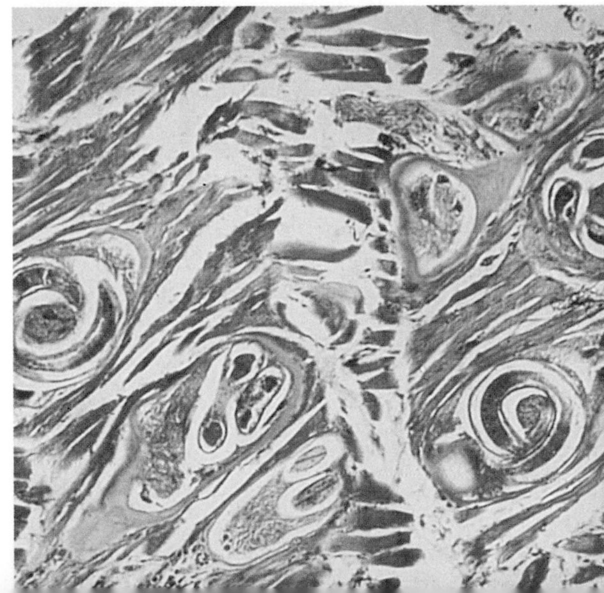

(f) *Trichinella spiralis* in tongue.

Plate 6

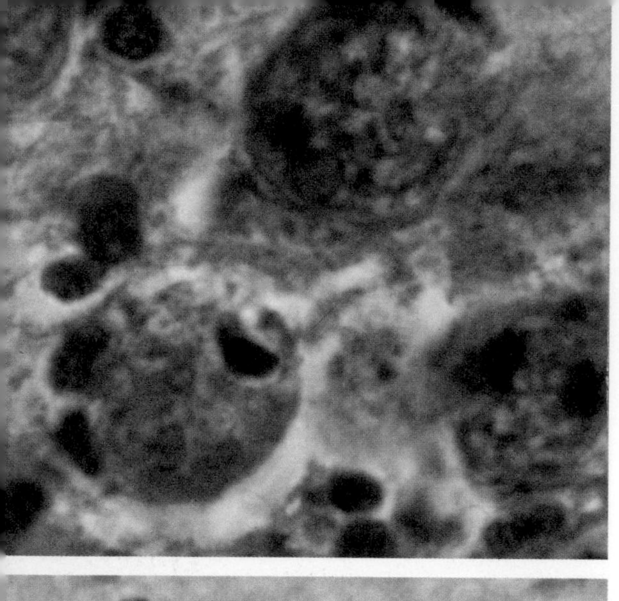

(a) *Entamobea histolytica* in the colon (H&E).

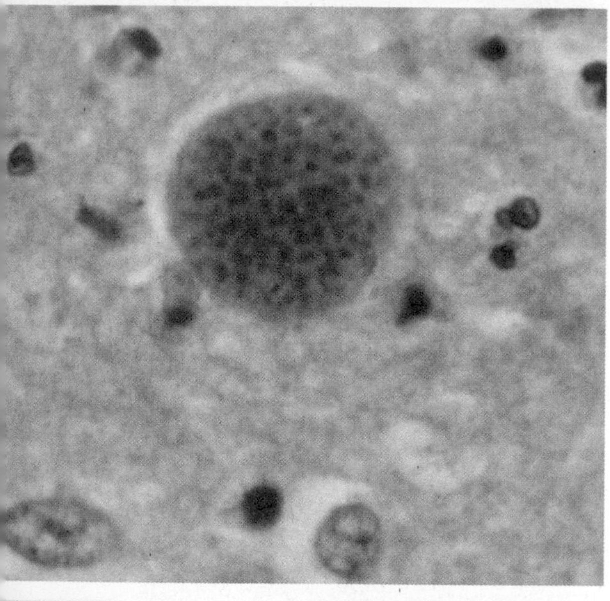

(b) *Toxoplasma gondii* zoites in the brain (H&E).

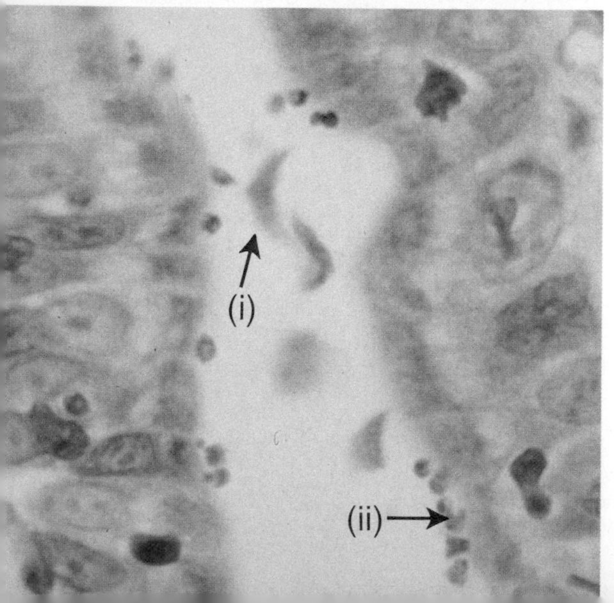

(c) Trophozoites of *Giardia lamblia* (i) and cyst of *Cryptosporidium parvum* (ii) in the villus.

(d) Microsporidia: section of small bowel showing numerous microsporidia in surface enterocytes (H&E).

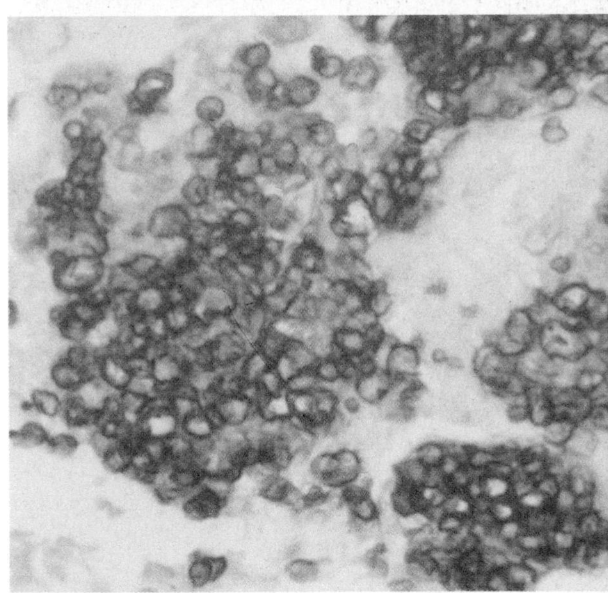

(e) *P. carinii* stained by immunoperoxidase method.

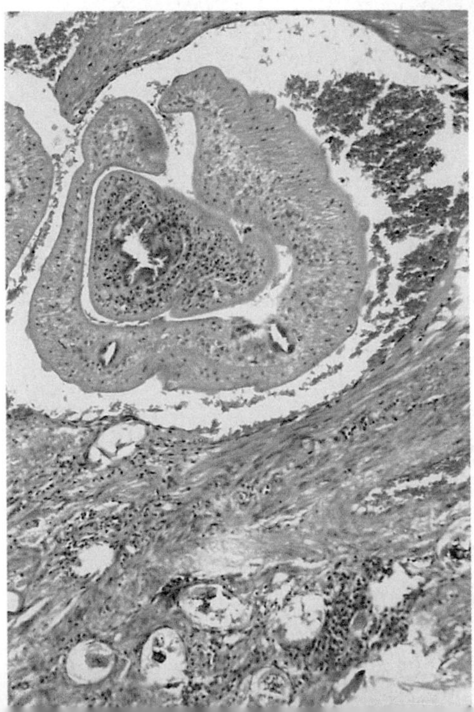

(f) Schistosomiasis of the cervix, showing adult male worm in the gynaecophoric canal of the female with ova in surrounding tissue.

1

Strategies for the diagnosis of parasitic infections

S. H. GILLESPIE and P. M. HAWKEY

1. Introduction

The organisms which are characteristically referred to as parasites are a heterogeneous group which range in size from microsporidia to complex multicellular organisms, such as *Taenia saginata*. Parasitic infections are found in all geographic areas and several, such as toxoplasmosis and toxocariasis, are common in temperate countries. Protozoa and helminths have historically been diagnosed and treated by a different group of doctors and scientists than other human pathogens, i.e. parasitologists and tropical disease specialists, rather than clinical microbiologists or infectious disease specialists. This division has arisen, in part, because of the tropical orientation of much parasitological investigation. Development of individual travel in the modern world has broken down the time barrier which used to stand between the developed and developing world. Increased numbers of journeys made to tropical countries have made infections, which might once have been thought of as exotic, commonplace. There is, therefore, a need for a greater awareness of the diagnosis of parasitological conditions amongst clinical microbiologists and infectious disease specialists.

2. Approach to the patient

In making a diagnosis of a parasitic infection, a full history is required, particularly the travel history which is considered in detail later. The history should include details of the presenting complaint, e.g. fever or weight loss. Many of the symptoms may be very subtle and thus repeated history taking may be beneficial, as the patient may remember important details or understand the significance of varying aspects on a second or subsequent consultation. The natural history of the complaint is of great importance. Symptoms may change over time, thus a patient who had recently been to Africa may remember a small itchy lesion on the lower leg, which was followed by the start of a febrile illness four to five weeks later, might suggest the diagnosis of acute schistosomiasis. Clearly, the presence of a fever on alternate days might point to the diagnosis of malaria, caused by *Plasmodium vivax* or *P. ovale*.

The presence of other key symptoms must be carefully sought. The most important of these is fever, and details of the degree and duration should be recorded together with any periodicity. In some conditions fever may have occurred as part of the early phase of infection, as in the case of schistosomiasis, so a history of fevers in the past which have subsequently resolved,

Table 1. Designation of abbreviations for places of acquisition used in Chapter 1

Abbreviation	Place of acquisition
AF	Africa
AM	America—(N) North, (S) South, (C) Central
AS	Asia
EUR	Europe
AUS	Australasia
WW	World-wide

Table 2. Parasitic infections causing persisting and relapsing fevers

Geographic distribution	Place
Focal	
Malaria	AF, AM (C,S), AS, EUR, AUS
Trypanosomiasis, African	AF
Trypanosomiasis, American (Chagas' disease)	AM (C,S)
Schistosomiasis (Katayama fever)	AF, AM (C,S), AS
Leishmaniasis, visceral	AF, AM (C,S,N), AS, EUR
Filariasis	AF, AM (C,S), AS, AUS
Loiasis	AF
Onchocerciasis	AF, AM (C,S), AS
Babesiosis	AM (C,N), EUR, (AF, AS?)
Angiostrongyliasis due to *Parastrongylus costaricensis*	AM
Widespread	
Amoebiasis	
Toxoplasmosis	
Toxocariasis (visceral larva migrans)	
Trichinellosis [a]	
Pneumocystis carinii infection [b]	
Cryptosporidiosis [b]	

[a] Increased frequency of infections reported in some immigrant groups in the United States because of food preparation habits. Infection can be acquired in the United States.
Strongyloidiasis hyperinfection syndrome in compromised hosts may be associated with recurring fevers, sometimes caused by bacterial infections.

[b] In immunocompromised individuals, especially those infected with human immunodeficiency virus.

should be recorded. It should be remembered that many patients express their fear of tropical disease by reporting fever, thus the temperature should be measured on presentation, and it may be necessary to admit a patient to observe whether fever is actually present. A list of parasitic infections which cause persistent fever is found in *Table 2*. *Table 1* lists the abbreviations used in this chapter for the distribution of agents.

2.1 Gastro-intestinal symptoms

Diarrhoea is an important symptom in infections caused by intestinal protozoa. The diarrhoea of amoebiasis is characteristically bulky and has an offensive odour. Blood staining is common, and symptoms are often chronic. In giardiasis, the stools are often bulky and fatty. Many patients complain of borborygmy, which may not abate after the acute attack. Watery diarrhoea is characteristic of patients infected with cryptosporidia or isospora. In most, this is self-limiting, but in severely immunocompromised patients, intractable diarrhoea can develop. Parasitic agents associated with diarrhoea are listed in *Table 3*.

Most intestinal helminth infections cause minimal gastro-intestinal symptoms, unless the worm load is heavy, when crampy abdominal pains may be found. Curiously, abdominal pain is a common symptom of toxocariasis, although this parasite does not have an intestinal stage in the human host. Tapeworms rarely produce clinical symptoms but occasionally patients may report passing segments in the stool. More disturbing for the patients is when segments escape *per ano* under their own muscular strength. Diarrhoea may develop during the intestinal stage of trichinosis and can be severe in heavy infections. This resolves without treatment as the adults are expelled. Bloody diarrhoea is a common symptom at the beginning of the egg-laying phase, during first attacks of schistosomiasis, but this symptom is rarely elicited except from patients living in endemic countries.

2.2 Respiratory symptoms

Cough and wheeze may develop during the migration of ascaris through the lungs. Toxocara, unable to complete its life cycle in man, is associated with prolonged cough and bronchospasm. Cough is one of the most frequent presentations of patients with pneumocystis infection. It is also a cardinal symptom of infection with the lung flukes such as *Paragonomiasis westermanii* when the sputum may be blood stained. In malaria, cough can develop during the acute stage of infection, leading to a misdiagnosis of pneumonia. This arises, in part, because of the presence of parasites in lung capillaries and, in part, because of the action of cytokines, such as TNF (tumour necrosis factor). A list of parasitic infections, in which fever and pulmonary infiltrations are seen, is listed in *Table 4*.

Table 3. Parasitic agents associated with diarrhoea

Diarrhoea and fever
Entamoeba histolytica[a]
Cryptosporidium[a]
Isospora belli
Schistosoma mansoni[a] and *S. japonicum*[a]
Trichinella spiralis[a]
Malaria[b]

Bloody diarrhoea
Entamoeba histolytica
Trichuris trichiura (trichuriasis)
Schistosoma mansoni and *S. japonicum*
Malaria[c]

Chronic diarrhoea ($\geq$ 3 weeks)
Entamoeba histolytica
Giardia lamblia[d]
Cryptosporidium[d]
Isospora belli[d]
Microsporidia (several genera, including *Enterocytozoan bieneusi*)
Trichuris trichiura
Hookworms (*Necator americanus* and *Ancyclostoma duodenale*)
Trichinella spiralis (in Canadian Arctic)
Schistosoma mansoni and *S. japonicum*
Strongyloides stercoralis[d]
Capillariasis (*Capillaria philippinensis*)[d]
Sarcocystis spp.[d] (sarcocystosis)
Trypanosoma cruzi (alternating diarrhoea, constipation)
Blastocystis hominis[e]

[a] May be associated with fever > 40°C.
[b] Acute malaria is associated with diarrhoea and other gastro-intestinal symptoms in 25% or more of patients.
[c] Bloody diarrhoea has rarely been reported in falciparum malaria.
[d] Malabsorption may accompany chronic diarrhoea.
[e] Pathogenicity questioned.

2.3 Neurological symptoms

The nervous system may be affected by parasitic infection. Patients may present with seizures due to the presence of space occupying lesions in the brain. For example, when man substitutes for the pig in the life cycle of *Taenia solium* infection, cysticerci can be found in the brain. The immune response to parasite antigens can provoke seizures. In amoebiasis metastatic brain abscess may be rarely encountered. In toxoplasmosis, almost all who are infected have asymptomatic lesions in the brain. It is only when immunity breaks down that CNS symptoms may result. Perhaps the most important of all neurological symptoms to detect is altered cerebral function of patients

Table 4. Parasitic causes of fever and pulmonary infiltrates

Geographic distribution	Place
Focal	
Filariasis	AF, AM (C,S), AS, EUR, AUS
Malaria (pulmonary oedema in severe falciparum)	AF, AM (C,S), AS, EUR, AUS
Gnathostomiasis [a]	AS (rare elsewhere)
Paragonimiasis [a,b,c]	AF, AM, AS, EUR, AUS
Schistosomiasis [a] (early, Katayama syndrome)	AF, AM (C,S), AS
Echinococcosis [b,c]	AF, AM, AS, EUR, AUS
Capillariasis hepatica [a,b]	AF, AM, AS, EUR
Widespread	
Pneumocystis carinii [e]	
Hookworm [a,b]	
Strongyloidiasis [a,b]	
Toxocariasis [a]	
Trichinellosis (*Trichinella spiralis*) [a]	
Toxoplasmosis	
Cutaneous larva migrans (rare infiltrate) [a,b,f]	
Ascariasis [a,b,e]	
Amoebiasis [e]	

[a] May cause fever and pulmonary infiltrates during larval migration (may also cause urticaria).
[b] Usually afebrile.
[c] Can cause cystic or cavitating disease.
[d] Pulmonary infection in immunocompromised hosts often reflects reactivation.
[e] Rare.

with acute *P. falciparum* malaria. Failure to recognize the seriousness of this development can result in the unnecessary death of the patient.

Eosinophilic meningitis can develop during infection with *Angiostrongylus cantonensis*. Primary amoebic meningitis is a rare and usually fatal condition which is acquired after swimming in water contaminated with the free-living *Naegleria fowleri* and *Acanthamoeba* spp. Meningoencephalitis is part of the pathogenic process of the late stages of African trypanosomiasis. Its presence indicates a poor prognosis and poses significant problems in treatment. A list of parasitic infections, which produce neurological symptoms, is found in *Table 5*.

Onchocerciasis is one of the most important causes of blindness, worldwide. This is, however, a late stage of infection which has been preceded by multiple attacks of ocular inflammation. Loiasis may be recognized when the patient notices the passage of a worm across the eye. In toxoplasmosis and toxocariasis, loss of vision occurs in the very young, and may go unrecognized, patients with HIV infection may also be similarly affected by toxoplasma. Some of the parasitic infections which can affect the eye are listed in *Table 6*.

Table 5. Parasitic infections causing fever and meningitis/encephalitis [a]

Infections	Place of acquisition
Malaria	AF, AM (C,S), AS, EUR, AUS
Trypanosomiasis, African [b]	AF
Trypanosomiasis, American (Chagas') [b]	AM (C,S)
Entamoeba histolytica (usually abscess) [c]	WW
Primary amoebic meningoencephalitis (*Naegleria*)	All continents
Acanthamoeba [b,c,d]	WW
Toxoplasmosis [b,d] (usually focal CNS infection)	WW
Strongyloidiasis (in compromised hosts) [g]	WW
Cysticercosis (*Taenia solium*) [f]	WW
Toxocariasis	WW
Anglostrongylus cantonenisis [f,g]	AF, AM, AS, [h] AUS
Gnathostomiasis (myeloencephalitis) [f,g]	AF, AM, AS, [h] AUS

[a] Some helminthic infections may cause focal neurologic changes, e.g. echinococcosis, fascioliasis, and schistosomiasis. Patients may have CSF pleocytosis but are often afebrile.
[b] May cause chronic meningitis (lasting four weeks or longer).
[c] CNS is rarely involved.
[d] Primarily in compromised hosts.
[e] Eosinophilic meningoencephalitis.
[f] May cause chronic meningitis (lasting four weeks or longer).
[g] Bacterial meningitis (often caused by coliforms) is a complication of strongyloidiasis hyper-infection syndrome.
[h] Most cases from Thailand and other areas of S.E. Asia.

2.4 Cutaneous symptoms

Pruritis, as in the case of swimmer's itch, is part of the natural history of acute schistosomiasis, but may also be a symptom of a wide-range of different infections, including scabies, onchocerciasis, strongyloidiasis, or cutaneous larva migrans. The localization of the itch, and any temporal relationship, should be sought (e.g. the characteristic itchy migrating lesions of larva currens, see Chapter 13). In many instances, such as cutaneous larva migrans, caused by dog hookworm, the history and cutaneous appearances are sufficiently characteristic for diagnosis. In others, such as mild onchocerciasis, the dermatological appearances can mimic a number of other conditions. In amoebiasis, the skin may be infected after the rupture of a liver abscess. This may prove destructive and difficult to treat. Parasitic infections which result in cutaneous manifestations are found in *Table 7*.

3. Travel history

The travel history might be better described as a geographic history as it emphasizes the need to investigate possible parasite exposure in the patient's country of origin. In the United States the subject of Tropical Medicine is sometimes known by the title Geographic Medicine. In patients who are

Table 6. Parasitic infections involving the eye

Disease/clinical features

1. Onchocerciasis (*Onchocerca volvulus*)
   Microfilariae in eye. Chronic conjunctivitis. Punctate and sclerosing keratitis. Anterior uveitis. Chorioretinitis. Optic atrophy.
2. Toxocariasis (*Toxocara canis, T. cati*)
   Larva in eye. Unilateral. Posterior or peripheral retinal granulomata. Anterior and posterior uveitis. Eosinophilic abscess of retina, vitreous membrane. May resemble tumour. *Baylisascaris procyonis* causes similar findings.
3. *Acanthamoeba* keratitis
   Usually follows trauma, use of contact lenses.
4. Leishmaniasis, cutaneous and mucocutaneous
   Probably direct inoculation of organisms from another lesion or extension of disease from lesion on eyelid. Interstitial keratitis occasionally ulcerative. Stromal opacification. Perforation of globe if treatment delayed. Nodules of cornea and sclera, anterior uveitis, and chorioretinitis reported with visceral leishmaniasis (Kala-azar).
5. *Toxoplasma gondii*
   Necrotizing retinitis. Granulomatous choroiditis. Papillitis. Anterior uveitis, particularly in AIDS patients.
6. Trichinellosis (*Trichinella spiralis*)
   Oedema of eyelids. Subconjunctival and retinal haemorrhages. Uveitis. Myositis of extraocular muscles (larvae in muscles).
7. Loiasis (*Loa loa*)
   Migration of worm (3–7 cm length), visible in subconjunctiva. May invade anterior chamber, vitreous, subretinal space. Rarely encysted in subconjunctival tissues. Painful oedema of eyelid.
8. Filariasis (*Wuchereria bancrofti; Brugia malayi; Mansonella* spp.)
   Conjunctivitis is described in patients with *W. bancrofti* and *B. malayi* infections. Changes may be from toxic-allergic reaction rather than invasion. Adult worm rarely found in anterior chamber and vitreous.
9. Hookworm infection (*Ancyclostoma* species)
   Migration of third stage larvae.
10. *Pneumocystis carinii*
    Rare cotton wool spots of the retina in patients with the acquired immunodeficiency syndrome (AIDS). Choroiditis in patient with disseminated extrapulmonary pneumocytosis.
11. Trypanosomiasis
    Unilateral oedema of palpebral conjunctivae (Romãna's sign); swelling of eyelids in 50% of children affected. Occurs when conjunctiva is route of inoculation. Dacryocystitis also reported.

normally resident in tropical countries, detailed knowledge of their travel or residence may be of considerable help, as the prevalence of infections can vary widely within one country (1).

The travel history must be detailed, including details of even short stopover

Table 7. Parasitic infections causing fever and skin lesions[a]

Geographic distribution/disease	Characteristics of skin changes
Focal	
Onchocerciasis	Papular, urticaria, nodules (scalp in AM, extremities in AF)
Loiasis	Urticaria (especially hands and forearms), migratory swelling (calabar)
Dracunculiasis	Local blister at site of worm, usually lower extremities, ulcer, urticaria
Filariasis (*Wuchereria bancrofti, Brugia malayi*)	Local acute lymphadenitis, chronic lymphoedema (legs, arms and scrotum), erythema nodusum (rare)
Schistosomiasis[b]	Urticaria (with Katayama fever); itchy maculopapules on trunk 2° to ectopic eggs, fistula, granulomas in vaginal area/perineum (especially *S. haematobium*)
Gnathostomiasis	Urticaria, creeping eruption (episodic, reoccurs in different location)
Widespread	
Ascariasis[b]	Urticaria
Cutaneous larva migrans[b]	Serpiginous, thin (2–3 mm), itchy, common, feet, legs, and hands
Fascioliasis	Urticaria, rare nodules
Hookworm infection[b]	Urticaria, papulovesicular rash
Strongyloidiasis[b]	Papular, urticaria, serpiginous (usually buttock, groin, or trunk)
Toxocariasis[b]	Urticaria, nodular rash (rare), trunk, lower extremities
Trichinellosis[b]	Urticaria, facial swelling (especially eyes)
Leishmaniasis,	
cutaneous/mucocutaneous	Papulae at bite, followed by crust covering ulcer, heals slowly leaving depressed scar. *L. braziliensis*—progressive ulceration, erosion of oro/nasopharynx
visceral	Nodule at bite (persists for months) papular, nodular infiltration of skin (post Kala-azar occurs after cure, hypopigmented or red macules on face)
Trypanosomiasis, African[c]	Erythematous, carcinate patches, wax and wane, prominent on trunk
Toxoplasmosis	Macular-papular (rare)

[a] Fever may be intermittent, low grade, or absent in many helminthic infections.

[b] May have urticaria, along with pulmonary infiltrates, fever, and cough during larval migration or non-human schistosomes.

[c] Primary chancre (dusky red indurated area 5 cm) may develop in African trypanosomiasis, and chagoma (painful indurated area 1–3 cm) may develop in American trypanosomiasis at the site of bite.

visits. It must also go back into the past, long enough to detect relevant exposure, for example, most cases of malaria arise within one year of return from a malaria endemic area, but rarely, the incubation period is longer. In the case of strongyloidiasis the time between exposure and seeking medical advice can be very long. Many prisoners of war, held in the Far East of Asia, during the Second World War, became infected with *Strongyloides stercoralis* while working on the Burma railway. Many of these patients were not diagnosed and treated until 30 or 40 years later. Although many patients had mild symptoms of larva currens, in some who became immunocompromised, the serious hyperinfection syndrome developed (see Chapter 13).

The travel history not only alerts the clinician to possible exposure to parasitic species, but may indicate variation in sensitivity to chemotherapeutic agents: malaria acquired in Thailand may exhibit multidrug resistance, including quinine.

4. General history

An account of hobby and leisure activities should be obtained. In a patient with undiagnosed eosinophilia, the recent acquisition of a dog may point to toxocariasis. A history of swimming in a river, or other water exposure in Africa, might indicate schistosomiasis. For infections which are highly localized, such as trypanosomiasis, a history of travel to game parks, where the disease is known to be endemic, may be important.

The occupation history may reveal vital details; sheep farmers, and others living in sheep farming districts, are more at risk of hydatid disease. Kennel maids, vets, and others with a close working relationship with whelping bitches, are more likely to be seropositive for toxocariasis.

Food is an important vehicle for parasitic infections. Undercooked meat is the main means of transmission of toxoplasmosis and trichinosis. Watercress grown in contaminated water is a vector for fasciola infection. In countries where there is not effective meat inspection process, cysticercosis, acquired by eating measly pork, may be common. Water, too, is an important vehicle of parasite transmission, both of helminths such as guinea worm, but more importantly, giardia and amoebic infection. In practice, however, it is rare that patients are able to be sufficiently precise about their water drinking habits, to provide useful diagnostic information.

A history of all relevant drugs should be taken. The diagnosis of malaria can not be excluded because patients have taken anti-malarial prophylaxis. The protection provided by prophylaxis is only partial and, moreover, patients may not have taken tablets as regularly as they would wish their doctor to believe. In travellers, it is useful to record illnesses which have occurred abroad, but the patient may now consider 'cured'. Intestinal amoebiasis is usually treated with metronidazole in most developing countries, and recurrent attacks may develop unless diloxanide is used to eradicate the cyst stage.

5. Clinical examination

The clinical examination of a patient with a parasitic infection should be thorough, as many infections lack characteristic signs. In the general examin-

Table 8. Parasitic infections causing lymphadenopathy

Filariasis
- *Brugia malayi* R, G
- *Brugia timori* R
- *Wuchereria bancrofti* R, G

Loiasis R
Onchocerciasis (*Onchocerca volvulus*) R, inguinal and femoral (hanging groin)
Opisthorchiasis (acute infection with *Opisthorchis felineus*) G
Schistosomiasis, acute (Katayama fever, usually caused by *Schistosoma japonicum* or *Schistosoma mansoni*) G
Leishmaniasis, cutaneous and mucocutaneous R (may be reaction to secondary bacterial infection of ulcerated area)
Leishmaniasis, visceral (*Leishmania donovani*) G
Toxoplasmosis (*Toxoplasma gondii*) R, G
Trypanosomiasis, African (*Trypanosoma brucei*; *T. gambiense*) R, G
Trypanosomiasis, American (Chagas' disease) (*Trypanosoma cruzi*) G

R indicates regional lympadenopathy.
G indicates generalized lympadenopathy.

ation, the skin must be carefully observed, as several parasitic infections have characteristic cutaneous manifestations. An example of this is the large nodules and thickened hyperkeratotic skin in the patient with onchocerciasis. In strongyloidiasis the skin changes are transient and it may be necessary to ask the patient to consult during an acute attack. Lymphadenopathy may be present in a number of conditions and some of these are listed in *Table 8*. The eyes should be examined, carefully, and patients with suspected onchocerciais should have a slit lamp examination.

During acute attacks of lymphatic filariasis, lymphatic vessels may be inflamed with surrounding oedema. Later in the course of the disease, permanent damage to the lymphatic vessels leads to obstruction and lymphoedema.

The presence of an enlarged liver, or spleen, should be sought. In amoebic liver abscess, the presence of hepatic tenderness may suggest that it is in danger of rupture. Hydatid cysts in the liver may be palpable. Splenomegaly is an important sign in acute malaria in returning travellers, but its absence by no means excludes the diagnosis. In endemic countries, the percentage of children with splenomegaly is used as a measure of the endemicity. The liver and spleen may be enlarged as a result of the presence of parasites within the cells of the reticulo-endothelial system, and in the case of leishmaniasis. Visceral leishmaniasis, because of a clinical picture of fever, weight loss, wasting, splenomegaly, and pancytopaenia, can be confused with malignancy, particularly as antibody tests may be negative (2). However, the tissue diagnosis is invariably positive (Chapter 8). In schistosomal infection, complicated by liver fibrosis, portal hypertension can result in splenomegaly. A

Table 9. Parasitic infections associated with fever and liver dysfunction,[a] including hepatosplenomegaly

Geographic distribution	Place
Focal	
Capillaria hepatica (develops into adult form in liver)	AF, AM, AS, EUR
Echinococcosis (cysts)	AF, AM, AS, EUR, AUS
Leishmaniasis, visceral	AF, AM (C,S,N), AS, EUR
Malaria	AF, AM (C,S), AS, EUR, AUS
Opisthorchiasis[b]	AM (S), AS, EUR
Schistosomiasis	AF, AM (C,S), AS
Trypanosomiasis, African	AF
Trypanosomiasis, American	AM (C,S)
Widespread	
Amoebiasis	
Ascariasis[b]	
Cryptosporidiosis (cholecystitis, cholangitis in compromised hosts)	
Fascioliasis[b] (*Fasciola hepatica*, rarely *F. gigantica*)	
Strongyloidiasis (with hyperinfection)	
Taeniasis (*Taenia saginata*)[b]	
Toxocariasis (visceral larval migrans)	
Pneumocystis carinii[c]	
Toxoplasmosis	

[a] Most helminth infections may be associated with granulomatous response in the liver. Fever may be low grade, intermittent, or absent.
[b] Mechanical obstruction of bile ducts, cholangitis.
[c] In the context of disseminated infection, pneumocystis can cause hepatitis in immunocompromised hosts, primarily AIDS patients.

Table 10. Parasitic infections causing fever and eosinophilia

Common infections	Rare infections
Hookworm infection (*Necator americanus, Ancyclostoma duodenale*)	*Capillaria hepatica* infection
Ascariasis	Paragonimiasis
Cutaneous larva migrans[a]	Opisthorchiasis
Schistosomiasis	Echinococcosis[a]
Onchocerciasis	Fascioliasis
Filariasis	Angiostrongyliasis due to *Angiostrongylus cantonensis* infection
Loiasis	Trichinellosis
Strongyloidiasis	Dracunculiasis
Toxocariasis (*Toxocara canis, T. cati*)	Cysticercosis

[a] Low grade or variable eosinophilia.

list of the causes of liver and splenic enlargement is found in *Table 9*. The results of a full blood count may reveal an eosinophilia, some of the more common parasitic causes of which are listed in *Table 10*.

References

1. Wilson, M. E. (1991). *A world guide to infections, diseases, distribution, diagnosis*. Oxford University Press, Oxford.
2. Oven, R. (1991). *J. Infect. Dis.*, **164**, 746.

Further reading

1. Beaver, P. C., Jung, R. C., and Cupp, E. W. (1984). *Clinical parasitology* (9th edn). Lea & Febiger, Philadelphia.
2. Warren, K. S. and Mahmoud, A. A. F. (1990). *Tropical and geographic medicine* (2nd edn). McGraw-Hill, New York.
3. Peters, W. and Gilles, H. M. (1989). *A colour atlas of tropical medicine and parasitology* (3rd edn). Wolfe, London.

2

Malaria

PETER L. CHIODINI and SHEILA CLARK

1. Introduction

More than 1.6 billion people live in malaria endemic areas. Diagnosis of malaria by microscopy is a vital laboratory procedure in endemic areas. In addition, given the substantial amount of travel from the developed world to the tropics there will remain a need to diagnose this imported infection in patients returning from the tropics to the temperate zone. Imported malaria is a common diagnosis in many developed countries. In 1991 there were 2332 reported cases of malaria in the UK, 1268 due to *Plasmodium falciparum*, with 12 deaths (11 due to *P. falciparum*).

1.1 Geographical distribution

The geographical distribution of malaria is shown in *Figure 1*.

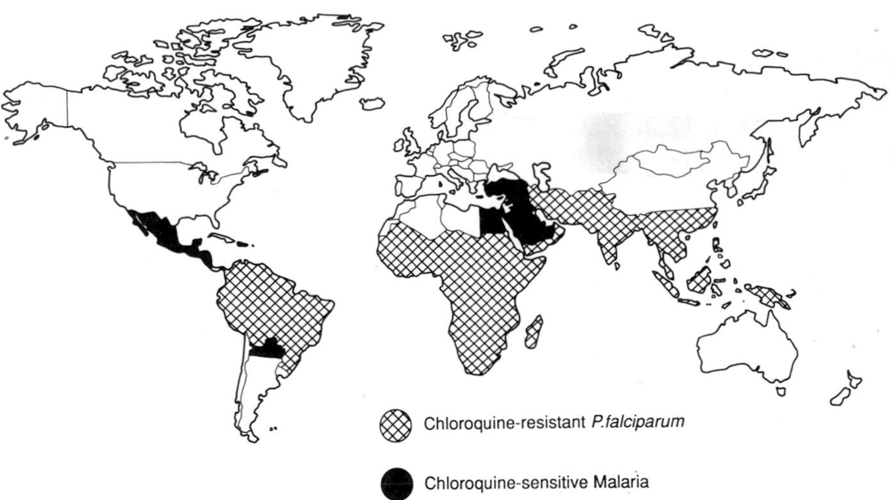

Figure 1. Geographical distribution of malaria and chloroquine-resistant *Plasmodium falciparum*, 1991. Reproduced with permission from Centers for Disease Control and Prevention, Atlanta, USA.

1.2 Life cycle

Infection is initiated following a bite from a female anopheline mosquito. Sporozoites liberated from the mosquito's salivary glands rapidly enter hepatocytes in the liver. There they may develop in two ways. In the case of *P. falciparum* and *P. malariae* the parasite develops to a pre-erythrocytic schizont which eventually ruptures to release merozoites into the bloodstream. In the case of *P. vivax* and *P. ovale*, some sporozoites develop into pre-erythrocytic schizonts while others lay dormant as hypnozoites. At a later time hypnozoites may become active, divide, and form schizonts and merozoites which can then initiate erythrocytic infection in the peripheral blood. It is this reactivation which is responsible for clinical relapse in this form of malaria.

A merozoite released from a hepatic schizont invades an erythrocyte, develops a vacuole, and forms the ring stage. The trophozoite (growth stage) enlarges, loses its vacuole, and forms pigment in its cytoplasm. Nuclear division follows (schizogony) and a mature schizont is eventually formed, consisting of merozoites, pigment granules, and a residue of waste material. Malaria pigment is formed within the food vacuole of the malaria parasite. The pigment is blackish-brown and thought to consist of insoluble monomers and dimers of haematin, plus ferriprotoporphyrin coupled to a plasmodial protein, and insoluble methaemoglobin.

Schizogony takes 48 hours for *P. vivax*, *P. ovale*, and *P. falciparum* (tertian malarias), and 72 hours for *P. malariae* (quartan malaria). The erythrocyte ruptures and merozoites are released from the schizont into the plasma, where they invade new erythrocytes.

Some merozoites do not develop into schizonts but differentiate instead into sexual forms, the female macrogametocytes and the male microgametocytes.

In the case of *P. vivax*, *P. ovale*, and *P. malariae*, at least two cycles of blood schizogony must take place before gametocytes are seen in the peripheral blood. However, in the case of *P. falciparum*, gametocytes are not seen in the peripheral blood until asexual parasites have been in the circulation for ten days.

1.3 Clinical features

The minimum incubation period for malaria varies according to species and is approximately as follows: *P. falciparum* 8 days, *P. vivax* 10 days, *P. ovale* 11 days, *P. malariae* 17 days (1). However, in the case of *P. ovale* and *P. vivax* the primary attack can be delayed by some months, e.g. nine months in some cases of *P. vivax* infection, due to the delayed activation of the hypnozoite stage. While most cases of malaria present in the first six months after return from an endemic area, some present more than one year after the patient was last in a malarious area. Diagnostic vigilance must therefore be maintained to ensure that these cases are not missed.

The clinical features of malaria are non-specific. This tendency of malaria

Table 1. Severe clinical features and complications of falciparum malaria, adapted from Warrell *et al.* (2)

Cerebral malaria (unrousable coma)
Impaired consciousness but rousable
Repeated generalized convulsions
Severe normocytic anaemia
Renal failure
Jaundice
Pulmonary oedema
Hypoglycaemia
Circulatory collapse, shock
Spontaneous bleeding/disseminated intravascular coagulation
Hyperpyrexia
Acidaemia/acidosis
Malarial haemoglobinuria
Prostration, extreme weakness

to mimic other infections has led to delay in diagnosis, which may have fatal results.

Clinical features include fever, rigors, anaemia, jaundice, and splenomegaly. These can occur with all four species of malaria parasite infecting humans. In the case of *P. falciparum*, more severe clinical manifestations may be present, as shown in *Table 1*.

It is evident that no aspect of the clinical picture of malaria is diagnostic and all the features, including the complications of *P. falciparum* infection, can be confused with other diseases.

1.4 Pitfalls in the diagnosis of malaria

Common misdiagnoses include influenza, hepatitis, gastro-enteritis, viral encephalitis, and psychosis. Chest diseases, e.g. pneumonia, pleurisy can also be mimicked. The pattern of fever is seldom reliable; the primary fever of falciparum malaria is irregular and often continuous. On occasions the temperature is found to be normal or below normal in cases of severe malaria, especially if the patient is shocked.

Important causes of missed malaria are:

- failure to take a travel history
- failure to obtain a history of blood transfusion
- failure to obtain a history of shared needles
- failure to obtain a history of residence near an airport
- false assumption that having taken prophylaxis excludes malaria infection

- false assumption that recent anti-malarial treatment excludes malaria infection

Thus, if a person has been geographically exposed to the infection and is unwell, the diagnosis of malaria (especially *P. falciparum*) must be excluded as a matter of urgency, irrespective of the clinical presentation.

2. Microscopy

The mainstay of malaria diagnosis is examination of stained blood films for malaria parasites.

2.1 Samples

In most instances, a peripheral blood sample is adequate for diagnosis. Finger prick is an alternative. Examination of the buffy coat obtained after centrifugation of the blood sample may provide increased sensitivity, and on occasions a bone marrow sample proves positive when several peripheral blood smears have been negative. However this is a rare occurrence and in the majority of cases the extra discomfort of bone marrow aspiration can be avoided by careful examination of peripheral blood samples. In obstetric practice, malaria parasites can be demonstrated by microscopy of cord blood or of placental impression smears. Finally, where a patient has died undiagnosed, post-mortem smears of grey matter enable the diagnosis of malaria to be confirmed by demonstrating the parasites of *P. falciparum* sequestered in capillaries or post-capillary venules.

2.2 The thin blood film

2.2.1 Preparation

Use clean, grease- and moisture-free slides to minimize the incidence of artefacts, and avoid clumping of red cells or detachment of blood films during staining. Handle slides by the edges to avoid placing finger marks on the surface.

Place a drop of blood, approximately 3 mm diameter on the microscope slide one third of the way from the labelled end, and use a second slide held at 45° as a spreader to distribute the blood smoothly and rapidly (a greater angle will result in too thick a smear, too thin if a smaller angle is employed). Air dry the blood film thoroughly.

2.2.2 Staining thin blood films

The standard method uses Giemsa stain (*Protocol 1*).

Protocol 1. Staining thin blood films with Giemsa stain

1. Fix the blood film in methanol for 1–2 min.
2. Prepare a 10% solution of Giemsa stain (e.g. BDH Laboratory Supplies) in phosphate-buffered saline solution pH 7.2, and use within 8 h.
3. Stain the slides in diluted stain for 20 min.
4. Rinse the slides in tap-water.
5. Blot dry, or air dry in a vertical position.

Staining with modified Field's stain permits rapid detection of malaria parasites but does not usually stain Schuffner's dots (*Protocol 2*).

Protocol 2. Staining thin blood films with Field's stain

1. Prepare a thin blood film as in Section 2.2.1.
2. Fix blood film in methanol for 1 min.
3. Wash off methanol with tap-water.
4. Cover the blood film with diluted Field's stain B (BDH Laboratory Supplies) (1:4 in buffered water at pH 7.2).
5. Immediately add an equal volume of Field's stain A.
6. Mix well and stain for 1 min.
7. Rinse the slide with tap-water, and place upright to drain and air dry.

Leishman's stain is methanol-based and thus is useful only for thin film examination. However, it is felt by some to be superior to other stains in demonstrating detail of malaria parasites (3) and thus has a place in aiding speciation of malaria parasites (*Protocol 3*).

Protocol 3. Staining thin blood films with Leishman's stain

1. Prepare a thin blood film as in Section 2.2.1.
2. Place six drops of Leishman's stain (BDH Laboratory Supplies) on the blood smear and spread over the film, which acts as initial fixative.
3. Allow the stain to fix the smear for approximately 20 sec. Take care not to allow the stain to dry up during that time.
4. Add 12 drops of buffer, pH 7.2 and mix on the slide.
5. Allow smear to stain for 20–30 min, then wash with buffer, pH 7.2.
6. Air dry the slide in a vertical position.

2.2.3 Examination of the thin blood film

Optimal morphology of malaria parasites is obtained in that part of the thin film where red blood cells are just overlapping (usually the lower third of the smear). However *P. vivax* and *P. ovale* (particularly mature forms) plus gametocytes of *P. falciparum* have a tendency to appear in the tail and edges of the blood films. Thus these areas should also be scanned as a routine. The thin film is examined under oil immersion microscopy, preferably with a × 100 objective, ideally with a flat field. In a satisfactorily stained thin film, erythrocytes appear pale straw to light grey in colour. The leucocytes have dark blue or purple nuclei, with lighter blue cytoplasm (mottled blue/grey in monocytes). Platelets appear blue or purple. The red blood cells containing malaria parasites are examined for their size (normal, enlarged, or small) and the presence or absence of stippling. Enlarged red cells with Schuffner's dots present suggests *P. vivax* or *P. ovale* (when the stippling is known as James's dots). However it is important to remember that stippling may not be present in red cells infected with young ring stages of *P. vivax* or *P. ovale*. It may also be absent if the blood film has been stained incorrectly; at pH 6.8 stippling would not be visualized and it is essential that the correct pH of 7.2 is used for staining blood films. In the case of *P. malariae* infection, infected cells may be smaller than normal. Cells containing late stage trophozoites of *P. falciparum* may contain irregular red/mauve dots which are larger but fewer in number than Schuffner's dots, and are termed Maurer's clefts.

The malaria parasites are recognized by the presence of blue staining cytoplasm, red to purple chromatin, and with the exception of young ring stages, by the presence of malarial pigment.

The parasites are observed for the stages present, the presence or absence of amoeboid trophozoites, the number of merozoites in any schizonts seen, the presence of gametocytes, and especially their shape. The characteristic features of malaria parasites in thin blood films are shown in *Table 2*, and examples of the most frequently seen forms are shown in *Plate 1*.

It is essential that films stained with Giemsa or Leishman's stain are examined in order to confirm the species of malaria parasite present. However, Field's stain remains a very useful screening method.

i. Estimation of parasitaemia in thin blood films

It is essential that the percentage parasitaemia is recorded if *P. falciparum* is diagnosed. This is undertaken by counting 1000 red cells in the thin film and counting the number of infected red blood cells, converting this to a percentage. It is important to note that the number of infected cells is recorded, **NOT** the number of parasites per 100 red blood cells.

ii. Artefacts

Before identifying a structure as a malaria parasite, the observer should make certain that the presence of the blue staining cytoplasm, red or purple

Table 2. Morphological appearance of malaria parasites in thin blood films (after WHO (4))

Stage	***P. vivax***	***P. ovale***	***P. malariae***	***P. falciparum***
Infected red cell	Enlarged, Schuffner's dots evident	Enlarged, James's dots evident; may be oval, with fimbriation	Normal or smaller than normal size	Normal size, Maurer's clefts may be evident
Early trophozoite (ring stage)	Quite large; one or two chromatin dots; may be two parasites per red cell	Compact, rarely see two parasites per red cell	Compact, rarely see two parasites per red cell	Small, delicate, often with two chromatin dots; accolé forms common; often two or more parasites per red blood cell
Late trophozoite	Large, amoeboid; pigment in fine rods	Small, not amoeboid; coarse pigment	Small and compact, often band shaped; coarse pigment	Moderate size, usually compact; granular pigment
Mature schizont	Large, with large merozoites (12–24); pigment coalescent	Smaller than *P. vivax*, 6–12 merozoites; pigment darker than in *P. vivax*	Small, with 6–12 large merozoites; classical 'daisy head' appearance; coarse pigment	Rare in peripheral blood, 8–26 small merozoites; pigment in a single mass
Gametocyte	Spherical and compact with a single nucleus; diffuse, coarse pigment	Similar to *P. vivax*, but smaller	Similar to *P. vivax* but smaller and less numerous; Schuffner's dots absent	Crescent shaped, with single nucleus

chromatin and, with the exception of ring stages, brown or black pigment are all present.

False positive diagnoses of malaria can be made by the observer confusing other cellular elements or their fragments with malaria parasites. For example platelets, particularly if superimposed upon red blood cells in thin films and clumps of platelets may be confused with parasites. Precipitated stain superimposed upon red blood cells may cause quite convincing artefacts. If debris from the patient's skin, or dust gets on to the film, this may produce a further source of confusion. During the drying process it is possible for bacteria, yeasts, and fungal spores to contaminate the film. Algae and other organisms may grow in staining solutions which have become contaminated and be introduced to an otherwise well produced film at the staining stage.

2.3 The thick blood film

2.3.1 Preparation

Protocol 4. Preparation of thick blood films

1. Add approximately 5 μl of blood to a clean slide with an applicator stick.
2. With the end of the applicator stick, quickly distribute the blood to make an even thick film about 1 cm^2. Avoid excessive stirring of blood. It should just be possible to read fine print through a thick film.
3. Label the slide. Allow the thick film to air dry (without heating the slide) in a horizontal position.

2.3.2 Staining thick blood films

Protocol 5. Method for staining thick blood films with Field's stain

Equipment and reagents

- One staining dish filled with Field's stain A
- One staining dish filled with Field's stain B
- Two dishes filled with clean water

Method

1. Dip the unfixed air dried slide into Field's stain A for 3 sec.
2. Wash gently by dipping (once) into clean water.
3. Dip into Field's stain B for 3 sec.
4. Wash as in step **2**.
5. Place slide upright in a draining rack to air dry.

Protocol 6. Method for staining thick blood films with Giemsa stain

1. Prepare a thick blood film as in *Protocol 4*.
2. Prepare a 3% solution of Giemsa stain in buffered water pH 7.2.
3. Apply the stain to the unfixed thick smear and stain for 30 min.
4. Remove the slides and wash in tap-water or buffered water pH 7.2.
5. Air dry the film in a rack.

2.3.3 Examination of thick blood films

Macroscopically the thick film should be light blue and semi-transparent. It is examined with a × 100 oil immersion objective. A minimum of 100 oil immersion fields must be examined but ideally the whole thick film should be scanned. The thick film will reveal white blood cells (WBC) and platelets but no RBC's as these are lysed during the staining process. In an optimally stained thick film the leucocyte nuclei appear deep purple with indistinct granulation in the cytoplasm. The background is mottled grey.

The malaria parasites, if present, are well defined but tend to be denser and more compact than in thin films. They are more difficult to speciate as the red cell characteristics (e.g. stippling) are usually absent. Thus, in the absence of details like size, shape, and stippling of host cell RBC's, it is important to examine the thin blood film for final species identification.

A satisfactorily prepared thick blood film, examined by a microscopist competent in malaria diagnosis, carries a sensitivity of approximately 20 parasites per microlitre, equivalent to 0.0004% parasitaemia (5).

2.3.4 Assessing level of parasitaemia

This is essential if *P. falciparum* is present. A variety of methods is available.

i. Counting malaria parasites in the thick blood film to estimate the number of parasites per microlitre

The malarial parasites are counted in relation to a predetermined number of white blood cells (WBC). Despite inaccuracies due to variation in number of WBC between individuals in health and a greater variation in ill patients, an average of 8000 leucocytes per microlitre is taken as standard and allows for reasonable comparison. If the precise WBC count is known for that patient a more accurate figure can be obtained.

(a) Two tally counters are required to count parasites and leucocytes separately.

(b) The equivalent of 0.25 μl of blood (about 100 fields using a × 100 oil immersion objective) should be examined in the thick film.

(c) 200 leucocytes are counted. If ten or more parasites are identified, the number of parasites per microlitre is recorded using the formula given below. If the number of parasites is nine or less the observer continues counting WBC's till 500 have been seen. The number of parasites per microlitre is calculated using the formula given below:

$$\frac{\text{number of parasites} \times 8000}{\text{number of leucocytes counted}} = \text{number of parasites per microlitre}$$

ii. The Earle and Perez method (6)

This counts the number of asexual parasites per known volume of blood (usually 5 μl) spread as a thick film. This is time-consuming and generally employed only in research studies.

iii. The 'plus' system

An alternative, but less precise, method to enumerate parasites in the thick blood film is the 'plus system'. The thick blood film is examined with an oil immersion objective and the results recorded using one to four pluses as shown below:

+ = 1–10 parasites per 100 thick film fields
++ = 11–100 parasites per 100 thick film fields
+++ = 1–10 parasites per thick film field
++++ = > 10 parasites per thick film field

This method suffers from the disadvantage that variation in the thickness of the thick film results in false variation in the parasite count.

2.3.5 Speciation of parasites in thick films

In thick films red cell characteristics are not usually available to aid the microscopist in speciation. Occasionally, however, Schuffner's dots can still be seen in the ghosts of the red blood cell. The characteristic gametocytes of *P. falciparum*, if present, provide a useful aid to speciation, *Plate 1b*. In early infections, however, when gametocytes may not be present, and when the ring stages are small, it may be difficult to speciate using a thick film alone.

2.3.6 Artefacts

The absence of formed red cells in the thick film makes it more difficult to distinguish artefacts from parasites as it is not possible to determine whether they are intracellular. Debris from red cells, notably chromatoid bodies present in severe anaemia may cause confusion in thick films. The other artefacts listed in Section 2.2.3 *ii* can also be a problem in thick film examination.

2.4 'Blood film negative' malaria

On occasions, there may be a strong clinical suspicion of malaria, but the blood films are reported negative by the laboratory. There are various possible explanations.

In areas where malaria is infrequently encountered misdiagnosis may occur (7). If the clinical suspicion of malaria remains, it is essential that apparently 'negative' films are reviewed and that further blood samples are taken until the diagnosis can be excluded. In this context, thrombocytopenia provides a useful clue. Thrombocytopenia of less than 80 000 per microlitre is common in acute *P. falciparum*, but also occurs in *P. vivax* infection. Microscopic diagnosis of malaria requires experienced microscopists regularly reviewing positive samples (8).

Sequestration of *P. falciparum* in the deep tissue capillaries and post-capillary venules may render the peripheral blood temporarily negative. Repeating the blood film twice daily will improve the chance of detecting malaria parasites as they are again released to the peripheral blood after schizogony. Anti-malarial chemoprophylaxis or partial treatment may temporarily render the blood film negative despite the patient being symptomatic. Sequential blood films should, therefore, be examined.

In negative blood films, the presence of malaria pigment (9) in peripheral blood mononuclear cells provides an important clue to the diagnosis.

2.5 QBC II system

Microscopic examination of Romanovsky stained thick and thin blood films is at present the most practical and reliable method of diagnosing malaria. But when the parasitaemia is low (e.g. 0.001% or less) the technique can be time-consuming and requires an experienced microscopist. Therefore, for rapid diagnosis of malaria, a new technique has recently been described using quantitative buffy coat (QBC) technology developed by Becton Dickinson (10). This technique is rapid but requires fluorescence microscopy.

In principle, the blood is centrifuged in an acridine-orange coated capillary tube in conjunction with an internal float. Malaria parasites take up acridine-orange and as the infected RBCs are less dense than uninfected cells they appear at the erythrocyte/granulocyte interface. Under UV illumination the acridine-orange staining parasite DNA fluoresces. The nuclei of malaria parasites appear much smaller and more compact than the nuclei of leucocytes which are 10–15 μm in size and diffuse. The cytoplasm of the malaria parasite appears red compared to the bright green of the nucleus.

The area within the white cell layer must also be examined in order to detect later stages in the asexual life cycle. Presence of malarial pigment is also detected here. This can be ingested pigment lying within white cells, or pigment contained within the intraerythrocytic malaria parasites themselves.

A summary of the method is given in *Protocol 7*, but the manufacturer's instructions must be consulted and followed when the technique is used.

Protocol 7. Examination of blood for malaria by QBC (Becton Dickinson)

Equipment

- Lancets, alcohol wipes
- QBC capillary tubes
- Haematocrit centrifuge [a]
- UV microscope [b]
- QBC float

Method

1. Fill the QBC capillary tube with blood.
2. The tube is rolled back and forwards for 5 sec to mix the blood with the contents of the tube.
3. Using forceps, a float is inserted in the capillary tube then cap the tube.
4. The tube is centrifuged for 5 min at 10 500 r.p.m.
5. The tube is removed from the centrifuge placed in the 'Paraviewer' and viewed under UV illumination using oil immersion.

[a] Battery operated centrifuges are available.
[b] An alternative is an UV adapter produced by the QBC manufacturer (Paralens®) which is a × 60 objective with UV illumination.

3. Detection of anti-malarial antibody

Antibodies to the asexual blood stages appear a few days after malaria parasites invade RBC's, and rise in titre over the next few weeks. These antibodies may persist for months or years in semi-immune patients in endemic areas where re-infection is frequent. However, in a non-immune patient treated for a single infection, antibody levels fall more rapidly and may be undetectable in three to six months or so. Re-infection or relapse leads to a secondary response with high and rapid rise in antibody titres.

Antibody detection cannot be a substitute for blood film examination in the diagnosis of an acute attack of malaria, but may help in prospective screening of blood donors and retrospective confirmation of malaria in residents of non-endemic areas recently treated empirically overseas. It is also useful in investigation of cases of tropical splenomegaly syndrome (hyperreactive malarial splenomegaly) (11). Antibodies to malaria parasites can be detected by various methods, the two most employed are the IFAT (*Protocol 9*) and the ELISA (*Protocol 10*) (12).

3.1 The indirect fluorescent antibody test (IFAT)

Antigens for this technique can be prepared from:

(a) Peripheral blood of infected patients (*P. falciparum*, *P. vivax*, *P. malariae*).

(b) Continuous *in vitro* culture of *P. falciparum* provides a useful source of antigen.

(c) Adapting *P. falciparum* to grow in primates (e.g. *Aotus* or *Saimiri* monkeys). However, supply is limited and this method is to be avoided if possible. The Simian parasite *P. fieldii*, from rhesus monkeys can be used instead of *P. falciparum*. *P. vivax* can be maintained in *Aotus* and *Saimiri* spp., especially if splenectomized. The Simian parasite *P. cynomolgi* from rhesus monkeys is an alternative source of antigen for serodiagnosis of *P. vivax* infection. *P. brasilianum* from *Aotus*, *Saimiri*, or *Cebus* monkeys is an alternative antigen where *P. malariae* cannot be obtained.

Protocol 8. Preparing malarial antigen for the IFAT

1. Collect 5 ml of citrated blood preferably from a patient with a parasitaemia > 3% (minimum 1%).
2. Centrifuge the blood at 2500 r.p.m. for 5 min.
3. Discard the supernatant and suspend the pellet in PBS, pH 7.2.
4. Repeat steps **1** and **2**, i.e. wash pellet three times with PBS.
5. Resuspend the packed cells in a small volume of PBS, approximately half the original blood volume.
6. Add a drop of the above preparation to each well of a Teflon coated slide.
7. Air dry the slide overnight and freeze at −20 °C (preferably −70 °C) until required.

Protocol 9. Method for indirect fluorescent antibody test

1. Remove antigen slides from the deep-freeze, dry, and label appropriately (each slide must contain a positive and a negative control).
2. Dilute the test sera 1:20 in PBS pH 7.2, add a 10 μl drop to the appropriate wells, and incubate in a moist chamber for 30 min at room temperature.
3. Wash the slides in phosphate-buffered saline (PBS) for 20 min with two changes of buffer, then air dry.
4. Dilute fluorescein labelled anti-human immunoglobulin (Wellcome)

Protocol 9. *Continued*

1:30 in PBS. Add a 10 μl drop to each antigen well. Incubate the slides in a humidified chamber at room temperature for 30 min.

5. Air dry the slides and add a drop of buffered glycerol to each well. Attach a coverslip and view the slides under a × 40 fluorescence objective.

   Bright green fluorescence denotes a positive result. The results are carefully compared with positive and negative controls.

6. If a serum is positive at the screening dilution of 1:20, test doubling dilutions of sera to determine the end-point titre of each positive sample.

The above test may also be performed using antigens of *P. vivax* or *P. malariae* to attempt species-specific serodiagnosis.

3.2 Enzyme-linked immunosorbent assay (ELISA) for antibody detection

ELISA for detection of anti-malarial antibody is available in kit form, e.g. the Launch diagnostics malaria antibody ELISA test kit which provides strips of *P. falciparum* antigen coated wells and the required reagents. A summary of the method is given in *Protocol 10*, but the manufacturer's instructions must be consulted and followed in detail when the kit is used.

Protocol 10. ELISA for detection of anti-malarial antibody

1. For each 16 well (2 × 8) *P. falciparum* antigen coated microstrip to be used prepare 105 ml PBS–Tween by adding 5 ml of 20 × PBS–Tween concentrate to 100 ml of distilled water.
2. Make a 1:10 dilution of reference positive serum, reference negative serum, and test samples in PBS–Tween.
3. Add 100 μl of the diluted samples to individual wells of the coated strip.
4. Cover the strip and incubate for 1 h at 37 °C in a humidified chamber.
5. 10 min before the end of incubation, prepare the diluted conjugate by adding 20 μl of concentrated conjugate to 3 ml of PBS–Tween and mix thoroughly.
6. Wash the strip at least three times with PBS–Tween.
7. Add 100 μl of diluted conjugate to each well. Cover the strip and incubate for 1 h at 37 °C in a humidified chamber.
8. 10 min before the end of the incubation, prepare the substrate by adding two OPD tablets to 6 ml distilled water, followed by one drop of 3% H_2O_2.

9. Wash the strip as in step **6**.
10. Add 100 μl of substrate solution to each well. Cover the strip and place in the dark at room temperature for 15 min.
11. Add 50 μl (one drop) of 2.5 M HCl to each well to stop the reaction and read the absorbance at 492 nm within 30 min.
12. Blank the reader against wells containing reacted substrate.
13. Read the absorbance of the reference positive and reference negative. They should give values of at least 0.8 and less than 0.1 respectively.

The cut-off to determine which samples are positive is defined as the reference negative absorbance +0.1. It is important to note that this test system is not a diagnostic method for active clinical malaria. The highest test values are expected with *P. falciparum* infections, with lower values in infections due to *P. vivax, P. ovale,* or *P. malariae* as cross-reaction is only partial.

Protocol 11. Enzyme-linked immunosorbent assay (ELISA) to detect *P. falciparum* antigens

Equipment and reagents

- Microtitration strips coated with anti-malaria monoclonal antibody (supplier PATH)
- Peroxidase labelled anti-malaria monoclonal antibody conjugate
- Conjugate diluent
- Tetramethyl benzidine solution
- TMB substrate buffer
- Washing solution: PBS–Tween, pH 7.5
- 1.25 M H_2SO_4
- 100 μl and 5 ml adjustable pipettes and tips
- Reference positive samples

Method

1. Add 100 μl blood haemolysate from specimens, reference positive, and negative controls, to the wells coated with anti-malarial monoclonal antibody and incubate at room temperature for 1 h in a humidified chamber.
2. After the incubation period, wash the wells three times with PBS–Tween and shake the plate dry.
3. Dilute the conjugate 1:1000 using the conjugate diluent, and add 100 μl of diluted conjugate to each well.
4. Incubate at room temperature for 1 h in a humidified chamber.
5. After incubation, wash wells with PBS–Tween as before.
6. For each 16 wells take 100 μl TMB in 2 ml of substrate buffer.
7. Add 100 μl of diluted substrate to each well and incubate at room temperature in the dark for 15 min. Include two blank wells.

Protocol 11. *Continued*

8. Stop the reaction with 100 μl of 1.25 M H_2SO_4.
9. Read the results within 30 min.
10. Read the optical density of all wells at 450 nm after blanking with the blank wells. Absorbance of reference positive should be over 0.5. Any result over 0.15 is reported to be positive.

In the future, methods to detect malaria parasites such as DNA probes (*Protocol 12*), RNA probes, polymerase chain reaction, and antigen detection assays such as radioimmunoassay or dot ELISA, may become available for use in the routine clinical laboratory for individual patient diagnosis. However, at present they are more applicable to field studies where the ability to process a very large number of samples in a day is a distinct advantage.

4. DNA probes

The method of Barker *et al.* (14) is described (*Protocol 13*). This method is specific for *P. falciparum* and able to detect 20–25 parasites per microlitre of blood.

Protocol 12. DNA probe for detection of *P. falciparum*

1. Add 200 μl of lysis mix (10 mM Tris–HCl pH 10, 50 mM EDTA, 200 μg/ml proteinase K, 0.1% Triton X-100) to each well of a microtitre plate.
2. Add 35 μl of heparinized blood to each well. Add positive and negative controls to each test run.
3. Incubate the plate for 1 h at 42 °C.
4. Transfer the samples to the (nylon-based) Genescreen Plus filtration membrane (Dupont NEN Research Products).
5. Air dry the filters for at least 30 min.
6. Denature the sample DNA for 10 min by placing the filtration membranes in 2 ml of 0.5 M sodium hydroxide and 1.5 M sodium chloride.
7. Neutralize the filters twice by placing them for 10 min each time in 1.5 ml of 1 M Tris–HCl pH 8.0, then dry them in air.
8. Hybridize the Genescreen filters overnight at 42 °C in hybridization solution:
   - 50% formamide
   - 5 × standard saline citrate (SSC): 0.56 M NaCl, 75 mM sodium citrate, 345 mM acetic acid
   - 5 × Denhardt's solution: 0.02% bovine serum albumin, 0.02% Ficoll 400, 0.02% polyvinyl pyrrolidone
   - 1% sodium dodecyl sulfate (SDS)

- 100 μg/ml denatured herring sperm DNA
- probe DNA: ^{32}P-radiolabelled pPF14 DNA (15), at a concentration of 5×10^5 c.p.m/ml hybridization solution. pPF14 contains 1 kb of *P. falciparum* DNA comprising tandemly arranged degenerate 21 bp repeats.

9. Wash the filters twice, for 5 min each time at room temperature in 2 × SSC, then twice for 30 min each at 65 °C in 2 × SSC and 1% SDS, then 30 min at room temperature in 0.1 × SSC.

10. Do *not* dry the filters before exposure to X-ray film.

Methods for processing large numbers of specimens for malaria diagnosis are necessary for field studies, and screening blood donations in endemic countries. The ELISA described in *Protocol 11* has been evaluated in developed and endemic countries. It has proved specific and at least as sensitive as thick film examination (13).

5. Polymerase chain reaction

The method of Barker *et al.* (16) is described.

Protocol 13. Polymerase chain reaction for detection of *P. falciparum*

1. Collect 20 μl blood samples in microcapillary tubes containing 5 μl of citrate solution (38 mM citric acid, 74 mM sodium citrate, 88 mM NaCl).
2. Add to each well of a microtitre plate 200 μl of Saponin lysis mixture (0.22% NaCl, 0.015% Saponin, 1 mM EDTA).
3. Transfer the lysed samples on to 903 paper (Schleicher and Schuell) using a Minifold vacuum filtration apparatus (Schleicher and Schuell) and a Nalgene hand vacuum pump.
4. Air dry the filters and cut out a 3 mm piece of filter using a biopsy punch.
5. Transfer the filter discs to 0.5 ml tubes containing 150 μl of PCR mixture.

   PCR mixture: 2.5 U of *Taq* I DNA polymerase (Cetus, or BioExcellence; PCR buffer [70 mM Tris pH 8.8, 20 mM $(NH_4)_2SO_4$, 2.5 mM $MgCl_2$, 1 mM DTT, 100 μg/ml of BSA, 0.1% Triton X-100]; 0.2 mM deoxynucleotides; 30–50 pmoles of oligonucleotide primers. Sequences of *P. falciparum* primers. These primers are degenerate and alternate nucleotides are given in brackets.

Protocol 13. *Continued*

186 AGGTC (TC) TAATT (TC) T (GAC) (GCT) TA (TA) C (CA) T
187 TA (TA) GT (TA) AG (GAT) (GAC) AA (GA) (TA) TA (GA) GACCT

The primers are specific for *P. falciparum* and are derived from the sequence of the probe pPF14.

6. Denature samples in the PCR mixture for 5 min at 94 °C and amplify for 30 cycles (3 min at 37 °C, 5 min at 72 °C, and 1 min at 94 °C).
7. Analyse PCR products either by Southern blotting (step **8**) *or* by dot blot hybridization (steps **9–11**).
8. Prepare Southern blots by resolving 20 μl of PCR product on 2% agarose gels, followed by Southern transfer on to Genescreen plus or Magna NT hybridization membranes.
9. Undertake dot blot hybridization using ^{32}P-labelled pPF14 as described in *Protocol 12*.
10. Alternatively, undertake dot blot hybridization with non-isotopic probes using Magna NT membranes. Label pPF14 probe DNA by incorporating digoxigenin-derivatized dUTP by PCR using a molar ratio of 0.35 dUTP: 0.65 dTTP. If the Genius kit (Boehringer-Mannheim) is used, undertake hybridization, washing, and binding of alkaline phosphatase-conjugated anti-digoxigenin antibodies according to the manufacturer's instructions.
11. Detect hybridization using the chemiluminescent substrate AMPPD (3-(2′-spiroadamantane)-4-methoxy-4-(3″-phosphoryloxy)-phenyl-1, 2-dioxetane (Tropix) according to the manufacturer's instructions. Use 2–4 h exposures to X-ray film.

Using the non-isotopically labelled probe following PCR amplification, it is possible to detect less than ten parasites in a 20 μl blood sample. The method is specific for *P. falciparum*.

References

1. Garnham, P. C. C. (1966). *Malaria parasites and other haemosporidia*. Blackwell Scientific Publications, Oxford.
2. Warrell, D. A., Molyneux, M. E., and Beales, P. F. (ed.) (1990). *Trans. R. Soc. Trop. Med. Hyg.*, **84** (suppl. 2), 1.
3. Shute, G. T. (1988). In *Malaria. Principles and practice of malariology* (ed. W. H. Wernsdorfer and I. McGregor), pp. 781–814. Churchill Livingstone, Edinburgh.
4. WHO. (1991). *Basic laboratory methods in medical parasitology*. World Health Organization, Geneva.
5. Bruce-Chwatt, L. J. (1984). *Lancet*, 795.
6. Earle, W. C. and Perez, M. (1932). *J. Lab. Clin. Med.*, **17**, 1125.

7. Chiodini, P. L. and Moody, A. H. (1989). *J. R. Soc. Med.*, **82**, 41.
8. Hawthorne, M., Chiodini, P. L., Snell, J. J. S., Moody, A. H., and Ramsey, A. (1992). *J. Clin. Pathol.*, **45**, 968.
9. Scheibel, L. W. and Sherman, I. W. (1988). In *Malaria. Principles and practice of malariology* (ed. W. H. Wernsdorfer and I. McGregor), pp. 219–52. Churchill Livingstone, Edinburgh.
10. Spielman, A., Perrone, J. B., Teklehaimanot, A., Balcha, F., Wardlaw, S. C., and Levene, R. A. (1988). *Am. J. Trop. Med. Hyg.*, **39**, 337.
11. Gillespie, S. H., and Chiodini, P. L. (1988). *Serodiagnosis Immunother. Infect. Dis.*, **2**, 157.
12. Voller, A. (1988). In *Malaria. Principles and practice of malariology* (ed. W. H. Wernsdorfer and I. McGregor), pp. 815–25. Churchill Livingstone, Edinburgh.
13. Taylor, D. W. and Voller, A. (1993). *Trans. R. Soc. Trop. Med. Hyg.*, **87**, 29.
14. Barker, R. H., Suebsaeng, L., Rooney, W., and Wirth, D. F. (1989). *Am. J. Trop. Med. Hyg.*, **41**, 266.
15. Barker, R. H., Suebsaeng, L., Rooney, W., Alecrim, G. C., Dourado, H. V., and Wirth, D. F. (1986). *Science*, **231**, 1434.
16. Barker, R. H., Banchongaksorn, T., Courval, J. M., Suwonkerd, W., Rimwungtragoon, K., and Wirth, D. F. (1992). *Am. J. Trop. Med. Hyg.*, **46**, 416.

3

Toxoplasmosis

JULIE D. JOHNSON and RICHARD E. HOLLIMAN

1. Introduction

The obligate intracellular protozoan, *Toxoplasma gondii*, is a recognized cause of lymphadenopathy or a clinical syndrome resembling glandular fever. Infection of immunocompromised individuals, including the fetus, patients with Hodgkin's disease, organ graft recipients, and the AIDS sufferer are prone to severe or even life-threatening disease. Routine serological assessment has been established for HIV infected persons and in cases of heart, heart/lung, or liver transplantation, while the place of antenatal screening is the subject of active consideration. Consequently, the diagnostic laboratory may receive requests for investigation of toxoplasma infection in a range of clinical settings and a large number of diagnostic assays have been developed to meet this challenge.

Antibody tests for toxoplasmosis can be classified into two major groupings: those using whole intact organisms (dye test, direct agglutination test, and fluorescent antibody test), and those using disrupted parasites as an antigen source (complement fixation test, enzyme-linked immunosorbent assay, latex agglutination test, indirect haemagglutination assay).

The antigens used in toxoplasma diagnostic assays come from either plasma or cytoplasmic membrane. In early infection the host immune response is directed towards the membrane antigens whereas the cytoplasmic antigens become progressively more important as antibody targets in chronic infection. Assays utilizing whole organisms as an antigen source are most reactive in early infection while tests incorporating disrupted parasites produce titres which rise more slowly during the course of the infection but persist for a greater time. The severity of a clinical illness is not associated with the magnitude of the antibody response, irrespective of the assay employed.

2. The dye test

The accepted reference assay for the measurement of toxoplasma specific antibody is the dye test of Sabin and Feldman (1).

The principle of the dye test is a complement-mediated neutralizing

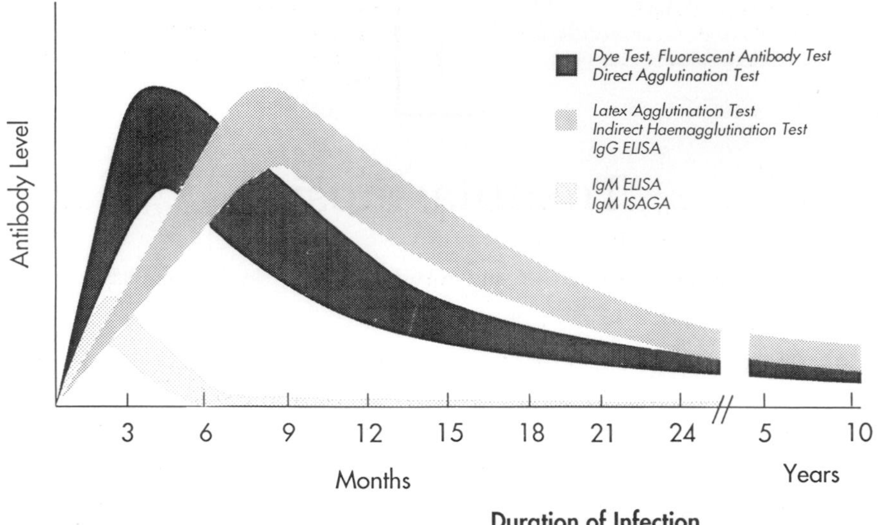

Figure 1. Variation of toxoplasma antibody test results with the duration of infection.

antigen–antibody reaction. Live trophozoites, the test sample, and complement are mixed and incubated at 37 °C for one hour after which time a vital stain, alkaline methylene blue is added (2). Specific antibody induces complement-mediated cytolysis of the parasites and the organisms are thus unable to retain the vital stain.

The dye test is highly specific and sensitive although low titre false positive reactions are seen in *Hammondia hammondii* infection or following blood transfusion, and false negative results have been demonstrated in immunosuppressed individuals. Reactivity with the dye test appears within one to two weeks of infection and titres rise to reach a peak within the following two months. The antibody levels decline gradually over many months or years, low titres often persist for life (see *Figure* 1).

Protocol 1. Production of antigen

Equipment and reagents

- 6–8 week old MF1 mice 25–30 g (toxoplasma antibody-free)
- Antibiotic saline: physiological saline (0.85% NaCl) containing 100 U/ml of penicillin and streptomycin, 12.5 U/ml heparin
- Penicillin and streptomycin: 1 g streptomycin, 1 million U penicillin in 100 ml sterile distilled water
- 5% bicarbonate buffer: 0.6 M $NaHCO_3$ (5 g), 0.2 ml 0.4% phenol red in 100 ml sterile deionized water saturated with CO_2
- Sterile viral transport medium: 10 ml Hanks B.S.S. (× 10), 90 ml sterile distilled water, 2 ml bicarbonate buffer, 1 ml penicillin and streptomycin
- Trophozoites of *T. gondii*

- Protective eye goggles[a]
- Fuchs–Rosenthal counting chamber
- Sterile scissors and forceps
- Alcohol
- Pasteur pipette and bulb
- Dissection board
- Physiological saline (0.85% NaCl)
- 5 ml sterile syringe and 0.6 × 30 mm hypodermic needle

Method

1. Dilute the trophozoites in viral transport medium to give an inoculum of 500 000 organisms/ml.[b]
2. Inoculate 0.5 ml of the suspension per mouse intraperitoneally.
3. Approximately 68 h after inoculation kill the mice.
4. Harvest the peritoneal exudate by flushing the peritoneal cavity with antibiotic saline.
5. Dilute the suspension with physiological saline to approximately 7 200 000 organisms/ml for use as the antigen in the dye test.[c]
6. The antigen must be shown to be free of mouse antibody (see *Protocol 2*).

[a] Wear eye goggles whilst handling live trophozoites of *T. gondii* to prevent accidental infection via the conjunctiva.
[b] This dose is critical as a lower dose results in a cellular exudate and a higher dose results in an exudate containing toxoplasma antibody produced by the mouse itself; neither is suitable for the dye test.
[c] The antigen must be continuously re-passaged in mice if the dye test is used as a routine diagnostic tool.

Protocol 2. Screening method for complement source and antigen source

Equipment and reagents

- Physiological saline (0.85% NaCl)
- Flat-well microtitre plate/s
- Inverted microscope
- Toxoplasma antigen (see *Protocol 1*)
- Positive control serum (pooled sera diluted to give a dye test titre of 1:256)
- Complement source[a]
- Disodium citrate[b]
- Methylene blue solution: saturated 1.6% (w/v) alcoholic solution of methylene blue 0.15 ml, 1.91% (w/v) sodium tetraborate 0.3 ml, 0.53% (w/v) sodium carbonate 9.7 ml, pH 11 buffer (filter before use)
- Plate mixer (optional)
- Clear adhesive tape
- Mechanical or hand diluter
- 37 °C incubator
- Automatic micropipettes and disposable tips
- 56 °C water-bath

Method

1. Use a flat-well microtitre plate and allocate one row per accessory factor tested. Place 25 μl of saline into wells 1 to 10 and well 12.

Protocol 2. *Continued*

2. Add 75 μl of saline to well 11.
3. Add 25 μl of the positive control to well 1, mix thoroughly, and double dilute through to well 10. Discard the last 25 μl.
4. Mix the complement thoroughly and add 50 μl to wells 2, 4 to 10, and 12.
5. Add 25 μl of toxoplasma antigen to every well. Final titres 1:16 (well 2) to 1:4096 (well 10).
6. Cover the plate with clear adhesive tape and mix thoroughly using a mechanical mixer or by tapping the sides of the plate.
7. Incubate the plate at 37 °C for 1 h.
8. Add 25 μl of alkaline methylene blue to wells 2 and 4 to 12.
9. Re-seal the clear adhesive tape, mix thoroughly, and re-incubate at 37 °C for 5 min.
10. Allow the plate to stand at room temperature for 10 min before reading using an inverted microscope with × 32 objective and × 10 eye-pieces.
11. Results:
    (a) Well 11 contains only saline, antigen, and dye and therefore represents 100% stained organisms.
    (b) Well 12 contains diluent, complement, antigen, and dye and should contain not less than 90% of toxoplasma organisms stained. If < 90% are stained then the complement contains toxoplasma specific antibody and can not be used.
    (c) The end-point is the dilution of the positive control showing 50% unstained toxoplasma organisms.
    (d) The complement source must give an end-point of 1:256 to demonstrate sufficient complement is present.
    (e) If all toxoplasma organisms are stained in every well there is no complement present in the complement source.

[a] Obtained from the National Blood Transfusion Service, this comprises fresh normal human serum or plasma which must be tested to show that it contains sufficient complement activity and no toxoplasma antibody. It must be stored frozen as complement activity declines at room temperature.

[b] 10% of plasma samples are suitable for use in the dye test as against 1% of serum samples. Addition of 5% disodium citrate to serum will improve the suitability for use to 10%.

Protocol 3. The toxoplasma dye test

Equipment and reagents

- See *Protocol 2*
- National control serum (pooled freeze-dried human serum from acute cases of toxoplasmic lymphadenopathy standardized against the WHO International control serum issued by the State Serum Institute, Copenhagen, Denmark
- Test samples [a]

Method

1. Use a flat-well microtitre plate and allocate one row per test specimen/control. Add 25 μl of saline into all wells.
2. (a) Where clinical details include ocular involvement, or immunosuppression due to AIDS or organ transplant, or if the specimen is fetal serum, amniotic fluid, or a CSF add 50 μl of the specimen into the first well of each row without the addition of saline.

   (b) For other test samples and the controls add 25 μl into the first well of each row.
3. Make serial doubling dilutions of the test sample/controls from wells 1 to 12. Discard the last 25 μl from well 12.
4. Add 50 μl of complement and 25 μl of toxoplasma antigen suspension to all wells of the rows that began with neat serum and to wells 2 and 4 to 12 of the rows that began with a 1:2 dilution.
5. Seal the plate/s with clear adhesive tape, mix thoroughly, and incubate at 37 °C for 1 h.
6. Add 25 μl of alkaline methylene blue to each well containing complement and antigen, mix thoroughly, and re-incubate at 37 °C for 5 min.
7. Allow the plate to stand at room temperature for 10 min before reading as in *Protocol 2*.
8. Results:

   (a) The end-point is the dilution of sample/controls showing 50% unstained toxoplasma organisms.

   (b) The positive control produces a dye test titre of 1:256.

   (c) The National Standard represents 1000 International Units per millilitre and either produces a dye test titre of 1:2000 or 1:4000.

   (d) The titres produced by the test samples may be expressed as International Units using the conversion (*Table 1*).

Protocol 3. *Continued*

(e) The dye test is the only test that can be quoted in International Units since it is standardized against the WHO International Control serum.

[a] With the dye test and all other assays outlined in this chapter test samples should be heat inactivated at 56 °C for 30 min as a precaution against the presence of HIV.

Table 1. Conversion of dye test titre to International Units

National std dye test = 1:200		National std dye test = 1:4000	
Dye test titre	**Units**	**Dye test titre**	**Units**
1/16 384	8000	1/16 384	4000
1/ 8192	4000	1/ 8192	2000
1/ 4096	2000	1/ 4096	1000
1/ 2048	1000	1/ 2048	500
1/ 1024	500	1/ 1024	250
1/ 512	250	1/ 512	125
1/ 256	125	1/ 256	62
1/ 128	62	1/ 128	31
1/ 64	31	1/ 64	16
1/ 32	16	1/ 32	7
1/ 16	7	1/ 16	4
1/ 8	4	1/ 8	2
1/ 4	2	1/ 4	

3. Fluorescent antibody test (FAT)

Outside of the United Kingdom the FAT is the most widely used procedure for the diagnosis of toxoplasmosis. It does not require live toxoplasma organisms and is available commercially through a variety of companies.

Killed trophozoites are fixed on to a slide and incubated with dilutions of the test sample. Using appropriate specific fluorescein labelled conjugates, IgG and IgM antibodies may be detected (2). In using IgM fluorescein conjugates care must be taken to avoid misinterpretation of fluorescence due to non-specific 'capping' of the trophozoites. It has been demonstrated that these false positive reactions involve expression of Fc receptors by toxoplasma and pre-treatment of the trophozoites with Fc abolishes this non-specific binding (3).

True fluorescence encompasses the whole organism. False positives may also occur with samples containing rheumatoid factor or anti-nuclear factor and false negative IgM reactions are observed with samples containing high titres of specific IgG. Fluorescent antibody tests for IgM are less sensitive than ELISA or agglutination assays and therefore results should be confirmed using more sensitive and specific assays.

Protocol 4. Fluorescent antibody test

Equipment and reagents

- U-well microtitre plates
- Phosphate-buffered saline pH 7.2 (PBS)
- Teflon coated 'multispot' microscope slides
- Veronal buffer pH 7.6
- Toxoplasma antigen from mouse peritoneal exudate (see *Protocol 1*)
- Fluorescein labelled anti-human immunoglobulin
- Buffered glycerol pH 9.2
- Positive and negative control sera
- Moist chamber or 'wet box'
- 37 °C incubator
- Micropipettes and disposable tips
- 56 °C water-bath
- Centrifuge
- Acetone
- Test samples (heat inactivated)

A. *Preparation of antigen coated slides*

These slides may either be obtained ready prepared commercially or may be 'home-made' if an antigen source is available.

1. Harvest the peritoneal exudate (*Protocol 1*) and test for the absence of antibody (*Protocol 2*).
2. Centrifuge the exudate, discard the supernatant and wash twice in PBS.
3. Dilute the trophozoites in PBS to a concentration of 8×10^6–10^7 organisms/ml.
4. Cover each well of the Teflon coated multispot slides and air dry.
5. Fix the slides in acetone for 10 min.
6. Air dry and store at −20 °C for use.

B. *Fluorescent antibody test*

1. Using a U-well microtitre plate make doubling dilutions of the test sample and controls in PBS from 1:2 to 1:64.
2. Remove the required number of slides from −20 °C and allow 2 min to thaw at room temperature.
3. Cover each successive spot on the antigen slide/s with the test sample, positive, and negative control dilutions.
4. Incubate in a moist chamber at 37 °C for 30 min.
5. Wash the slide/s gently in running tap-water for 10 min and air dry.
6. Dilute the conjugate to its optimal dilution determined by manufacturer's recommendation or chequerboard titration with PBS, and cover each antigen/sample spot.

Protocol 4. *Continued*

7. Incubate the slide/s in a moist chamber at 37 °C for 30 min.
8. Wash in gently flowing tap-water for 10 min and air dry.
9. Mount the slide(s) in buffered glycerol and examine by fluorescent microscopy.
10. Results: the titre is the highest dilution at which the fluoresce of the whole toxoplasma organism is still evident.

4. Complement fixation test (CFT)

Warren and Russ (1948) first described a complement fixation test using the chorio-allantoic membrane of hens eggs infected with *T. gondii* as an antigen source (4). Subsequently, by the use of parasites obtained from mouse peritoneal inoculation, the sensitivity of this assay was improved (5), but the importance of the antigen preparation coupled with complex procedures and strict standardization of the reagents have lead to a lack of commercially available CFT kits. Therefore CFT is not the test of choice for the non-reference laboratory and is indeed rarely used.

5. Haemagglutination test

The haemagglutination test (6,7) involves fixation of toxoplasma cytoplasmic and membrane-bound antigen to pyruvic aldehyde-treated sheep or turkey red cells which act as carrier particles. The protein of the antigen sticks to the red cells and the sensitized cells agglutinate in the presence of toxoplasma specific antibody. This test was first used by Jacobs and Lunde in 1957 and is still commercially available although its sensitivity and specificity is inferior to the dye test.

6. Latex agglutination test

In this reaction latex particles are sensitized with a preparation of sonicated trophozoites containing both cytoplasmic and membrane-bound antigens and the pattern of agglutination is observed when the specimen to be tested is added and incubated for 12 hours. The latex agglutination test is available commercially or may be prepared in the laboratory (*Protocol 5*). Compared to the dye test it has a sensitivity of 99% but a specificity of 81% and produces false positives in 1–2% of cases due to the reaction of non-specific IgM. It should be considered as a screening test for toxoplasmosis but not as a replacement for the dye test.

Protocol 5. Latex agglutination test

Equipment and reagents

- U-well microtitre plates
- Test samples (heat inactivated)
- Diluent buffer solution: 0.2 M 2-amino-2-methyl-1-propanol HCl buffer
- Positive and negative controls
- Latex beads, 0.9 μm (Sigma Chemical Co. Ltd.)
- Trophozoites of *T. gondii* (see Protocol 1)
- Magnifying mirror for microtitration plates (optional)
- Plate mixer (optional)
- 56 °C water-bath
- Mechanical or hand diluter
- Clear adhesive tape
- Micropipettes and disposable tips
- 0.2 M ammonium chloride buffer pH 8.2
- Glycine buffer pH 8.2 + 0.1% sodium azide
- 37 °C incubator
- 0.2 M ammonium chloride buffer + 50% sucrose
- Borate buffer pH 8.7 + 4 g bovine serum albumin + 1 g NaN_3 per litre

A. *Preparation of latex/antigen suspension coated using the method of Tsuboda and Ozawa* (8)

1. Add 100 μl of 0.2 M ammonium chloride buffer (pH 8.2) to 10 mg of latex beads suspended in 200 μl of glycine buffer (pH 8.2) containing 0.1% sodium azide.
2. Add 25 μg of *T. gondii* antigen per milligram of latex particles (see *Protocol 9*).
3. Mix thoroughly and incubate at 37 °C for 1 h.
4. Add 100 μl of ammonium chloride buffer containing 50% sucrose, mix thoroughly, and incubate overnight at 4 °C.
5. Wash the suspension twice by centrifugation, and resuspend the sedimented beads in 1.5 ml of borate buffer (pH 8.7) containing 4 g of bovine serum albumin, and 1 g of NaN_3 per litre.

B. *Performance of latex agglutination test*

1. Use U-well microtitre plates and allocate one row per test sample/controls. Add 25 μl of diluent into all wells.
2. (a) Where clinical details include ocular involvement, or immunosuppression due to AIDS or organ transplant, or if the specimen is fetal serum, CSF, or amniotic fluid add 50 μl of the specimen into the first well of each row without the addition of any buffer.

   (b) For other samples add 25 μl of the test sample/control into the first well of each row.
3. Make serial doubling dilutions of the samples and controls from wells 1 through to 12. Discard the last 25 μl.
4. Mix the latex suspension thoroughly and add 25 μl to all wells of the rows that began with neat serum, and to wells 4 and 6 through to 12 of the rows that began with a 1:2 dilution.

Protocol 5. *Continued*

5. Cover the plate/s with clear adhesive tape and mix thoroughly.
6. Incubate the plate on a horizontal surface at room temperature for at least 12 h.
7. Read the plates using a magnifying mirror for microtitration plates or against a dark background.
8. Results:
   (a) A negative reaction is observed as a small distinct button of sedimentation in the centre of the well.
   (b) A positive reaction is observed as agglutination of the latex suspension.
      i. The agglutination may appear as a large plaque which may have dropped into the well giving an irregular, torn effect (+++ agglutination).
      ii. A large plaque of agglutination spread throughout the well (++ agglutination).
      iii. A small plaque of agglutination with a small button (+ agglutination).
      iv. All samples producing a positive latex agglutination should be examined by the dye test.
   (c) The titre is the highest dilution of the sample/controls showing an agglutination reaction. The results are expressed as a titre.

7. Latex slide agglutination test

Early attempts at producing slide agglutination tests for the detection of toxoplasma specific immunoglobulins were of low sensitivity. However, recently a commercially available slide agglutination test has been compared to the dye test for the detection of toxoplasma specific IgG and has proven to have a sensitivity of 98.7% and a specificity of 95.8%. Polystyrene latex particles are coated with *T. gondii* soluble antigen and mixed with test sample on a slide and after five minutes rotation the suspension is examined for visible agglutination. The slide agglutination test is therefore suitable as a screening assay for toxoplasmosis but not as a replacement for the dye test. It is recommended that sera from immunocompetent patients showing positive agglutination at ≥1:16 and at neat sera for immunocompromised patients are examined by the dye test.

8. Direct agglutination test

Fulton and Turk (9) were the first to describe a direct agglutination test which involved the reaction of specific antibody with formalin fixed trophozoites to form a visible agglutination pattern. However, its specificity was low due to the binding of non-toxoplasma specific IgM, sensitivity was lower than the dye test, and numerous trophozoites were required.

Couzineau and Baufine-Ducrocq (10) and Desmonts and Remington (11) increased the reproducibility of this method by using mouse sarcoma cells to grow larger numbers of trophozoites and by pre-treating sera with 2-mercaptoethanol to remove cross-reacting IgM. By rupturing the walls of the sarcoma cells with the enzyme trypsin, increased yields of free parasites are obtained with the added advantage that the cytoplasmic antigens are exposed increasing the sensitivity of the assay.

Using the dye test as a reference the sensitivity and specificity of the direct agglutination test have been found to be 96% and 98% respectively, but the semi-quantitative method does not correlate with the dye test.

Recently a direct agglutination test has been described to differentiate acute and chronic disease. By using acetone fixed trophozoites in the agglutination method and by comparison of the results with a formalin fixed assay it is evident that in acute infection, the ratio of formalin fixed to acetone fixed reactivity is smaller than in chronic latent disease (12).

It is thought that the treatment of trophozoites with different agents results in alterations of the antigens available for antibody detection.

Protocol 6. Production of antigen

Equipment and reagents

- Alkaline buffer pH 8.7: 0.12 M (7.02 g) NaCl, 0.05 M (3.09 g) H_3BO_3, 24 ml 1 M NaOH, 4 g BSA made up to 1 litre with distilled water, sodium azide 1 g
- Formalin, diluted 1:5 in PBS (6% formaldehyde solution)
- Phosphate-buffered saline pH 7.2 + 0.05% trypsin
- 37 °C water-bath
- Microscope
- Trophozoites of *T. gondii* and/or sarcoma cells
- Centrifuge
- Phosphate-buffered saline (PBS)
- 56 °C water-bath
- Micropipettes and disposable tips

Methods

1. To obtain a satisfactory volume of antigen for the direct agglutination test either:
   (a) Follow *Protocol 1*.
   (b) Cultivate the RH strain of toxoplasma along with mouse TG 180 sarcoma cells (12).
   (c) Use one of the commercially available direct agglutination test kits which provide formalin treated toxoplasma obtained from mouse ascitic fluid.
2. To formalin fix and sensitize the trophozoites obtained from step **1a**

Protocol 6. *Continued*

and **b** adjust the concentration of organisms to 3×10^7 organisms/ml with PBS. Centrifuge the sarcoma cells and/or antigen at 500–600 *g*, discard the supernatant, and resuspend the deposit in PBS–trypsin.

3. Incubate in a water-bath at 37 °C under continuous agitation. Examine microscopically at 5 min intervals until the sarcoma cells disrupt.
4. Centrifuge the suspension for 10 min at 500–600 *g* and discard the supernatant.
5. Resuspend the sediment in PBS and repeat the centrifugation process.
6. Suspend the parasites in 6% formaldehyde solution and incubate at 4 °C for at least 16 h.
7. Centrifuge and resuspend in PBS for a total of four times to remove all cell debris and formaldehyde.
8. Suspend the parasites in alkaline buffer (pH 8.7) to the original 3×10^7 organisms/ml and store at 4 °C for use.

Protocol 7. Direct agglutination test

Equipment and reagents

- U-well microtitre plates
- 2-mercaptoethanol (2-ME) diluted in PBS to 0.2 mol/litre: 0.35 ml 2-ME + 25 ml PBS freshly made and stored in the dark (may be used for up to one month)
- Test samples (heat inactivated)
- Positive and negative controls
- 32 °C incubator or even room temperature[a]
- Clear adhesive tape
- Plate mixer
- Formalin fixed antigen suspension (see *Protocol 6*)
- Magnifying mirror for microtitration plates (optional)
- Micropipettes and disposable tips
- 56 °C water-bath

Method

1. Use a U-well microtitre plate and allocate one row per sample/control tested. Add 50 μl of fresh 0.2 M 2-ME/PBS into every well.
2. (a) Dilute the test sample/control 1:20 using PBS/2-ME and add 50 μl to the first well of each appropriate row and make serial doubling dilutions from well 1 through to well 12. Discard the final 50 μl from well 12.

   (b) Alternatively if screening is to be performed before titration, two dilutions, i.e. 1:20 and 1:500, should be tested to avoid false negative results due to the prozone phenomenon.
3. Mix the antigen suspension well and add 50 μl into every well.
4. Cover the plate with clear adhesive tape and mix thoroughly.

5. Incubate the plate overnight in a 32 °C incubator.[a]
6. Reading: plates may be read at 16, 24, 48, or even 72 h as long as they have not dried.
7. Read the plates on a magnifying mirror for microtitration plates or against a dark background.
   (a) A smooth button at the bottom of the well is recorded as negative.
   (b) A complete carpet of agglutination is recorded as positive (+++).
   (c) Intermediate readings of ++, +, and ± are also noted.
   (d) The results are expressed as the reciprocal of the final dilution of sample/control to exhibit agglutination.

[a] It is recommended that an incubator set as 32 °C is used for incubation since the pattern of agglutination and sensitivity of the test are greatly modified when working at different temperatures

9. Enzyme-linked immunosorbent agglutination assay (ELISA)

Numerous systems have been developed based on ELISA methodology for the detection of specific antibodies to *T. gondii* since it was first described in 1976 (13, 14). Early systems concentrated on the detection of IgG and involved fixation of toxoplasma antigens derived from disrupted trophozoites on to a solid phase. After incubation with the test sample to allow binding of specific antibody the subsequent addition of anti-human IgG conjugated to an enzyme and of the enzyme substrate facilitates detection of the immune complex by a colour change. This can be made quantitative by strict standardization of reagents. However, due to the lack of availability of suitable antigens these immunodiagnostic assays were slow to appear and when compared directly against the dye test antibody levels did not show good correlation. The antibody class capture assay described by Duermeyer for the detection of IgM in human serum for hepatitis A (15) has been adapted for the study of toxoplasmosis by several groups (16, 17). The solid phase is coated with anti-human IgM and after incubation with the test sample capture of the IgM on to the solid phase is detected by the addition of an antigen indirectly labelled with an enzyme through a complex with monoclonal antibody to toxoplasma. This will form a complex with any specific IgM from the original sample and on addition of the chromogenic enzyme substrate the immune complex is detected using a spectrophotometer.

An ELISA system has been developed (18) to measure the antigen binding avidity of toxoplasma specific IgG. In early infection low avidity antibodies are formed and as the course of infection progresses so the avidity of specific antibody increases. This method is still under evaluation.

Many commercial assays are available for the detection of toxoplasma specific IgG and IgM but their sensitivity and specificity should be independently assessed by reference laboratories before consideration of usage in a non-reference laboratory.

Protocol 8. Enzyme-linked immunosorbent assay (ELISA)

Equipment and reagents

- Falcon flexible PVC microtitration plates
- Coating buffer—Carbonate/bicarbonate buffer pH 9.6: Na_2CO_3 0.015 M (1.5 g/litre), $NaHCO_3$ 0.023 M (2.92 g/litre), adjust to pH 9.6 (may be used for two weeks if stored at 4 °C)
- Mechanical or hand washer
- Tetramethylbenzidine (TMB): dissolve 100 mg TMB in 10 ml of DMSO (store at room temperature in a dark bottle)
- 2 M sulfuric acid
- 6% H_2O_2
- Citric acid/sodium acetate buffer pH 6:0.1 M sodium acetate (CH_3COO Na) anhydrous 16.4 g/2000 ml, 0.1 M citric acid (C(OH) (COOH) $(CH_2COOH)_2$ H_2O) 2.1 g/100 ml (add the citric acid to the sodium acetate solution to bring pH to 6.0, distribute in 100 ml volumes, autoclave, and store at room temperature)
- Phosphate-buffered saline Tween (PBST): 1000 ml phosphate-buffered saline + 0.5 ml (0.05% v/v) Tween-20
- Spectrophotometer
- Micropipettes and disposable tips
- Test samples (heat inactivated)
- 56 °C water-bath
- Phosphate-buffered saline (PBS)
- 37 °C incubator
- Moist chamber or 'wet box'
- Light-proof box
- TMB substrate (for one plate): 15 ml acetate buffer pH 6.0, 150 μl TMB, 15 μl 6% (v/v) H_2O_2

Reagents specifically for IgM ELISA

- Diluent: 10 mM phosphate-buffered saline containing 0.05% (v/v) Tween-20 (PBST) 38 ml, 20% (w/v) bovine serum albumin (BSA) 2 ml (freshly made)
- Polyclonal rabbit anti-human IgM
- Antigen/conjugate C1E3-horse-radish peroxidase at optimum dilution
- Standard serum (100 EIU)
- Positive and negative controls

A. *Preparation of antigen*

1. Harvest the antigen from mouse peritoneal exudate (see *Protocol 1*).
2. Wash the trophozoites three times in PBS by centrifugation at 700 *g* for 10 min.
3. Resuspend the washed parasites in sterile distilled water in the ratio of 250 μl of sterile distilled water to 10^8 organisms/ml.
4. Subject the suspension to three cycles of freezing in liquid nitrogen and thawing at 37 °C.
5. Centrifuge at 700 *g* for 10 min, recover the supernatant, and store at −20 °C for use.
6. Conjugate the monoclonal antibody C1E3 (specific for a major surface membrane antigen of *T. gondii*) with horse-radish peroxidase as described by Isaac and Payne (19). The optimum working dilution is established by chequerboard titration. Store the conjugate at −20 °C.
7. The antigen/conjugate are mixed just prior to use.

B. *IgM ELISA method*

1. Dilute the anti-human IgM 1:1000 (this should be checked by chequerboard titration) by adding 12 μl of anti-human IgM to 12 ml of coating buffer pH 9.6.
2. Mix well and aliquot 100 μl into each well of a flexible PVC microtitration plate.
3. Cover with clear plastic tape or a lid and incubate in a moist chamber at 37 °C for 1 h.
4. Wash the plate thoroughly five times with PBST using a mechanical or hand washer. Tap out the residual solution on to absorbent paper and re-cover the plate with the lid. The plate should NEVER be allowed to dry out.
5. Prepare 1:1000 dilutions of the test samples/controls in PBST/BSA.
6. Aliquot 100 μl of each dilution into duplicate wells.
7. Add 100 μl of PBST/BSA into two wells to function as the antigen/conjugate and substrate controls. Standard serum, positive, and negative controls should also be added.
8. Incubate the plate, covered, in a moist chamber at 37 °C for 1 h.
9. Wash the plate thoroughly as in step **4**. Tap out the residual fluid on to absorbent paper and cover with a lid.
10. Dilute the antigen/conjugate in PBST/BSA to the specified dilution; 12 ml is sufficient for one plate, a typical dilution being 1:30.
11. Add 100 μl of antigen/conjugate to all wells apart from the substrate control. Add only 100 μl of PBST/BSA to the substrate control.
12. Incubate the plate covered in a moist chamber at 37 °C for 1 h.
13. Repeat the wash cycle of step **4**.
14. Prepare the TMB substrate just before use.
15. Immediately and rapidly add 100 μl of the substrate solution to every well. Mix the plate by gently tapping the sides and incubate at room temperature in a light-proof box for at least 30 min.
16. Stop the reaction by adding 25 μl of 2 M H_2SO_4 to each well.
17. Measure the absorbance at a wavelength of 450 nm blanking the plate against the substrate control well using a spectrophotometer.
18. Results are expressed in enzyme immunoassay units as a percentage value of the National control serum (20). The mean absorbance reading at 450 nm is used to calculate the EIU for each sample with the expression:

$$\text{EIU} = \frac{\text{test absorbance} - \text{negative absorbance}}{\text{100 EIU absorbance} - \text{negative absorbance}} \times 100$$

Protocol 8. *Continued*

19. Interpretation of specific IgM levels:
- a unit value of $\leqslant$ 25 is considered negative
- a value of 26–34 is considered a doubtful positive
- 40–100 is positive
- $>$ 100 strong positive

The standard serum used must represent 100 EIU and standardization and controls are essential for qualitative and quantitative assay.

Protocol 9. Detection of toxoplasma specific IgG using ELISA

Equipment and regents

- See reagents for ELISA (*Protocol 8*)
- Rabbit anti-human IgG conjugated to horse-radish peroxidase
- Diluent: PBST + 1% casein hydrolysate (PBST-C)

A. *Preparation of antigen*

1. Harvest the antigen from mouse peritoneal exudate (see *Protocol 1*).

2. Wash the trophozoites three times in PBS by centrifugation at 700 *g* for 10 min.

3. Resuspend in the ratio of 500 μl of sterile distilled water to 10^8 organisms/ml.

4. Subject the suspension to three cycles of freezing in liquid nitrogen and thawing at 37 °C.

5. Centrifuge at 700 *g* for 10 min, discard the supernatant, and replace with an equal volume of PBS.

6. Resuspend the pellet and centrifuge/wash for a total of three times.

7. Macerate or sonicate the cells for 15 min and store at −70 °C.

B. *IgG ELISA method*

1. Dilute the antigen suspension in coating buffer. This is usually at 1:200 dilution.

2. Dispense, incubate, and wash the plate (see *Protocol 8*, steps 2–4).

3. Using PBST-C dilute the test samples 1:100.

4. Aliquot 100 μl of each dilution into duplicate wells.

5. Add 100 μl of PBST-C to two wells to function as conjugate and substrate controls. Standard serum, positive, and negative controls should be included.

6. Incubate the plate covered in a humidified chamber at 37 °C for 30 min.
7. Wash (see *Protocol 8,* step 4).
8. Dilute the rabbit anti-human IgG conjugated to horse-radish peroxidase to optimum dilution (determined by initial titration, typically 1:64 000 in PBST-C).
9. Add 100 μl to every well except the substrate control, add 100 μl PBST to substrate control.
10. Cover with a lid and incubate in a moist chamber at 37 °C for 30 min.
11. Wash (see *Protocol 8,* step 4).
12. Prepare and add substrate, stop the reaction, and read (see *Protocol 8,* steps 13–16).
13. (a) The conjugate and substrate controls should have absorbance values < 0.1
    (b) Negative control < 0.1.
    (c) Test result < 0.05 absorbance = negative.
    (d) > 0.1 absorbance = positive.
    (e) The test is expressed in enzyme immunoassay units (EIU) using the National control serum.

10. Immunosorbent agglutination assay (ISAGA)

The unique IgM ISAGA test was developed by Desmonts *et al.* (21) in order to eliminate the need for an enzyme conjugate, as in the IgM ELISA, and to combine the simplicity of an agglutination test. However, agglutination is subjective to a degree and testing in large batches gives optimal results.

The ISAGA involves an initial IgM capture step using a monoclonal antibody to the CH_2 domain of the human μ-chain. This reduces the incidence of false negative reactions associated with the presence of excess toxoplasma IgG, and false positive results due to rheumatoid factor or anti-nuclear antibody (which are known hazards of the conventional ELISA or indirect immunofluorescent antibody test), and cross-reactivity with IgA and IgE.

Microtitre plates are coated with anti-human IgM and test sera added and incubated to allow binding of immunoglobulin-M. The presence of specific IgM is demonstrated by the subsequent agglutination of entire fixed trophozoites. An ISAGA involving antigen-tagged latex particles has also been developed (22). Serological tests that utilize whole toxoplasma trophozoites as antigens produce a more accurate reflection of the antigenic stimulation of the immune system induced in acute infection.

It has been demonstrated that the ISAGA detects specific IgM with greater sensitivity than the DS-ELISA, conventional ELISA, or fluorescent antibody methods, and that this increased sensitivity coupled with exceptional specificity results in the detection of specific IgM for a protracted period of time, usually 12 to 24 months after initial infection of the immune competent person. As a result the ISAGA may produce a positive result when testing the pregnant woman although her initial exposure to toxoplasma pre-dated conception. Less sensitive IgM tests should be used to estimate the duration of infection when a pregnant woman is found to be ISAGA reactive. Toxoplasma infection of immune compromised patients such as the fetus, neonate, and AIDS victim may be associated with a low level IgM response. In these circumstances, a highly sensitive IgM assay such as ISAGA is of greater clinical value than less sensitive tests.

The ISAGA is available commercially but for the diagnosis of recent toxoplasma infection additional tests must be performed.

Protocol 10. Immunosorbent agglutination assay (ISAGA)

Equipment and reagents

- Microtitration plate (U-well)
- Anti-human IgM (μ-chain specific monoclonal antibody)
- Test sera (heat inactivated)
- Positive and negative controls
- Phosphate-buffered saline (PBS) pH 7.2
- Tween-20
- Toxoplasma antigen (see *Protocol 1*)
- Bovine serum albumin (BSA)
- Magnifying mirror for microtitration plates
- Alkaline buffer pH 8.7: 0.12 M (7.02 g) NaCl, 0.05 M (3.09 g) H_3BO_3, 24 ml 1 M NaOH, 4 g bovine serum albumin, 1 g NaN_3 made up to 1 litre with distilled water
- 0.1 M carbonate buffer pH 9.8
- Micropipettes and disposable tips
- 37 °C incubator
- 56 °C incubator

Method

1. Dilute the IgG fraction of rabbit anti-human IgM (μ-chain specific) in 0.1 M carbonate buffer (pH 9.8) and add 100 μl per reaction well required as previously described (17).
2. Incubate the plates overnight at 4 °C.
3. Wash the wells three times for 5 minutes each in PBS containing 0.05% Tween-20.
4. Post-coat the wells with 1% BSA in PBS containing 0.05% Tween and incubate for 1 h at 37 °C.
5. Wash the plates again as in step **3**, dry, and store at 4 °C.
6. Make a 1:100 dilution of the test samples/controls in PBS. For neonatal and fetal samples, CSF specimens, and amniotic fluid a 1:20 dilution should be used.
7. Add 100 μl of each diluted test sample/controls into three pre-coated wells, cover with a lid, and incubate in a moist chamber at 37 °C for 1 h.

8. Wash the plate in PBS containing 0.05% Tween-20 and twice in ordinary PBS.
9. Dilute the tachyzoites in alkaline buffer (pH 8.7) to obtain a final concentration of 3.3 to 3.6 × 10^7 organisms/ml and mix thoroughly.
10. Dispense the antigen for each set of three wells: 100 μl into the first well, 150 μl into the second well, 200 μl into the third well.
11. Cover the plate and incubate in a moist chamber at 37 °C overnight.
12. Reading:
    (a) Read the ISAGA using a magnifying plate reader and good natural light.
    (b) The antigen control should have total sedimentation of the antigen (button).
    (c) The positive control should have agglutination of the antigen in a mat covering the base of the well.
    (d) By strict standardization of reagents and good controls a quantitative score may be given; see *Figure 2*.
    (e) For each set of three wells add up the values obtained with the three antigen concentrations.

Example: 100 μl antigen		150 μl antigen		200 μl antigen		ISAGA index
4	+	3	+	2	=	9

    (f) Interpretation
    ISAGA index; 0–5 : negative reaction
    6–8 : borderline reaction
    9–12: positive reaction

A matt agglutination covering the base of the well is recorded as positive and a button of sedimentation is negative. The results may be quantified from 0–4 using *Figure 2*.

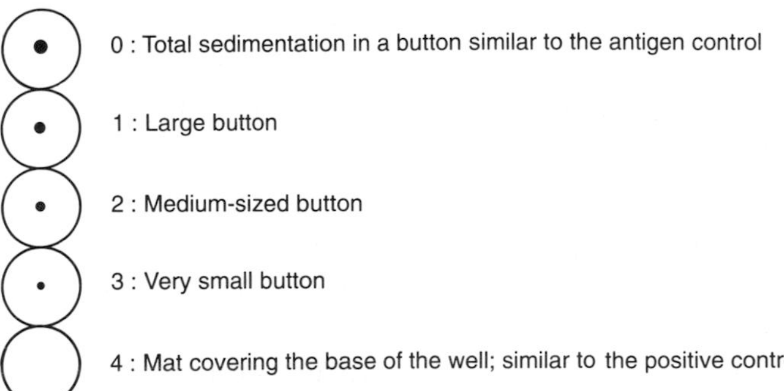

Figure 2. Agglutination patterns in ISAGA.

11. Antigen detection tests

The detection of circulating or localized antigens may be useful in the diagnosis of toxoplasmosis in immunosuppressed patients and congenital infections. *T. gondii* was first detected by Raizman and Neva (23) using '*in vitro*' diffusion methods. Other methods described include ELISA (24) and latex agglutination systems (25).

12. Isolation of *Toxoplasma gondii*

T. gondii can be isolated from tissues and tissue fluids by intraperitoneal injection into mice, inoculation of tissue culture (26), and the chorio-allantoic membranes of eggs. The latter method lacks sensitivity and is rarely used except to harvest antigen for diagnostic tests where a high degree of sensitivity is not needed. Antigen detection has not been widely used in clinical laboratories due to the relative lack of sensitivity of these assays. Parasite isolation and molecular biological techniques are favoured. Tissue culture produces results more rapidly than animal inoculation, however, findings vary with the cell type employed and the level of sensitivity of the technique is inferior to that achieved by animal inoculation.

Intraperitoneal inoculation of mice is the method of choice but is rarely performed outside of reference laboratories.

Developmental methods for the detection of toxoplasma nucleic acid include DNA probes (27) and the polymerase chain reaction (28, 29). They have the advantage that they provide a more rapid diagnosis and do not require animal inoculation. In comparison to current isolation techniques such investigations are only reliable when the integrity of the specimen can be ensured. PCR examination of bone marrow, tissue biopsy material, and peripheral blood produces useful results but investigation of the placenta, amniotic fluid, fetal blood, and cord blood may be associated with misleading findings due to contamination of the sample with maternal blood.

Although isolation of the organism indicates infection with *T. gondii* it does not prove that the organism is causing a current infection. Toxoplasma-antibody free cats have been used when large quantities of tissue need to be examined. The animal is fed with the tissue and the faeces examined for the oocysts of *T. gondii* (30).

Protocol 11. Animal inoculation and incubation

Equipment and reagents

- 6–8 week old MF1 mice toxoplasma-antibody free
- Antibiotic saline: 0.85% NaCl containing 100 U/ml of penicillin and streptomycin, 12.5 U/ml heparin
- Pestle and mortar
- 5 ml sterile syringe and 0.6 × 30 mm hypodermic needle
- Class I exhaust protective cabinet (EPC) to BS 5726

- Tissue/tissue fluids for inoculation
- Sterile scissors and forceps
- Dissection board
- Alcohol
- Small bore glass Pasteur pipette and bulb

Method

1. Material for inoculation must arrive in the laboratory within 24 h of removal.
2. Fluids should be centrifuged at 400 *g* for 10 min and the deposit inoculated directly. Tissues for inoculation should be sent to the laboratory dry or in antibiotic saline; DO NOT FREEZE.
3. Grind the tissue in a pestle and mortar in an EPC with as little antibiotic saline as will make a suspension suitable for intraperitoneal inoculation into mice.
4. All tissue/fluids received should be accompanied by a serum specimen or evidence of a positive toxoplasma serology result.

The protocol for examining mice is set out in *Figure 3*.

13. Alternative diagnostic procedures

The histological appearance of tissues infected with toxoplasma may be characteristic and aid differentiation from Hodgkin's disease, sarcoidosis, and leishmaniasis. The characteristic findings are follicular hyperplasia and collections of mononuclear cells, most often at the periphery of the node. The causative organisms are rarely seen and the normal architecture of the node is usually preserved.

T. gondii may be demonstrated in formalin fixed, paraffin-embedded tissues by immunoperoxidase staining (31). The value of histology is limited but has proven useful in monitoring heart transplant recipients.

Diagnostic skin tests (32) have been developed using purified secretory/excretory antigen obtained from tissue culture but have limited applications due to the delay in developing a response after exposure to *T. gondii*.

Immunoblotting ('Western blotting') (33) facilitates the study of the antigenic composition of organisms and the dissection of the quality and quantity of the antibody response to these organisms. This technique has been applied to toxoplasma but individual variation in the qualitative and quantitative recognition of antigens has limited its use as a diagnostic tool so far.

Development and evaluations of assays to detect *T. gondii* specific immunoglobulins E (34) and A (35) involving ELISA technology and immunocapture are currently in process with encouraging results.

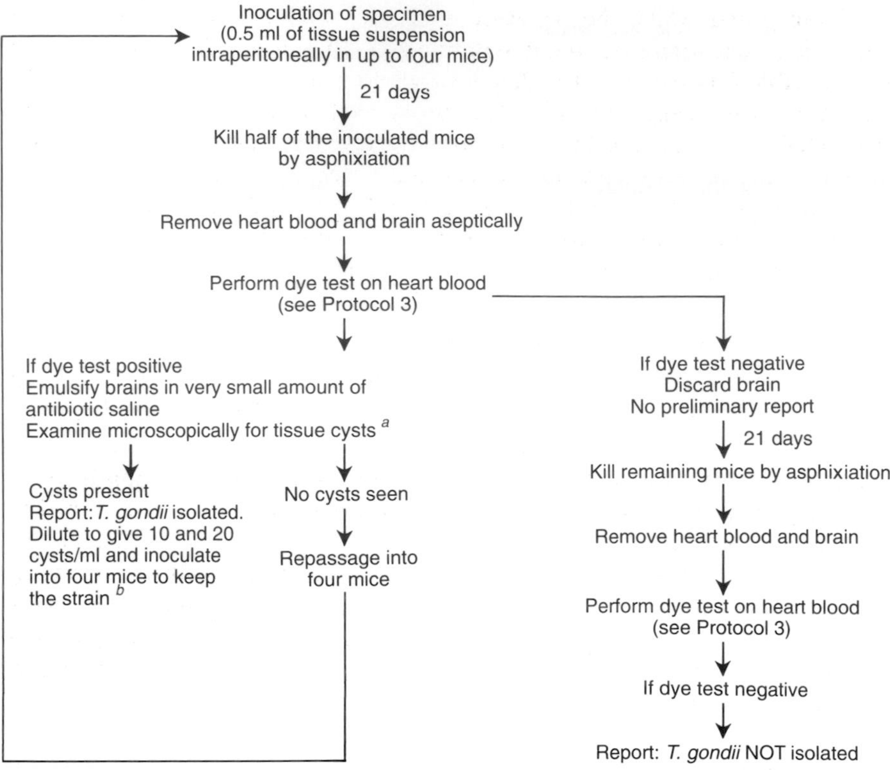

Figure 3. Flow chart for isolation of *T. gondii* by animal inoculation. [a]Tissue cysts grow intracellularly as the bradyzoites divide by endodyogeny and vary in size. Young cysts may be as small as 5 μm and contain only four bradyzoites whereas older ones may have a diameter of 50 μm and contain hundreds of organisms. [b]For maintenance of tissue cysts in mice, these animals should be inoculated subcutaneously with brain homogenate every 3–6 months.

14. Diagnostic strategy

The selection of an appropriate test for suspected toxoplasma infection depends on the clinical context of the case under investigation. Separate strategies can be defined for a number of distinct clinical situations. Immunocompetent patients with lymphadenopathy, glandular fever-like illness, or chorioretinitis may be investigated. In addition those contemplating conception and pregnant women may require assessment. Immunosuppressed patients requiring toxoplasma testing include the fetus, the neonate, the organ graft recipient, and the HIV infected individual.

14.1 Immunocompetent patients

Most cases are investigated using serological methods. Due to the rapidity of the immune response and delay in considering the diagnosis, a rising IgG titre is seldom noted whilst the persistence of IgG after acute exposure makes diagnosis based solely on immunoglobulin-G titres unreliable. The absence of detectable IgG excludes the diagnosis whilst measurement of specific IgM indicates more recent infection. The more sensitive the IgM assay the more protracted the detectable IgM response. It should be remembered that concurrent toxoplasmosis and malignancy have been reported. When lymph node biopsy or excision has been performed to exclude malignancy, histological examination of the tissues may reveal characteristic features of toxoplasma infection, particularly if immunohistochemical studies are employed.

14.2 Pre-conception assessment

Following the confirmation of acute toxoplasma infection a woman may seek advice as to when pregnancy can proceed in safety. One approach to this problem is to advise delay until the risk of parasitaemia is likely to be negligible or lost altogether. Arbitrary periods from one to 12 months have been suggested but to defer pregnancy for six months represents a reasonable compromise. Alternatively, serial IgM tests may be performed to document loss of IgM response. Undoubtedly this constitutes a highly conservative approach as the duration of IgM production exceeds the persistence of parasitaemia. Individual cases require assessment on their merits and an appropriate course of action should be chosen to meet the patient's own perception of an acceptable risk of infection.

14.3 Antenatal screening for toxoplasmosis

Routine serological assessment to identify women at risk of delivering congenitally infected infants is performed in a number of countries including France and Austria. The advisability of undertaking a similar scheme in the UK has not been established but is the subject of active research. The optimum method of detecting acute infection acquired during pregnancy is to demonstrate seroconversion in serial samples using a dye test. Recent infection is then confirmed by the measurement of toxoplasma specific immunoglobulin-M. Women found to lack specific immunoglobulin-G should be offered health education to reduce the incidence of primary infection and re-tested at periods throughout the remainder of the pregnancy. Women with chronic latent infection (IgG positive IgM negative) can be reassured as congenital infection is only associated with active parasitaemia during the pregnancy.

Patients with recently acquired infection require specialized management and should have the diagnosis confirmed by a reference unit. Antenatal screening using an IgM assay alone is problematic as many IgM tests have poorly defined sensitivity and specificity. Due to the persistence of the IgM response, the presence of detectable IgM does not necessarily indicate infection acquired after conception.

14.4 Fetal assessment

Investigation of the fetus *in utero* has been developed to detect cases of congenital infection associated with maternal toxoplasmosis (36). A combination of ultrasound guided cordocentesis is undertaken. Fetal blood and amniotic fluid are assessed by haematological parameters, liver function tests, parasite isolation, and measurement of specific and non-specific IgM levels. Immunoglobulin-M assays of maximal sensitivity (e.g. ISAGA) must be used but even then less than half of infected infants will have detectable IgM. Parasite isolation should be attempted by culture of the fetal blood clot and spun deposit from the amniotic fluid in tissue culture, giving a rapid but less sensitive result, and by animal inoculation, producing a highly sensitive result which may be delayed for 20–45 days. In view of the risk of fetal loss induced by cordocentesis, active fetal investigation is only justified when the risk of congenital infection is thought to be great. The incidence of fetal loss after cardiocentesis depends on the experience of the operator but is usually 1–2%. Cordocentesis is considered when the risk of congenital infection is estimated to exceed 5% and the mother is prepared to undergo a termination of pregnancy or change of therapy if the fetal blood shows evidence of toxoplasmosis.

14.5 Diagnosis of congenital infection in the post-natal period

Severely affected infants can be diagnosed on the results of clinical and radiological investigations demonstrating hydrocephalus, cerebral calcifications, and choroidoretinitis. Isolation of the parasite from the placenta or a neonatal blood sample is diagnostic but negative findings do not exclude infection. As congenital infection is associated with acute maternal infection, the absence of a positive dye test and IgM (ISAGA) in the mother's blood rules out the diagnosis. If the mother is shown to have recent infection, the presence of specific IgM in the neonatal circulation is diagnostic of congenital infection unless placental damage has allowed a significant volume of maternal blood to reach the child. The half-life of IgM is only five days, antibody acquired in this manner is quickly lost. The absence of detectable IgM does not, however, exclude congenital infection and IgG studies are required. Specific IgG in the infant's circulation may be actively produced or passively acquired by transplacental transfer. The half-life of IgG is about 30 days so that antibody of maternal origin is progressively removed and should not be detected in the child's blood beyond the age of six to ten months, depending on the original titre. Persistence of IgG indicates infection of the infant. Serological assessment at intervals of two months after birth are required to establish the status of the child as quickly as possible and to permit active therapy if indicated.

14.6 Ocular toxoplasmosis

Retinal disease is associated with excystation of previously latent toxoplasma with resultant cellular damage. Although a definitive diagnosis rests on the isolation of the parasite from ocular tissues, such samples are rarely available. Serological investigation must utilize a highly sensitive IgG assay as the absence of specific immunoglobulin-G excludes the condition. The presence of specific IgG and compatible clinical findings form the basis for the diagnosis in most cases. Conventional IgM assays are negative during an exacerbation of retinal toxoplasmosis although initial studies suggest more sensitive tests may be reactive reflecting a secondary IgM response.

14.7 Toxoplasmosis and AIDS

A minority of cases of toxoplasmosis with AIDS represent primary infection and elevated IgG levels with IgM production can be demonstrated using any reliable assay. Most disease results from a secondary reactivation of quiescent cysts within the cerebral tissue. In such cases IgM can not be measured and the IgG levels are stable without gross elevation. The absence of specific immunoglobulin-G is not compatible with the diagnosis of cerebral toxoplasmosis in AIDS. If cerebrospinal fluid (CSF) and serum are obtained, comparison of the ratio of specific and non-specific antibody levels in the two samples may demonstrate local production of toxoplasma specific antibody in the central nervous system. Alternatively, trophozoites may be visualized in the CSF. When brain biopsy is undertaken, immunohistochemical examination and demonstration of parasitic nucleic acid can be used to confirm the diagnosis.

14.8 Toxoplasmosis and organ transplantation

When a donated organ containing viable toxoplasma cysts is implanted into a recipient lacking previous exposure to the parasite, life-threatening infection may result. The likelihood of infection occurring is related to the likelihood of the transplanted organ containing viable parasites. *T. gondii* is found in the heart, liver, kidney, and bone marrow with decreasing frequency. Centres undertaking heart or liver transplants should assess all donor and recipient pairs for the presence of toxoplasma specific IgG. When a seronegative recipient of a seropositive donor is demonstrated, prophylactic anti-parasitic therapy is indicated. When severe infection does occur in these patients a rising IgG titre with IgM production is detected. Conversely, the rare instances of toxoplasma infection in bone marrow transplant recipients are most often associated with reactivation of the patients' own quiescent infection. Rising antibody levels and IgM production are rare. Parasite isolation, antigen detection, or demonstration of toxoplasma nucleic acid is required in such instances.

15. Conclusions

The varied clinical presentations of toxoplasmosis produce distinct requirements of methods used for investigation. A knowledge of the attributes of individual assays permits the application of a suitable diagnostic assay to each clinical case. A suggested scheme for the selection of appropriate tests for a range of toxoplasma infections is presented in *Figure 4*. As novel assays for toxoplasmosis are developed each will require careful consideration to ensure optimal benefit to the infected patient.

	Dye test (IgG and IgM)	Latex agglutination test (IgG and IgM)	Direct agglutination test (IgG)	IgG ELISA	IgM ELISA	ISAGA (IgM)	Non-serological methods
Lymphadenopathy 'glandular fever'					+	+	
Pre-conception status and antenatal screening		+	+	+			
Acute infection in pregnancy	+				+	+	
Fetal and neonatal assessment	+					+	
Ocular disease		+	+	+		?	+
HIV positive individual		+	+	+			
Cerebral disease and AIDS	+					?	+
Pre-transplant screening (donor and recipient)			+	+			
Infected heart/lung/liver recipient					+	+	
Infected bone marrow recipient							+

Figure 4. Diagnosis of toxoplasma infection.

References

1. Sabin, A. B. and Feldman, H. A. (1948). *Science*, **108**, 660.
2. Fleck, D. G. and Kwantes, W. (1980). *Public Health Lab. Serv. Monograph*, **13**, London, HMSO.
3. Budzko, D. B., Tyler, L., and Armstrong, D. (1989). *J. Clin. Microbiol.*, **27**, 959.
4. Warren, J. and Russ, S. B. (1948). *Proc. Soc. Exp. Biol. Med.*, **67**, 85.
5. Fleck, D. G. and Payne, R. A. (1963). *Mon. Bull. Minist. Health Public Health Lab. Serv.*, **22**, 97.

6. Jacobs, L. and Lunde, M. N. (1957). *J. Parasitol.*, **43**, 308.
7. Lunde, M. N. and Jacobs, L. (1959). *J. Immunol.*, **82**, 146.
8. Tsuboda, N. and Ozawa, H. (1977). *Jpn. J. Parasitol.*, **26**, 276.
9. Fulton, J. D. and Turk, J. L. (1959). *Lancet*, **ii**, 1068.
10. Couzineau, P. and Baufine-Ducrocq, H. (1970). *Ann. Biol. Clin.*, **28**, 411.
11. Desmonts, G. and Remington, J. S. (1980). *J. Clin. Microbiol.*, **11**, 562.
12. Danneman, B. R., Winston, C. V., Thulliez, P., and Remington, J. S. (1990). *J. Clin. Microbiol.*, **28**, 1928.
13. Voller, A., Bidwell, D. E., Bartlett, A., Fleck, D. G., Perkons, M., Oladehin, B. (1976). *J. Clin. Pathol.*, **29**, 150.
14. Wreghitt, T. G. and Morgan-Capner, P. (ed.) (1990). *ELISA in the clinical microbiology laboratory*. Public Health Laboratory Service 61, Colindale Avenue, London.
15. Duermeyer, W. and Van der Veen, J. (1978). *Lancet*, ii, 684.
16. Naot, Y. and Remington, J. S. (1980). *J. Infect. Dis.*, **142**, 757.
17. Payne, R. A., Isaac, M., and Francis, J. M. (1982). *J. Clin. Pathol.*, **35**, 892.
18. Hedman, K., Lappalainen, M., Seppaia, I., and Makela, O. (1989). *J. Infect. Dis.*, **159**, 736.
19. Isaac, M. and Payne, R. A. (1982). *J. Med. Virol.*, **10**, 55.
20. Turunen, H., Vuorio, K. A., and Leinikki, P. O. (1983). *Scand. J. Infect. Dis.*, **15**, 307.
21. Desmonts, G., Naot, Y., and Remington, J. S. (1981). *J. Clin. Microbiol.*, **14**, 486.
22. Remington, J. S., Eimstad, W. M., and Araujo, F. G. (1983). *J. Clin. Microbiol.*, **17**, 939.
23. Raizman, R. E. and Neva, F. A. (1975). *J. Infect. Dis.*, **132**, 44.
24. Van Knapen, F. and Panggabean, S. O. (1977). *J. Clin. Microbiol.*, **6**, 545.
25. Suzuki, Y. and Kobayashi, A. (1985). *Jpn. J. Parasitol.*, **34**, 149.
26. Hughes, H. P., Hudson, L., and Fleck, D. G. (1986). *Int. J. Parasitol.*, **4**, 317.
27. Savva, D. (1989). *Microbiology*, **58**, 165.
28. Savva, D., Morris, J., Johnson, J. D., and Holliman, R. E. (1989). *J. Med. Microbiol.*, **32**, 25.
29. Burg, J. L., Grover, C. M., Pouletty, P., and Boothroyd, J. C. (1989). *J. Clin. Microbiol.*, **27**, 1787.
30. Dubey, J. P. and Streitel, R. H. (1976). *J. Am. Vet. Med. Assoc.*, **169**, 1197.
31. Conley, F. K. and Jenkins, K. A. (1981). *Infect. Immunol.*, **31**, 1184.
32. Rougier, D. and Ambroise-Thomas, P. (1985). *Lancet*, ii, 121.
33. Partanen, P. and Turunen, H. J. (1984). *J. Clin. Microbiol.*, **20**, 133.
34. Pinon, J. M., Toubas, C., Marx, G., Mougeot, G., Bonnin, A., Bonhomme, A. *et al.* (1990). *J. Clin. Microbiol.*, **28**, 1739.
35. Stepick-Biek, P., Thulliez, P., Araujo, F. G., and Remington, J. S. (1990). *J. Infect. Dis.*, **162**, 270.
36. Daffos, F., Forestier, F., Capella-Pavlovsky, M., Tulliez, P., Aufrant, C., Valenti D. *et al.* (1988). *N. Eng. J. Med.*, **318**, 271.

4

Pneumocystis carinii

ALASTAIR DEERY

1. Introduction

A preliminary description of this unicellular eukaryotic organism was given by Chagas in 1909 and then Carini in 1910. Both thought the observed cysts to be a stage in the life cycle of *Trypanosomes*. Delanoes in 1912 correctly identified that the organism was associated with a distinct infection in rats not infected with *Trypanosomes* and christened it *Pneumocystis carinii*, after the earlier Brazilian worker. The organism is an opportunistic pathogen causing disease exclusively in immunocompromised persons and pre-eminently in those with the acquired immunodeficiency syndrome (AIDS). Other groups of patients sporadically affected include those with congenital immunodeficiency states including cellular immune impairment, immunosuppressive therapy after organ transplantation, chemotherapy for neoplasia whether for 'solid' tumours or for leukaemias and lymphomas, and corticosteroid therapy for 'autoimmune disease' and various illnesses.

An infective stage of the organism has not been identified, as with *Cryptococcus*. No environmental niche is known. Airborne infection is the identified method of spread yet the disease is not transmitted between individuals. Reactivation of latent infection is presumed from serological studies which indicate that most persons develop antibodies to cyst wall antigens at a very young age. Apart from rare exceptions, the disease is confined to the lungs. Experimental evidence, largely in rats, supports the view that impaired T lymphocyte function is a potent inducer of reactivation.

Symptoms of infection are not specific, may evolve slowly or suddenly appear, and take the form of fever (pyrexia), dyspnoea, and tachypnoea. These may be difficult to disentangle from the usual prodromal signs of developing AIDS. Classical radiographic features observed on plain chest radiographs include bilateral diffuse reticulo-nodular shadowing, or opacities beginning in the lower lung fields and becoming denser to include all fields.

The pathology of the pneumonia caused has been extensively reviewed (1), and the characteristic microscopic pattern consists of a foamy, vacuolated, 'exudate' that proceeds to fill the alveoli, alveolar ducts, and bronchioles of the affected lung or lungs. The 'exudate' is actually almost entirely composed of agglomerated 'cysts' and 'trophozoites'. Other more atypical but rarer patterns of disease are described.

Perhaps mostly because of its initial misrecognition in rats also infected with *Trypanosomes*, the organism has largely been presumed to be a protozoan. Ultrastructural studies, whilst elucidating some details in the putative reproductive cycle of the organism and confirming its anchorage to type I pneumocytes, have failed to resolve its correct taxonomy. A single recent study by transmission and scanning electron microscopy addresses this question directly and concludes in favour of it being a fungus of primitive type (2). The most important and convincing evidence to date arises from a comparative study of phylogenetic relationships utilizing nucleotide sequencing of small subunit ribosomal RNAs (16S-like rRNAs). This study offers evidence of *Pneumocystis* being clearly related to fungi and demonstrates its genetic dissimilarity from the diverse and distinct phylogenetic lineages apparent amongst protozoa (3).

Ultrastructure studies reveal the cell wall of the cysts to be fungal-like in having a thin plasma membrane bounded by a thicker capsule. Conventional PAS and silver stains ably stain the organism walls—in both techniques the fungal wall components are oxidized to aldehydes which are then demonstrated by Schiff's reagent or methenamine silver solution respectively.

At no identified stage is the organism capable of movement. No structures such as cilia, flagella, tubules, or Golgi apparatus are present. The nomenclature for the identified replicative cycle forms remains, by tradition, 'protozoal'. The steps themselves are none the less still obscure. The 'cysts' are the most frequent tissue form identified, are 4–7 μm in diameter, and contain as many as eight (though usually fewer) 'intracystic bodies' or 'sporozoites' each 1–2 μm in diameter. These develop within the cyst and either just prior to, or following its rupture, collapse and their consequent release, transform into unicellular 'trophozoites' which may be between 2 μm and 8 μm in diameter. These 'trophozoites' are thought to develop into new cysts with thicker capsulated cell walls and derive more 'sporozoites' for the cycle to revolve again.

If the organism is indeed a fungus then the more appropriate terminology might identify the 'cysts' as truncated mycelial forms, the 'sporozoites' as endospores, and the developing 'trophozoites' and 'pre-cysts' as maturing mycelia. The infective form must remain unidentified (*Figure 1*).

2. Sample collection

Serological methods of detecting infection have been unhelpful. Cell-free culture of the organism has not been possible. The diagnosis has come to depend on the morphological recognition of the organisms in either cell or tissue samples, obtained by various techniques, from the lower respiratory tract, i.e. the bronchiolar and alveolar space. Various investigators are

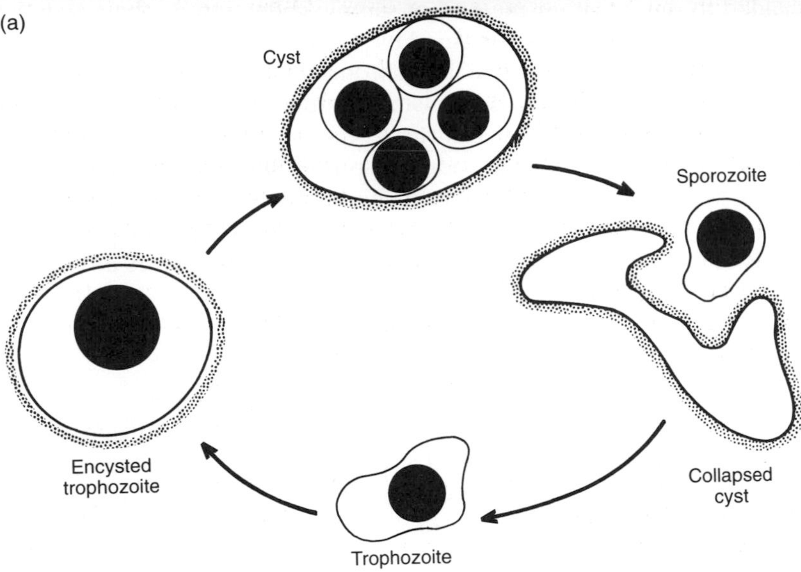

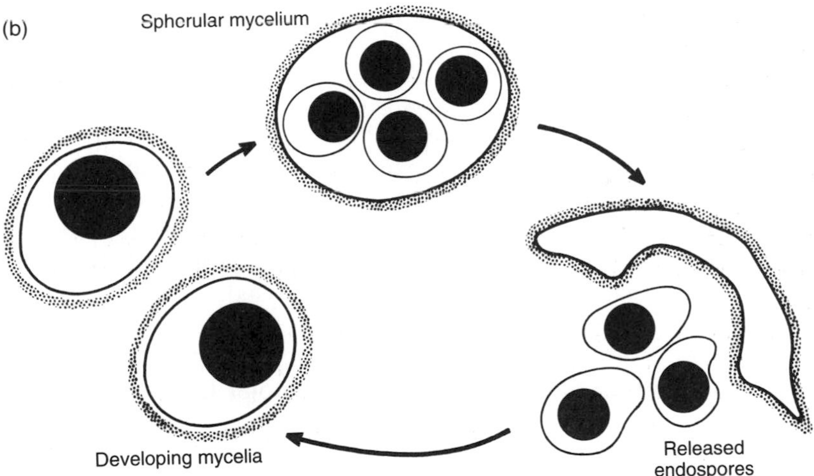

Figure 1. (a) Life cycle of *P. carinii*—protozoal nomenclature. (b) Tissue forms of *P. carinii*—suggested fungal nomenclature.

persuaded to one or other method of sample collection by their own experience. The highest yields are obtained by open lung biopsies arguably rivalled by bronchiolo-alveolar lavage. Transbronchial biopsies are less effective. Simple bronchial washings and assisted sputum collection (induced sputum collection) provide the lowest returns.

All cytological methods, i.e. induced sputum samples, bronchial washings obtained at bronchoscopy, and bronchiolo-alveolar lavage fluids must be prepared to high standards to give the best results. Commonly, it is in these methods of subsequent handling of fluid specimens that errors are made, due to poor technique, with resultant loss of sensitivity.

2.1 Bronchiolo-alveolar lavage fluid

Segmental washings of lung employing a small calibre bronchoscope, correctly placed in a segmental bronchus and with the use of warmed saline solution, represents the most effective method of sampling a wide area of the bronchiolo-alveolar space (*Protocol 1*). In young persons, the relatively large calibre of the selected bronchoscope by comparison with the segmental bronchus may limit the quality of the sample, which is then diluted by bronchial mucus with attendant exfoliated bronchial epithelial cells from larger airways. This factor rather than the underlying pathology probably explains some of the quoted differences in yields between AIDS and non-AIDS patients. The latter are often young leukaemics or marrow transplant patients with smaller calibre airways than the usual early adult AIDS victim.

2.2 Induced sputum

The use of ultrasonic rather than jet nebulizers is a prerequisite for reasonable yields from this admittedly minimally invasive technique (*Protocol 2*). The basic principal involved is to stimulate coughing and expectoration of sputum by irritant bronchial injection of sodium chloride mist. Sputum specimens normally contain an alveolar macrophage sample and the hoped for 'exudate'. Bronchial mucus must be cleared or lysed.

Protocol 1. Preparation of bronchiolo-alveolar lavage fluids

Equipment and reagents

- Class I safety cabinet[a]
- Shandon cytospin
- Cytospin cuvettes, filter cards, and clips for the above
- Frosted end microscope slides
- Balanced isotonic strength saline (BISS), e.g. RPMI 1640, Hepes buffered (Sigma)[b]
- 30% bovine serum albumen (BSA)[c]
- Centrifuge
- Screw-capped centrifuge tubes or plastic Universal containers
- Pasteur pipettes
- Absolute methanol
- Formol–alcohol: 4 ml of 37% (w/v) aqueous formaldehyde, 96 ml absolute ethanol
- Aerosol spray cytological fixative[d]

Method

1. Transfer sample to screw-capped centrifuge tube or plastic Universal container. Centrifuge at 1400 *g* for 5 min. Decant supernatant.
2. Resuspend the deposit in BISS and centrifuge again at 1400 *g* for 5 min; decant supernatant.
3. Resuspend the deposit in BISS to give a faintly turbid cell suspension.[e]
4. Add one drop 30% BSA per 2 ml of cell suspension.
5. Label slides and assemble with cytospin cuvette, filter card, and clip.[f]
6. Place the assembled cuvettes in the rotor head and add two drops of cell suspension per cuvette; secure lid.
7. Place the head assembly into the centrifuge. Spin at 850 r.p.m. for 3 min, low acceleration.
8. Remove head assembly, remove cuvettes singly, disassembling each. Immediately fix slides for Papanicolaou staining in formol–alcohol for 15 min, then drain spray with aerosol fixative and leave to air-dry (see *Protocols 4A* and *4B*).

For May–Grunwald Giemsa staining, rapidly air dry and fix in fresh absolute methanol (see *Protocol 7*).
For Grocott's hexamine silver technique or PAS, rapidly air dry and fix in formol–alcohol for 15 min, drain, and spray with aerosol fixative; leave to air dry (see *Protocols 5* and *6*).

[a] Apart from centrifugation, all stages must be carried out under exhaust protection.
[b] The use of BISS enables specimens to be held at 4°C for 24 h or more and show little degeneration.
[c] 30% BSA serves both as an 'adhesive' and to reduce cell rupture on air drying.
[d] The use of formol–alcohol gives more consistent fixation and better morphology than aerosol fixative alone. The subsequent aerosol fixation and air drying aids in cell retention.
[e] The most critical part of the technique is in the production of a cell suspension of correct cell concentration. Generally, this improves with experience. As a guide, the average lavage requires between 5–15 ml of BISS. This gives a cell count of approximately 3 to 5 $\times 10^6$ cells/ml. Another guide is the appearance of the air dried preparations, a transparent disc of cells should be readily seen. Purulent lavage specimens may need to be diluted twice (i.e. resuspend, withdraw 1 ml, and dilute this further).
[f] Generally, six slides are sufficient: three Papanicolaou, one May–Grunwald Giemsa, and two air dried for special stains.

Protocol 2. The method for (induced) sputum

Reagents

- Mucolytic reagent: 2% solution 3-methyl-cysteine in BISS[a]
- Fixative: formol–alcohol

Method

1. Add a volume of mucolytic reagent equal to twice the sample volume and mix well (vortex).
2. Incubate for 15 min to 2 h, depending on sample viscosity, at 37 °C. Agitate and examine periodically.[b]
3. Centrifuge at 1400 *g* for 5 min, decant supernatant.
4. Resuspend deposit in 10 ml BISS, centrifuge at 1400 *g* for 5 min; decant supernatant.
5. Resuspend deposit in 10 ml BISS containing six to ten drops 30% BSA.
6. Centrifuge again at 1400 *g* for 5 min; decant supernatant.
7. Either:
   (a) Prepare direct smears and wet fix in formol–alcohol.
   (b) Resuspend in the appropriate amount of BISS containing 5% BSA and make cytocentrifuge preparations. Wet fix slides in formol–alcohol.

[a] Mucolytic reagent will keep for several days at 4 °C.
[b] The mucolytic reagent–sample mixture can be left for up to 18 without significant cell damage.

Protocol 3. Removal of red blood cells from cell suspensions

Equipment and reagents

- Centrifuge
- Screw-capped centrifuge tubes or plastic Universal containers
- Pasteur pipettes
- Disposable 5 or 10 ml pipettes
- BISS (*Protocol 1*)
- Cell separation medium, e.g. Lymphoprep (Nycomed) or Histopaque (Sigma)

Method

1. Transfer sample to screw-capped centrifuge tube or plastic Universal container; spin at 1400 *g* for 5 min.

2. Decant supernatant and resuspend in 5–15 ml BISS.
3. Either:
   (a) Into a screw-capped container, place 5–8 ml cell separation medium; using a Pasteur pipette, carefully layer the cell suspension on top of cell separation medium.[a]
   (b) If necessary transfer the cell suspension to a screw-capped container, fill a pipette with 5–8 ml cell separation medium and place the pipette through the cell suspension to touch the bottom of the container, then gently run in the cell separation medium. The cell suspension will rise to the top.
4. Spin at 450 *g* for 20 min.
5. Using a Pasteur pipette, remove the cell containing BISS layer from above the cell separation medium, transfer to another container.[b]
6. Spin the red cell-free cell suspension at 1400 *g* for 5 min; decant the supernatant.[c]
7. Proceed from *Protocol 1*, step 3.

[a] Whichever method is adopted, it is important that the cell suspension and cell separation medium should remain as separate and distinct as possible.

[b] The cells will be at, or just above (1–2 mm), the interphase. The majority of red blood cells will have passed through the cell separation medium and be at the bottom of the container.

[c] If any cell separation medium is collected together with the cell-rich BISS layer, then the cells should be resuspended in 10–15 ml BISS and step **6** repeated to remove the cell separation medium, which may otherwise interfere with staining.

3. Staining techniques

Stains are usually selected to provide either the broadest spectrum diagnostic yields of the variety of opportunist and other pathogens that might be encountered, or else selected and directed to obtaining the most specific identification of an individual organism's characteristics.

3.1 Papanicolaou staining

The haematoxylin of the haematoxylin and eosin (H&E) or Papanicolaou stains will optimally identify all the various forms of *P. carinii* (*Figure 2*) in addition to other fungi such as *Aspergillus*, *Mucor*, *Histoplasma*, and *Candida*. The Papanicolaou stain is the most appropriate for cytological material and is the preferred stain for regular use (*Protocol 4A* and *4B*).

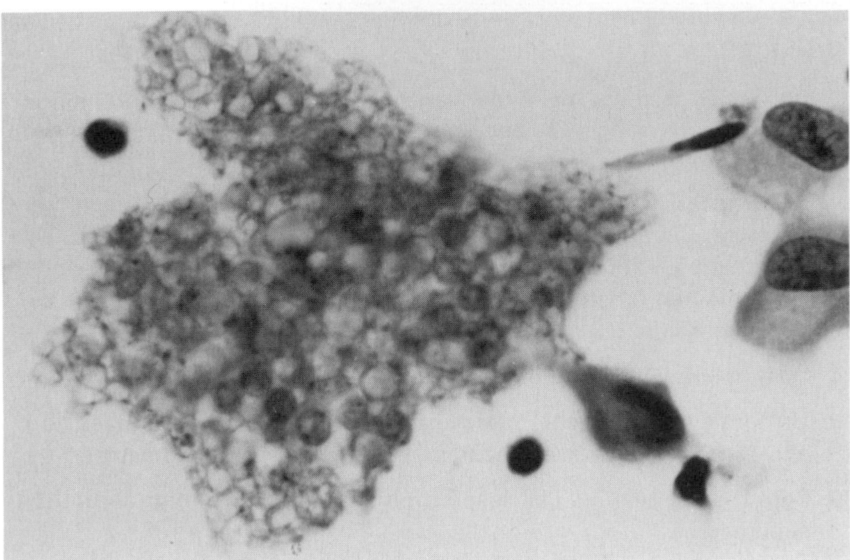

Figure 2. Papanicolaou stain of alveolar casts in BAL fluid, demonstrating cysts, trophozoites, and nuclei.

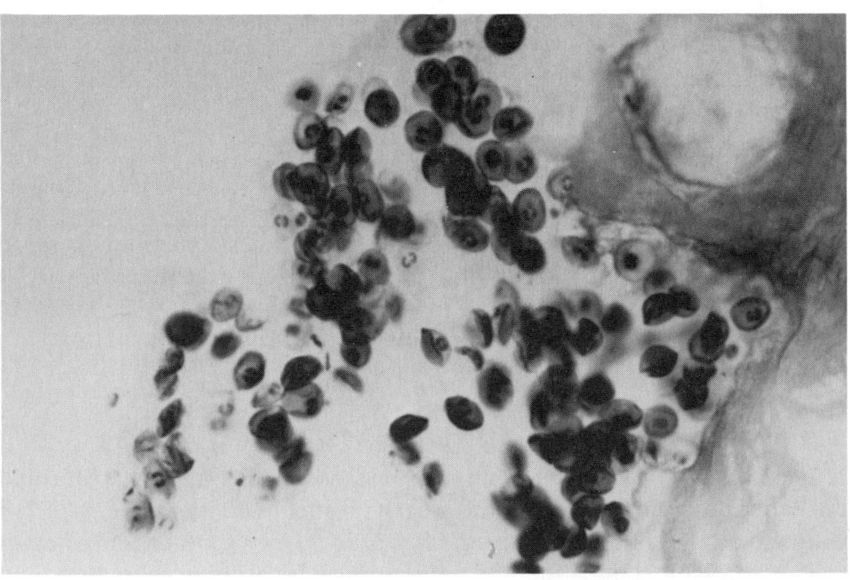

Figure 3. Grocott stain of cysts only, including collapsed forms, within an alveolar cast. Trophozoites are not stained.

Protocol 4. Papanicolaou staining for cytospin preparations

Equipment and reagents

- Staining machine[a]
- Staining dishes and racks
- 70% alcohol
- 95% alcohol
- Absolute alcohol
- 0.25% hydrochloric acid in 70% alcohol
- Xylene or equivalent
- Water
- Running tap-water
- Harris' haematoxylin[a]
- Papanicolaou stain OG6[a]
- Papanicolaou stain EA50[a]
- Mounting medium (e.g. DPX)
- No.1 coverslips

A. *Sequence and times using a staining machine*[b]

1. 95% alcohol	30 sec
2. 70% alcohol	30 sec
3. Water	1 min
4. Harris' haematoxylin	2 min 30 sec
5. Running tap-water	30 sec
6. 0.25% acid alcohol	10 sec
7. Running tap-water	3 min[c]
8. 70% alcohol	30 sec
9. 95% alcohol	30 sec
10. 95% alcohol	30 sec
11. 95% alcohol	30 sec
12. OG6	1 min
13. 95% alcohol	30 sec
14. 95% alcohol	30 sec
15. 95% alcohol	30 sec
16. EA50	2 min 15 sec
17. 95% alcohol	30 sec
18. 95% alcohol	30 sec
19. Absolute alcohol	30 sec
20. Absolute alcohol	30 sec
21. Absolute alcohol	1 min
22. Xylene	30 sec
23. Xylene	1 min

Protocol 4. *Continued*

24. Xylene 1 min

25. Mount from xylene using synthetic resin under no. 1 coverslip.

B. *Sequence and times using handstaining*

1.	70% alcohol	30 sec
2.	Water	1 min
3.	Harris' haematoxylin	4 min
4.	Running tap-water	30 sec
5.	0.25% acid alcohol	25–30 sec (dipping)
6.	Running tap-water	3 min[b]
7.	70% alcohol	1 min
8.	95% alcohol	1 min
9.	95% alcohol	1 min
10.	OG6	1 min[c]
11.	95% alcohol	1 min
12.	95% alcohol	1 min
13.	EA50	2 min 30 sec

14. Follow *Protocol 4A,* from step 17.

[a] This staining sequence is designed for the Shandon Varistain 24–3 and stains supplied by Orthodiagnostics. The use of other machines or stains will require adjustment of times. Stains should be filtered before use, and stains and reagents changed as required (dependent on through put).

[b] This schedule is designed for thin smear preparations; thick preparations will require longer in the pre-haematoxylin water and in all alcohols beyond step 9, in *Protocol 4A,* to be roughly doubled or trebled.

[c] This assumes running tap-water is suitably alkaline to 'blue' the haematoxylin. In areas where this is not so, or where running tap-water is unavailable, an equivalent time in Scott's tap-water substitute followed by distilled water is recommended.

3.2 The Grocott stain

The most frequently used stain for confirmation of *Pneumocystis* in tissue pathology is Grocott's (Gomori's) hexamine (methenamine) silver stain (GMS). Many believe this stain to be the ultimate high contrast technique and certainly, when carefully applied, it offers absolutely reliable identification of 'cysts' but not 'trophozoites' or 'sporozoites' (*Figures 3, 4* and *Protocol 5*).

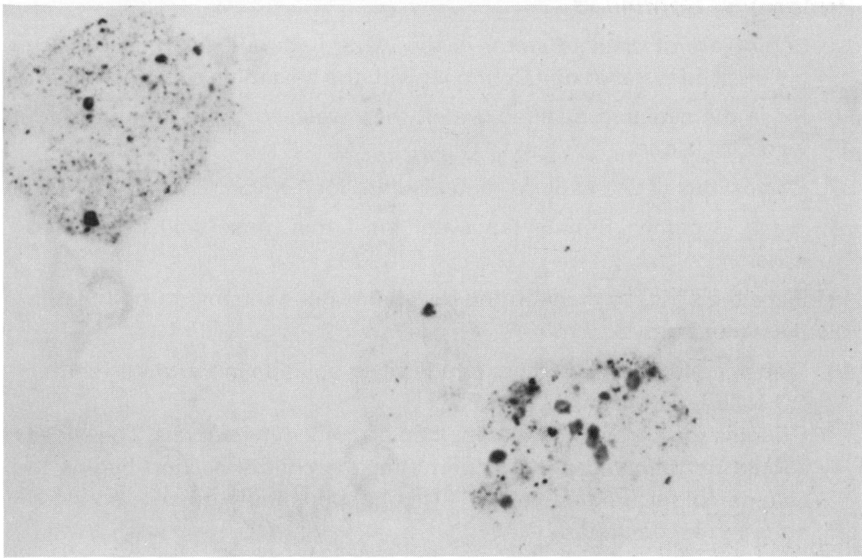

Figure 4. Grocott stain showing cysts and degenerate cysts within alveolar macrophages also containing anthracotic pigment.

Protocol 5. Grocott's hexamine silver technique

Equipment and reagents

- Water-bath at 56°C
- Coplin jars[a]
- Measuring cylinders
- 70% alcohol
- Absolute alcohol
- Distilled water
- Xylene or equivalent
- Coverslips (no.1)
- Formol–alcohol (*Protocol 1*)
- 5% aqueous silver nitrate
- 3% aqueous methenamine (hexamine)
- 5% aqueous borax
- 2% aqueous sodium thiosulfate
- 5% aqueous chromic acid
- 0.1% aqueous gold chloride
- 0.2% light green in 0.2% acetic acid
- 2% sodium metabisulfite
- Control paraffin section
- Plastic forceps or plastic Spencer–Wells clamps

Method

1. Fix air dried smears in formol–alcohol 15–30 min; dewax paraffin control section in xylene or equivalent.
2. Rinse slides in absolute alcohol.
3. Rinse slides in 70% alcohol.
4. Place slides in distilled water for 2 min, drain well.
5. Oxidize in 5% chromic acid for 1 h and at the same time place two

Protocol 5. *Continued*

Coplin jars of distilled water in the water-bath, after 40 min replace the distilled water in one Coplin jar with the hexamine silver solution.[b]

6. Rinse the slides in distilled water, then wash in gently running tap-water for 1 min.
7. Place slides in 2% sodium metabisulfite for 1 min.
8. Wash in gently running tap-water for 1 min, rinse well in distilled water.
9. Place the slides in the warmed distilled water-containing Coplin jar in the water-bath for 2 min.[c]
10. Transfer slides to heated hexamine silver solution in the water-bath—DO NOT USE METAL FORCEPS.
    Examine the slides after 10 min, then at 1 or 2 min intervals. The slides should be removed about 1 min after the control section begins to change colour (golden-yellow). This happens fairly quickly, so close attention is required.[d]
11. Rinse in warm distilled water, then in room temperature distilled water, several changes over 2 min.
12. Tone in 0.1% gold chloride for 5 min.
13. Rinse in distilled water, place in 2% sodium thiosulfate for 2 min.
14. Wash in gently running tap-water for 2 min.
15. Counterstain in 0.2% light green in 0.2% acetic acid for 1 min.
16. Wash in distilled water for 1 min.
17. Place in 70% alcohol for 1 min.
18. Dehydrate in absolute alcohol: three changes, 1 min each.
19. Clear in xylene or equivalent: three changes, 1 min each.
20. Mount under a no.1 coverslip using a synthetic resin.

[a] If possible plastic Coplin jars should be used in the water-bath—glass jars may crack.

[b] Prepare the hexamine silver solution immediately before use: to 25 ml of 3% methanamine, add 1.25 ml of 5% silver nitrate and mix. Then add 3 ml of 5% borax and mix. Add 25 ml distilled water and mix well.

[c] Placing slides in warmed distilled water prevents them from chilling the hexamine silver solution.

[d] The usual advice is to remove slides when the control section is the 'colour of toast'—if that is followed for smears, then fungal elements will stain black and be difficult to distinguish from carbon debris and red blood cells (which by this stage will also have started to colour).

3.3 The PAS stain

Periodic acid–Schiff staining (PAS) for carbohydrates will identify the 'cyst' and 'trophozoite' walls but will also stain free mucus in secretions present

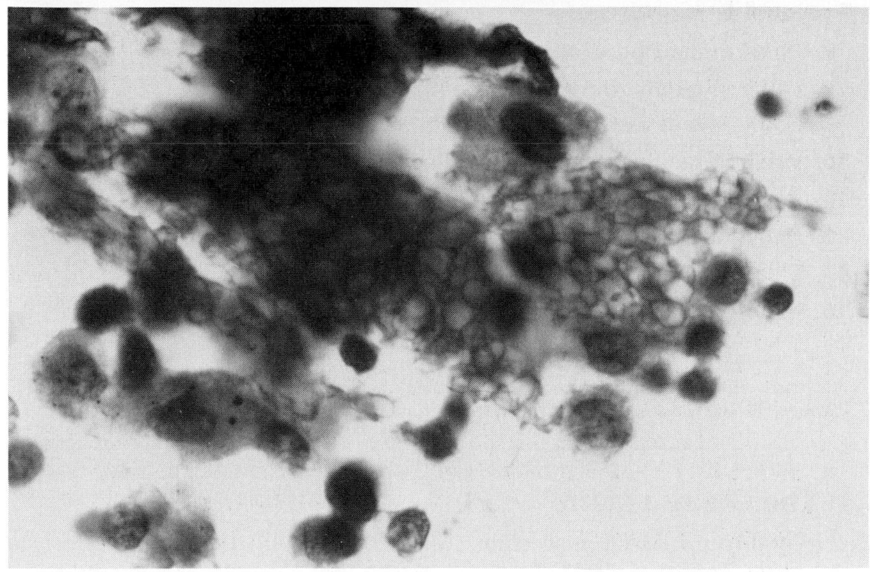

Figure 5. PAS stain demonstrating cyst and trophozoite walls. Bronchial mucus is also stained.

and mucus within bronchial epithelial cell cytoplasm. This is not a preferred stain, but is included for comparison of results (*Figure 5* and *Protocol 6*).

Protocol 6. Periodic acid–Schiff staining for carbohydrates

Equipment and reagents

- Staining rack
- Running tap-water
- Periodic acid solution[a]
- Schiff reagent
- Mayer's haemalum
- Distilled water
- 70% alcohol
- Absolute alcohol
- Formol–alcohol (*Protocol 1*)
- Xylene or equivalent
- No.1 coverslips
- Synthetic mounting resin

Method

1. Fix smears in formol–alcohol: 10 min.
2. Rinse in 70% alcohol.
3. Rinse in distilled water, several changes over 2 min.
4. Oxidize smears in periodic acid solution: 5 min.
5. Wash smears in distilled water, several changes over 2 min, drain well.
6. Cover smears with Schiff's reagent, two changes, 5 min each.

Protocol 6. *Continued*

7. Rinse in distilled water.
8. Wash in gently running tap-water: 10 min, drain well.
9. Counterstain with Mayer's haemalum: 1 to 2 min.
10. Wash in gently running tap-water: 2 min.[b]
11. Rinse in 70% alcohol.
12. Dehydrate in absolute alcohol: three changes 1 min each; drain well.
13. Clear in xylene or equivalent: three changes, 1 min each.
14. Mount under no.1 coverslip using a synthetic resin.

[a] 1 g periodic acid in 100 ml distilled water.

[b] If tap water is not sufficiently alkaline to 'blue' the haemalum, use Scott's tap-water substitute or similar, rinsing with distilled water before and after use.

3.4 The Giemsa stain

The May–Grunwald Giemsa stain (MGG), will stain the 'sporozoites' and nuclei of the 'trophozoites' violet, while the cytoplasm of the 'trophozoites' may appear blue. The 'cyst' wall is not stained but can often be delineated against a stained mucoid background (*Figure 6* and *Protocol 7*).

Modified rapid Giemsa stains such as 'Diff-Quik' (American Hospital Supplies) may also be employed.

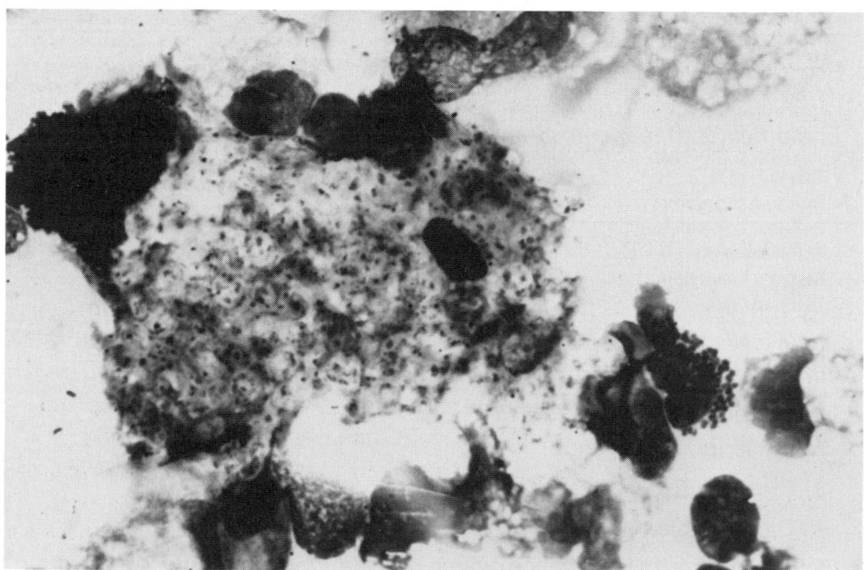

Figure 6. May–Grunwald Giemsa stain demonstrating nuclei of sporozoites and trophozoites. 'Ghost' cyst outlines can be discerned against the mucoid background.

Protocol 7. The May–Grunwald Giemsa stain

Equipment and reagents

- Absolute methanol[a]
- May–Grunwald stain (stock)[a]
- Giemsa stain (stock)[a]
- pH 6.5 (Giemsa) phosphate buffer[a]
- Measuring cylinders
- Coplin jars
- Xylene or equivalent
- Fluff-free blotting-paper
- No.1 coverslips
- Synthetic mounting resin

Method

1. Fix air dried preparations in fresh absolute methanol: 15 min.
2. Stain in May–Grunwald working solution.[c]
3. Rinse briefly in pH 6.5 buffer.
4. Stain in Giemsa working solution: 20 min.[c]
5. Rinse in pH 6.5 buffer.
6. Differentiate in pH 6.5 buffer: two changes, 2 min 30 sec each.
7. Blot dry, then leave to thoroughly air dry.
8. Clear in xylene or equivalent: 1 min.
9. Mount under no.1 coverslip using synthetic resin.

[a] These should be purchased (or aliquoted) in small (500 ml) quantities as all absorb moisture from the atmosphere which will impair their performance.

[b] All fixation, staining, and differentiation is conveniently carried out in Coplin jars (50 ml).

[c] Working solutions should be prepared immediately before use, used once (possibly twice with another batch of slides immediately afterwards), and discarded. Working solutions: May–Grunwald—equal parts of stock solution and pH 6.5 buffer (25 ml: 25 ml); Giemsa—1:10 stock solution in pH 6.5 buffer (5 ml: 45 ml). The working solutions' staining efficiency falls with time.

3.5 Other methods of demonstration

The orange-G in the Papanicolaou stain will autofluoresce in ultraviolet light, emitting a bright greenish fluorescence (4). Many of the 'cysts' will contain two central reniform (kidney-shaped) or comma-shaped areas of particularly brilliant fluorescence (*Figure 7*). These are undoubtedly the correlate of the parenthesis-like wall structures identifiable in not over-cooked Grocott stains (*Figure 8*). Both methods are identifying the eccentric thickened plaque of cell wall material demonstrable by transmission electron microscopy.

A high degree of sensitivity is possible using immunocytochemical methods of demonstrating the organism with a monoclonal antibody to an 82 kd parasite component (5), the appearance of a 'cyst' stained thus is shown in *Plate 2a*.

In my experience of paralleling most of these techniques in more than 300 positive identifications of *Pneumocystis carinii*, there is no better method

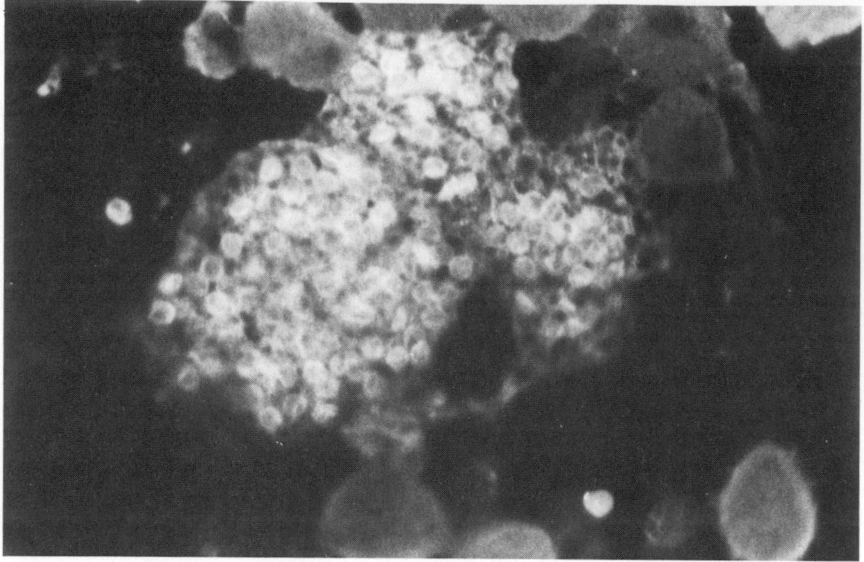

Figure 7. Papanicolaou stain viewed by ultraviolet light, showing autofluorescence of cysts with brilliant central crescents.

than Papanicolaou staining without any flourishes. The most important aspects rather rest with the satisfactory clinical obtaining of the alveolar fluid specimen (BAL preferred) and subsequent preparation of consistently good, even cytospin smears, free of all debris. The diagnosis is then very simple with very few exceptions, given the considerable numbers of alveolar 'casts' and fragmented 'casts' usually seen. The situations where only a very few cysts are present within a satisfactory sample are in fact vanishingly rare. Within macrophage-poor, induced sputum samples, these occasional organisms might well be thought missable with all but good immunocytochemical technique. However, the literature reports no improvement on conventional staining, despite increased efforts and costs.

3.6 Summary of diagnostic staining patterns of *Pneumocystis* organisms

(a) The haematoxylin of the Papanicolaou stain stains the 'cyst' and 'trophozoite' walls blue-green, and some stain will penetrate the organisms to stain the nuclei of 'sporozoites' and 'trophozoites'.

(b) The GMS or Grocott silver stain will stain the 'cyst' walls black and show the thickened eccentric part of the cyst wall either as an edge-on disc or paired comma-shaped central structures.

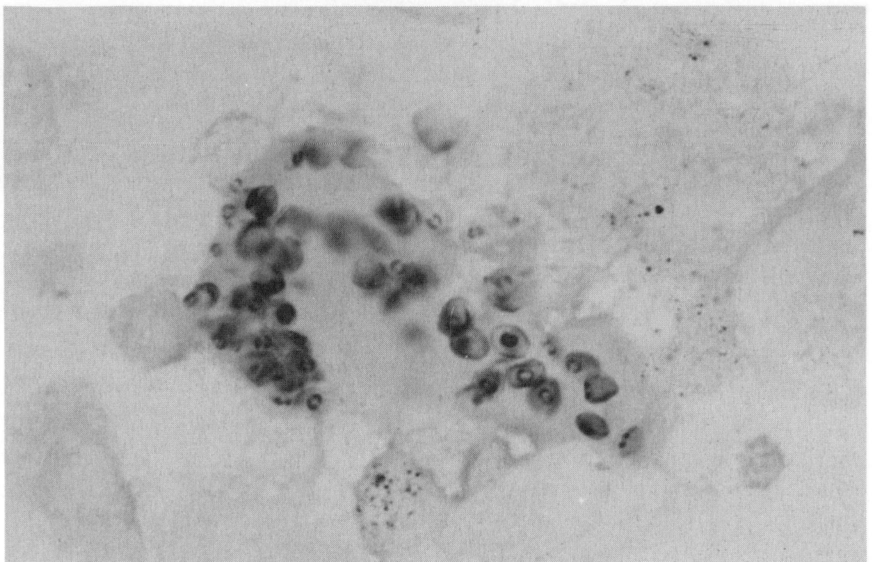

Figure 8. Grocott stain of cyst walls with paired, comma-shaped central structures. These thickened cyst wall plaques can also be seen end-on as two dots, or a single edge-on disc.

(c) The PAS stain for carbohydrates will stain the 'cyst' and 'trophozoites' walls blue-purple.

(d) The MGG or Giemsa stain or modified rapid variants will stain the nuclei of 'sporozoites' and 'trophozoites' violet and the cytoplasm of 'trophozoites' blue.

4. New techniques

Molecular techniques, employing *in situ* hybridization are being developed, but will almost certainly not be applied routinely in diagnosis. The polymerase chain reaction (PCR) when combined with DNA hybridization has been reported as a more sensitive diagnostic technique than immunofluorescence (6, 7). Equally certainly, this will identify a very much larger population without pneumocystis pneumonia. These techniques may expand our epidemiological understanding, however. They offer the potential to identify nuclear or mitochondrial genetic material and therefore, possibly, all forms of the organism including the putative 'latent' form, if it exists in normal lungs. Searches of lung tissue with anti-cyst wall antigen antibodies and special conventional cyst wall stains such as GMS can not achieve this. PCR studies might finally bring us full circle to looking for an environmental source of primary infection.

References

1. Watts, J. C. and Chandler, F. W. (1991). In *Pathology annual* (ed. P. P. Rosen and R. E. Fechner), Vol. 26, part 1, pp. 93–138. Appleton and Lange, East Norwalk, Connecticut, USA.
2. Haque, A., Plattner, S. B., Cook, R. T., and Hart, M. N. (1987). *Am. J. Clin. Pathol.*, **87**, 504.
3. Edman, J. C., Kovacs, J. A., Masur, H., Sant, D. V., Elwood, H. J., and Sogin, M. L. (1988). *Nature*, **334**, 519.
4. Ghali, V. S., Garcia, R. L., and Skolon, J. (1984). *Hum. Pathol.*, **15**, 907.
5. Elvin, K. M., Bjorkman, A., Linder, E., Huerlin, N., and Hjerpe, A. (1988). *Br. Med. J.*, **297**, 381.
6. Malin, A. S. and Miller, R. F. (1992). *Rev. Med. Microbiol.*, **3**, 80.
7. Olsson, M. *et al.* (1993). *J. Clin. Microbiol.*, **31**, 221.

5

Intestinal protozoa

H. V. SMITH

1. Collection and examination of faeces for the presence of protozoan parasites

Examine the stool macroscopically and record whether it is formed, soft, unformed, or liquid or it contains evidence of blood or mucus. Stools with evidence of blood or mucus may contain the developmental or reproductive stages of protozoa and are examined with the minimum of delay by direct microscopy to ensure that these stages are still intact and motile. Where possible, blood or mucus should be examined separately as they are more likely to contain trophozoites.

Formed stools without any evidence of blood or mucus are normally examined following concentration within 24 hours of passage, and are stored at 4 °C until then. When long storage or transit times, which can result in the deterioration of protozoan morphology are anticipated, the use of a preservative should be considered.

1.1 Micrometry

In diagnostic parasitology, definitive diagnosis of intact organisms often necessitates the measurement of their size and shape. The measurement of microscopic objects (< 1 mm) is achieved by means of a stage micrometer in conjunction with an eye-piece micrometer. Objects are measured in System International (SI) units, and the standard unit of measurement for conventional microscopy is the μm (0.001 mm). The stage micrometer consists of a 76 × 26 mm glass slide which has a millimetre scale, graduated in microns. The eye-piece micrometer is a disc of transparent glass or plastic bearing a graduated scale which is placed in one of the eye-pieces of a binocular microscope. The scale is usually 1 cm in length and is subdivided into millimetre intervals. When the microscope is focused on the object to be measured, both the scale on the eye-piece micrometer and the image of the object are seen simultaneously in focus. The standard scale on the stage micrometer is usually one or two millimetres.

Protocol 1. Calibration using the eye-piece and stage micrometers

1. Place the graticule in the eye-piece by unscrewing the lower component of the eye-piece and placing it into the open tube. It must be seated correctly before the lower component is screwed back on to the eye-piece.
2. Ensure that the diameter of the graticule is similar to the internal diameter of the lower lens tube. Do not touch the surface of the graticule—hold it by its edges. Make sure it is dust and grease-free.
3. Focus the eye lens on to the graticule by adjusting it until the scale on the graticule is sharp.
4. Insert eye-piece micrometer, with its scale already in focus, and the right way up, into the microscope.
5. Select the lowest power objective lens (e.g. × 10 objective) and focus the microscope on the stage micrometer, rotating the eye-piece and positioning the stage micrometer until the scales of the eye-piece micrometer and the stage micrometer lie parallel and close to, or overlapping, each other (*Figure 1*).
6. Count the number of intervals on the stage micrometer that correspond exactly to a whole number of divisions on the eye-piece micrometer.
7. Divide the value observed on the stage micrometer by the number of divisions counted on the eye-piece micrometer scale to determine the value of each division on the eye-piece micrometer scale.
8. Repeat the above for each objective lens.[a]
9. Keep a permanent record of the calculation of the value for each of the divisions on the eye-piece micrometer for each objective in close proximity to, or attached on to, the body of the microscope (e.g. a piece of cardboard stuck to the front of the microscope).

[a] You will notice that the value calculated in millimetres for each of the divisions on the eye-piece micrometer will be different for objectives of different magnifications, with values calculated for actual length being smaller for each of the divisions of the eye-piece micrometer with increasing magnification.

When measurements are to be made, the appropriate objective lens is chosen and the number of divisions corresponding to the length or breadth of the image of the object are read on the scale of the eye-piece micrometer.

2. Concentration techniques for the identification of protozoan parasites

Typically, the stages of the parasite life cycle present in faeces are the environmentally robust transmissive stages which do not multiply outside the

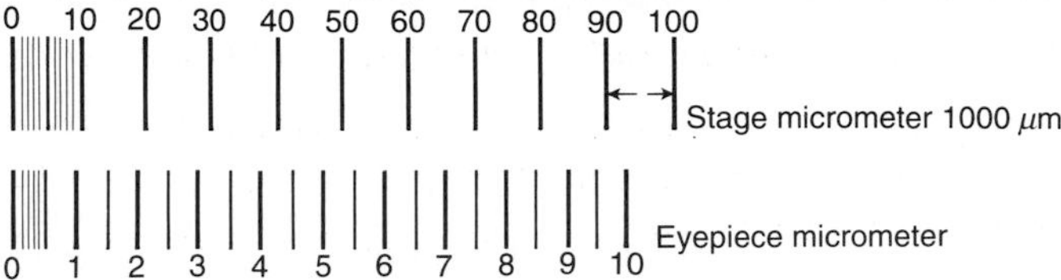

Figure 1. Eye-piece and stage micrometer scales in parallel (*Protocol 1*).
Example
For each objective lens:

x eye-piece divisions $= y$ μm (on the stage micrometer)

1 eye-piece division $= \frac{y}{x}$ μm

body of the host. In instances of florid diarrhoea, the reproductive stages may be voided. With the exception of the reproductive trophozoite stages of a few intestinal protozoa, which can be expanded *in vitro*, the number of parasites voided in the stool will be the maximum number detectable. Methods for the preferential concentration of parasitic stages in suspensions of faeces have been devised to separate any parasites present from the bulk of the faeces, such as bacteria and undigested food particles. The efficiency of such methods is dependent on the density on the parasite(s) sought and the robustness of the parasite in question. Whereas protozoan cysts, helminth ova, and larvae can withstand concentration procedures, the reproductive and developmental stages of protozoa can not. In addition, certain protozoan parasites have no recognized cyst stage. In order to identify these stages, the direct examination of wet films or permanently stained smears of stools is recommended.

2.1 Sedimentation

Microscopic parasites that are heavier than bacteria and undigested food particles in an aqueous stool suspension settle more rapidly. By emulsifying a stool in tap-water, and settling by gravity, protozoan cysts and helminth ova can be concentrated. However, food particles of similar density will settle at similar rates.

2.2 Sedimentation by centrifugation

Parasites will settle more rapidly if the stool suspension is centrifuged, however, partly digested food particles will also sediment, reducing test sensitivity. To overcome this problem, larger food particles can be removed prior to centrifugation by filtering the emulsified stool through a sieve with an aperture size large enough for parasites to pass through, but which retains the larger food particles. As this process is more efficient than sedimentation by gravity, a smaller faecal sample (500 mg–1 g, i.e. pea sized) is sufficient. The efficiency of detection is increased by adding formalin for fixation and preservation of parasites, and ether to remove fats and oils. After centrifugation, a fatty plug, which may adhere to the inner walls of the tube, can be seen at the interface of the two liquids (*Figure 2*). The ether layer, the fatty plug, and the formalin below it are discarded and the pellet examined.

Many modifications to this procedure have been advocated, and the following protocol, based on the method of Allen and Ridley (1), is a typical method. This method concentrates cysts and eggs 15- to 50-fold, dependent upon the parasite sought.

Protocol 2. Formol ether concentration for ova and cysts

Equipment and reagents

- 15 ml conical glass centrifuge tubes
- Disposable wooden applicator sticks
- Sieve (425 μm aperture size, 38 mm diameter[a])
- Pyrex beaker[b]
- Centrifuge with 15 ml swing-out buckets
- Glass microscope slides (76 × 26 mm)
- Coverslips (22 × 32 mm)
- Diamond marker
- Bright-field microscope with × 10 and × 40 objective lenses
- 10% formalin (10% of 40% formaldehyde in water)
- Diethyl ether (or ethyl acetate)
- Lugol's iodine: dissolve 10 g potassium iodide in 100 ml distilled water, then add 5 g iodine crystals (store in a dark glass bottle, out of direct sunlight, stable for several weeks)

Method

1. Sample approximately 500 mg–1 g faeces with an applicator stick, including material from the surface and interior of formed stools, and place in a clean 15 ml conical centrifuge tube containing 7 ml of 10% formalin. If the stool is liquid, dispense about 750 μl into the centrifuge tube.
2. Break up the sample thoroughly and emulsify with an applicator stick.
3. Filter the resulting suspension through the sieve into a beaker and pour the filtrate back into the same tube. Debris trapped on the sieve is discarded. Sieve and beaker are washed thoroughly in running tapwater between samples.
4. Add 3 ml of diethyl ether or ethyl acetate (flammable, perform in well ventilated area) to the formalinized solution, and mix on a vortex mixer.
5. Transfer the contents to a centrifuge tube and centrifuge the tube at 750 *g* for 60 sec, higher speed or longer times rupture helminth ova.
6. Loosen the fatty plug with a wooden stick, by passing the stick between the inner walls of the tube and the plug. Discard the plug and the fluid both above and below it by inverting the tube, allowing only the last one or two drops to fall back into the tube. Resuspend the pellet by agitation.
7. Pour the whole, or the majority of the resuspended pellet on to a microscope slide, or transfer the resuspended contents on to a microscope slide, with a Pasteur pipette, apply a coverslip, and examine for

the presence of parasites using the $\times$ 10 objective lens. Too large a pellet is indicative of one or more of the following: centrifuging above the recommended speed and/or time, insufficient shaking, taking too large a faecal sample.

8. Identify any definite morphological features under the $\times$ 40 objective. If protozoan cysts of the correct size and shape can be seen, but no diagnostic inclusions can be recognized, add a drop or two of Lugol's iodine either to the fluid at the edge of the coverslip, and re-examine the preparation when the iodine has diffused into the fluid under the coverslip (about 5 min), or to the resuspended pellet from another concentrate prior to applying the coverslip. Lugol's iodine stains nuclei and glycogen masses in cysts yellow to brown. Lugol's iodine preparation should be viewed within 15 min of preparation, otherwise over-staining of cyst inclusions will occur.

9. Assess the numbers of parasites present and record as scanty, moderate, or numerous.

[a] 425 μm aperture size, 38 mm diameter is equivalent to 36 mesh British Standard (BS 410–86) or 40 mesh American Standard (ASTM E11–81).

[b] The skirt of the sieve should fit neatly into the rim of the beaker.

A commercial device for concentrating helminth ova, larvae, and protozoan cysts according to a modification of the formalin–ether method of Ritchie is available, sold as the Fecal Parasite Concentrator (FPC, Evergreen Scientific), it is an enclosed system, and consists of two polypropylene tubes, a flat-bottomed tube used for emulsifying the stool, and a conical tube used for centrifugation, with an interconnecting sieve. The comprehensive method states that both fresh and preserved (10% formalin, merthiolate–iodine–

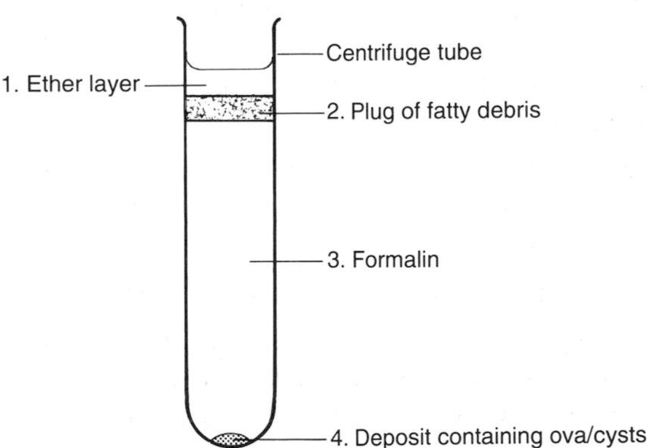

Figure 2. The various layers seen in a conical centrifuge tube after centrifugation. 1. Diethyl ether or ethyl acetate; 2. faecal debris and fat; 3. formalin; 4. sediment containing parasitic ova, larvae, and cysts.

formalin, polyvinyl alcohol, and sodium acetate–formalin) stool specimens may be used.

2.3 Flotation

The specific gravity of helminth ova and larvae, and protozoan cysts are in the range 1.050–1.150 and the flotation principle utilizes a liquid medium denser than the parasites so that they rise to the surface and can be skimmed from the surface film. A successful flotation fluid must not only be heavier than the parasites, but must not produce damaging shrinkage. Concentrated aqueous NaCl solution (S. G. 1.120–1.200) have been employed, and ova of the common intestinal helminths are not damaged by this process but protozoan cysts become badly shrivelled or open up. The optimal time to examine specimens obtained from brine flotation is 5–20 minutes after flotation. For these reasons, other flotation fluids such as sucrose solutions have been advocated.

Protocol 3. Sucrose flotation of parasites

Equipment and reagents

- 15 ml test-tubes, wooden applicator sticks
- Microscope slides (76 × 26 mm)
- Bright-field microscope with × 10 and × 40 objective lenses
- Sucrose solution (dissolve 910 g of sucrose in 1 litre distilled water, S.G. 1.180)
- Lugol's iodine (*Protocol 2*).

Method

1. Transfer 1 g of faeces with an applicator stick to 3 ml of sucrose solution in a test-tube and mix thoroughly.
2. Add, with gentle stirring, sufficient sucrose solution to form a positive meniscus at the top of the test-tube.
3. Remove any large particles from the surface and, if necessary, add more sucrose solution to maintain the positive meniscus.
4. Gently place one surface of a coverslip[a] on to the positive meniscus. Leave for 20 min, then lift the coverslip vertically, together with its hanging drop, and place on to a clean microscope slide.
5. Examine for the presence of parasites, using the × 10 objective lens. Identify any definitive morphological features under the × 40 objective. If no morphological features seen, see *Protocol 2*, step 8.
6. Assess the numbers of parasites present, record as *Protocol 2*.

[a] The dimensions of the coverslip should be larger than the diameter of the rim of the centrifuge tube so that it can be placed to rest manually, with ease, on the rim. Take great care not to disturb the meniscus. Alternatively, a wire loop bent at right angles can be used to remove several drops of the surface film.

2.4 Microscopical examination of a sample

The sample must be examined in a systematic manner. Observation should commence using the × 10 objective ensuring that the entire coverslip or sample is viewed. Commence in the upper left-hand corner of the sample, working across the slide from left to right, one field width at a time, until the upper right-hand edge of the sample is reached. When observing protozoa, the fine focus should be adjusted continuously so that the depth of the sample is also scanned. Protozoan cysts are refractile under bright-field microscopy. When a suspicious object is located, it is inspected under high power (× 40) magnification and either verified or disregarded.

3. Characteristics of intestinal protozoa

The classical approach to the diagnosis of parasitic diseases of man has been to identify the various stages in the life cycle present, on the basis of morphology. For the intestinal protozoa, mentioned below, both the reproductive and developmental, and the transmissive stages are sought as the detection of different stages can increase the likelihood of diagnosis. The diagnostic stages for flagellate and ciliate protozoa are the trophozoite and cyst (when present in the life cycle), and the oocyst for the coccidia. These stages occur in faeces and can be sought for by examination of a wet mount or a permanently stained smear. Wet mounts can be faecal suspensions or concentrates and may be unstained (saline or formalin) or stained (iodine, which is primarily a stain for cysts, or other temporary stains). Concentration techniques are unsatisfactory for trophozoites, and the direct examination of emulsified stools or the examination of permanently stained smears is necessary. The characteristics used to identify intestinal flagellates are as follows:

Trophozoites

- shape
- motility in saline preparations
- number of nuclei
- other features (e.g. ventral sucker, undulating membrane, cystosome)

Cysts

- shape
- size
- number of nuclei
- presence of other organelles

Not all of the above features will be seen in a single preparation, therefore, both unstained and stained preparations should be examined.

There is only one ciliate parasite of man, *Balantidium coli*, and being the largest protozoan parasite, both trophozoite and cyst are easily seen. The characteristics used to identify intestinal coccidia occur in the transmissive stage, the oocyst.

3.1 *Giardia intestinalis*

3.1.1 Life cycle and morphology

Three morphologically different *Giardia* spp. are recognized, *G. agilis*, in amphibians, *G. muris* in rodents, birds and reptiles, and *G. duodenalis*) in humans, other mammals, birds, and reptiles (8). Parasites infecting the small intestine of human beings are referred to as *G. lamblia* or *G. intestinalis*. The life cycle is direct (*Figure 3*), requiring no intermediate host, and the parasite exists in two distinct morphological forms, namely the reproductive trophozoite which parasitizes the enterocytes of the upper small intestine, and the

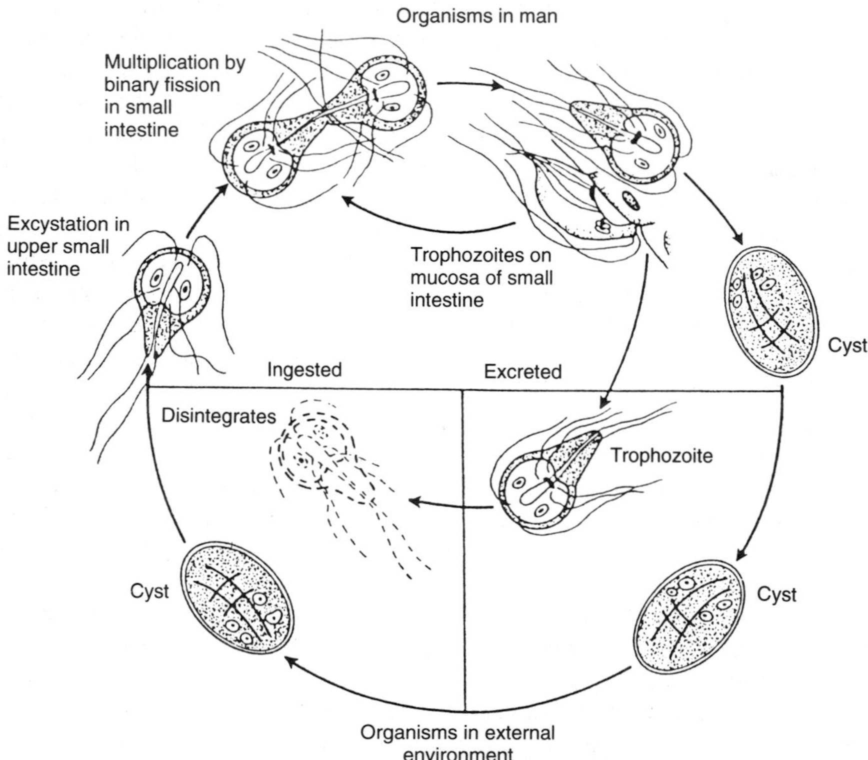

Figure 3. Diagram of the life cycle of *Giardia intestinalis* (redrawn from Figure 1, Meyer and Jarroll, *Am. J. Epidemiol.*, **111**, 1980).

environmentally-resistant cyst, voided in the faeces, which is the infective stage (*Plate 2b*).

The motile trophozoite exhibits forward movement during which the organism tends to rotate around its longitudinal axis displaying both a tumbling movement resembling that of a falling leaf and an up and down movement referred to as 'skipping'. Exposure to bile salts and alkaline pH, as the trophozoite passes down the small intestine induces the trophozoite stage to encyst, whereby it becomes rounded, forming the binucleate immature cyst. Mature cysts contain four nuclei located at one pole and other structures found within the trophozoite (i.e. axostyles and median bodies) (*Plate 2b*).

Transmission is via the faecal-oral route and by water, especially with community water systems (2).

3.1.2 Symptoms

The clinical presentation ranges from acute to chronic disease and asymptomatic infection. The prepatent period is on average 9.1 days (3). In most people, the disease is self-limiting, the acute phase being normally short-lived and followed by a chronic phase, which is the commonest presentation of symptomatic disease. Typical symptoms include diarrhoea, flatulence, upper intestinal cramps, abdominal distension, nausea, and weight loss, together with signs of malabsorption (e.g. steatorrhoea, disaccharidase deficiency and vitamin B12 malabsorption) (4). Such symptoms usually disappear following effective treatment. In rare cases symptoms may occur sporadically for years.

Stools are often loose or watery in the acute stage and may be intermittently in the chronic stage, and may contain only trophozoites. Therefore, it is important to examine, immediately, a wet film of a freshly-passed (hot) stool specimen in an attempt to identify intact motile organisms, or to preserve an aliquot in polyvinyl alcohol (PVA) fixative, or merthiolate–iodine–formaldehyde (MIF) stain and fixative for conventional staining and examination later. The use of permanent conventional stains can aid the identification of parasitic protozoa, and differentiate related species. In addition, permanently stained slides serve as a record to document an infection or the presence of a parasite. Both PVA and MIF provide good preservation of the morphology of trophozoites and cysts. An asymptomatic cyst passing stage has also been documented with prevalence rates varying from 13%–76% however, its duration is unknown (5, 6).

Cyst excretion can be intermittent, and some infected persons may be low rate cyst excretors (7). In addition, symptoms may be present before parasites can be detected in stool, and repeated examinations on a weekly basis may be necessary until the infection becomes patent (8). For these reasons, timing of stool collection is important. Cysts can be detected in a single stool sample in between 35%–50% of cases, whereas between six and ten specimens are required to achieve a detection rate of 70%–90% (9). Microscopic examination of a single stool sample can not exclude infection, therefore, at least three stool specimens should be examined before other diagnostic procedures. In severe infections, up to 14 billion parasites can occur in a diarrhoeal stool, whereas in a moderate infection, up to 300 million parasites can occur (10). Where parasites are numerous, direct smear examination in saline or Lugol's iodine may be sufficient (*Plate 2b*). Generally, concentration of cysts by the formol ether method should be performed (*Protocol 2*).

The sensitivity of microscopic examination can be increased by immunofluorescence assays using monoclonal antibodies (Mabs) (*Protocol 4*). These commercial kits utilize Mabs which recognize surface-exposed epitopes of the cyst, and the fluorescence visualized defines the maximum dimensions of the cyst. Both the direct and indirect immunofluorescence procedures are available. Indirect fluorescence is more time-consuming, but the use of a second antibody increases the assay sensitivity. For maximum sensitivity, concentration of the sample, prior to immunofluorescence detection, is recommended. Although this method is more time-consuming than bright-field microscopy, translucent cysts and cysts with poor morphology can be detected, and this is especially useful for environmental samples. A disadvantage of immunofluorescence on dried smears is that the organelles within the cyst can become distorted, thus reducing the potential for definitive identification. If the test result is negative, giardiasis cannot be excluded, and further stool samples should be obtained and tested.

Protocol 4. Identification of *Giardia* cysts in stools by immunofluorescence following concentration

Equipment and reagents

- Multiwell (4) microscope slides (Henley)
- Coverslips (22 × 64 mm)
- Adjustable automatic pipette (5–25 μl) and disposable tips
- Coplin jar or similar
- Humidified chamber
- Fluorescence microscope with filter system for FITC (maximum excitation wavelength 490 nm, mean emission wavelength 530 nm) equipped with × 20 and × 40 (dry) objective lenses suitable for fluorescence
- Acetone or methanol for fixation if formalin is found to be unsuitable
- 150 mM phosphate-buffered saline (PBS) pH 7.2
- Materials usually provided with the kit: FITC labelled anti-*Giardia* monoclonal antibody (provided at the working dilution) containing Evans blue and sodium azide, glycerol-based mounting medium containing a photobleaching inhibitor

Method

1. Pipette 25 μl of emulsified stool or formol ether concentrate (*Protocol 2*) on to, and spread over, a well of a multispot slide which corresponds to the identity code of the patient.
2. Air dry the slide at room temperature.
3. If formalin fixation proves to be unsuitable, fix the slide for 1–5 min in acetone or methanol and air dry.

4. Place 25 μl of the FITC labelled monoclonal antibody (at the predetermined working dilution) on to the fixed air dried specimen. Include a *known* negative and positive control.
5. Incubate the slide(s) horizontally in the dark in a humidified chamber for 30 min at 37 °C.
6. Rinse the slide in a gentle stream of water (e.g. with wash bottle).
7. Drain the excess moisture from the slide and add two or three drops of the mounting medium supplied[a] and apply a coverslip.
8. Scan the smear using × 20 objective lens. Confirm any cyst-like object[b] using the × 40 objective lens.
9. Assess the numbers of cysts present, record as scanty, moderate, or numerous.

[a] If mounting medium is not supplied, a mixture of 50% non-fluorescent glycerol: 50% 150 mM PBS pH 7.2 (v/v) is suitable.

[b] Specific fluorescence localized on the cyst wall, on objects measuring 8–12 μm long and 7–10 μm wide, should be demonstrable in the positive control. Specific fluorescence is apple-green in colour, background fluorescence is red (due to the presence of Evans blue which reduces non-specific fluorescence). Non-specific fluorescence is yellow. Always refer to the positive control to ensure that the size, shape, and colour of the putative cyst are consistent with those of the positive control.

Antibodies raised to *Giardia*-specific antigen(s) can be used to detect *Giardia*-specific antigen in faeces. Both counter-immunoelectropheresis (CIE) and enzyme-linked immunosorbent assays (ELISA) have been used for this purpose (11, 12).

Techniques for detecting genus-specific or species-specific DNA sequences have promised much as diagnostic tools, but are cumbersome and lack sensitivity when compared with microscopy. Two DNA probes for the diagnosis of *G. intestinalis* have been reported (13, 14). PCR, together with a DNA probe has been used to detect a single *Giardia* cyst and differentiate *G. duodenalis* from other species (15).

When trophozoites or cysts are not found following the examination of a reasonable number of stool samples, and giardiasis is suspected clinically, the examination of duodenal or jejunal fluid may be indicated. The specimen to be analysed for the presence of trophozoites by microscopy or *in vitro* culture can be obtained with an endoscope, in which case it will be a liquid sample, or with Enterotest® (see Chapter 9, *Protocol 6*). Another alternative is small bowel biopsy (*Plate 6c*). *In vitro* culture does add significantly to the chance of making a diagnosis. *In vitro* culture is also useful for studies of:

- the biochemistry and immunochemistry of trophozoites
- the characterization of isotype-specific responses in clinical and subclinical giardiasis by ELISA, SDS–PAGE, and Western blotting.

- trophozoite–drug interactions
- the development of rapid detection assays
- the analysis of the *Giardia* genome

3.1.3 *In vitro* culture and subculture of trophozoites

G. intestinalis is an aerotolerant anaerobe, and the axenic culture of trophozoites in a medium containing both thiol-reducing agents (*Protocol 5*), such as cysteine and mammalian bile, led to the formulation of a medium which supports the growth of a variety of *G. duodenalis* isolates from humans and other mammals (16). Cysteine, and other thiol-reducing agents, protect trophozoites from the lethal effects of oxygen; this effect is enhanced by ascorbic acid. However, only the former is capable of supporting the growth of trophozoites. In addition, cysteine is required for both the initiation of attachment of trophozoites to a solid phase (e.g. glass or plastic) *in vitro*, and their subsequent adherence (17). Keister's modification of TYI-S-33 (30) supplemented with either 10% (v/v) sterile bovine or equine serum is capable of supporting the growth of trophozoites. Either plastic or glass tissue culture tubes can be used. They are filled to 90%–95% of their capacity to minimize the gas volume above the surface of the medium, and are incubated at 35 °C either vertically or at a shallow angle (about 5 ° from the horizontal). During growth *in vitro*, trophozoites attach to the walls of the culture vessel forming monolayers which become confluent by the end of the logarithmic phase of growth. Unattached, motile trophozoites can be seen swimming in the medium.

Cultures can be instigated from trophozoites in jejunal juices. Intestinal

Protocol 5. *In vitro* culture and subculture of trophozoites

Equipment and reagents

- 2 litre beaker
- Magnetic stirrer and flea
- pH meter
- Whatman No. 1 filter-paper or equivalent (32 cm diameter) with suitable filter funnel and stand
- Sterile filtration unit (consisting of an in-line 0.45 μm membrane filter with inlet and outlet tubes, the outlet tube being clamped)
- Peristaltic pump and two lengths of compatible tubing (ensure that both pump and tubing are clean)
- 20 sterile 100 ml screw-capped bottles (e.g. Duran bottles)

Basic medium (Keister Modification of TYI-S-33)

- K_2HPO_4 2.0 g
- KH_2PO_4 1.2 g
- Casein digest peptone 40.0 g (e.g. BBL Cat. No. 097023)
- Yeast extract 20.0 g (e.g. Difco Bacto 0127-02)
- Glucose 20.0 g
- NaCl 4.0 g
- Cysteine–HCl monohydrate 4.0 g
- L-Ascorbic acid 400 mg
- Ferric ammonium citrate 45.6 mg
- Dehydrated bovine bile 2.0 g (e.g. Bile Bacteriological, Sigma B-8381)

Method

1. Weigh out and dissolve the above ingredients in 1 litre of distilled water using a magnetic stirrer.

2. When the components are in solution, adjust the pH to 7.0 with 1 M NaOH.
3. Make the volume of the solution up to 1800 ml with distilled water, and filter through Whatman No. 1 filter-paper or equivalent.
4. Observing sterile procedure in a class II hood, filter sterilize the medium through the 0.45 μm membrane filter using a peristaltic pump.
5. Dispense 90 ml of medium into sterile 100 ml bottles, store at −20°C.

When complete medium is desired for culture, thaw (at 57 °C) the required number of bottles of basic medium needed for subculturing for one or two weeks, and add the recommended volumes of heat-inactivated serum and antibiotics as indicated below.

Complete medium

6. For each 100 ml of complete medium add 10 mL of sterile heat inactivated (56 °C for 30 min) bovine or equine serum to 90 mL of sterile basic medium.[a]
7. Sub-culture the parasites when they become confluent on the inside wall of the culture vessel.[b]
8. Take 2–3 mL of the medium to inoculate the next flask.[c]

[a] Sterile complete medium can be stored for two weeks at 4 °C.

[b] Timing of subculture is dependent on seeding density used to initiate culture and is usually required twice a week.

[c] If there are few trophozoites in the medium, adherent organisms can be detached by chilling and used to initiate subculture.

fluids are likely to contain organisms which can multiply by *in vitro* (*Protocol 6*). If the culture tube containing the trophozoites and contaminants is incubated horizontally, or at an angle of 5° from the horizontal, the trophozoites will settle on to the warm lower inner surface of that tube and attach in that position. Although bacterial multiplication is more rapid than that of trophozoites, overgrowth of resistant bacteria is reduced by rotating the culture tube through 180° so that the adherent trophozoites are attached on to what becomes the upper inner surface of the tube. This encourages the resuspended organisms to separate from the adherent trophozoites by sedimentation and, once separated, the medium containing the contaminants can be discarded and the culture replenished with fresh complete medium. Alternatively, the culture can be incubated vertically, and the free-swimming, contaminant-free trophozoites near the surface can be harvested, and transferred to a fresh culture tube containing complete medium with added antibiotics where necessary. This process may have to be repeated, dependent on the antibiotic resistance pattern of the contaminants present. Eventually, using the two selection processes outlined above, axenic cultures of trophozoites can be obtained. At this stage, the additional antibiotics can be withdrawn from the formulation of the medium.

Protocol 6. *In vitro* culture of trophozoites from jejunal aspirates

Equipment and reagents

- 15 ml sterile culture tubes
- Sterile Pasteur pipettes and teats
- Centrifuge with 15 ml swing-out buckets
- Inverted microscope with × 10 and × 20 objective lenses
- Laminar flow hood
- 35 °C incubator.
- Complete medium containing added antibiotics: penicillin 100 U/ml, streptomycin 100 µg/ml, vancomycin 20 µg/ml, and clindamycin 20 µg/ml

Method

1. Warm 20 ml of complete medium containing added antibiotics to 35 °C.
2. Place the specimen of intestinal fluid in a sterile culture tube or similar container and centrifuge at 500 *g* for 2 min. Aspirate the supernatant to waste, being careful not to disrupt the pellet.
3. Resuspend the pellet thoroughly in a minimal volume of complete medium containing added antibiotics, and transfer the suspension to a sterile culture tube. Add sufficient of the same medium to fill the tube to 90%–95% of its capacity.
4. Incubate cultures at 35 °C either horizontally, or at an angle of 5 ° from the horizontal. Examine the inner surface of the tube for adherent trophozoites and the medium for free-swimming trophozoites with the × 10 and × 20 objective lenses of an inverted microscope, daily for a week.[a]
5. When attached trophozoites are seen, rotate the culture tubes through 180 °.[b]
6. Repeat step **4**.[c]
7. Re-feed the culture every three to four days by decanting the old medium and replacing it with fresh sterile complete medium.[d]
8. When the culture is free of contaminants, withdraw the additional antibiotics from the formulation of the medium, and initiate axenic cultures.
9. Examine the contents of the culture tube after 24 h with the × 10 and × 20 objective lenses of an inverted microscope to determine whether the trophozoites are multiplying.

[a] If no trophozoites are seen after a few days, it is unlikely that the trophozoites in the intestinal fluid have adapted to the culture medium.

[b] This permits the expansion of the trophozoite isolate on the tube surface whilst diluting the contaminants in the vicinity of the trophozoites by causing them to sediment to the opposite side of the tube.

[c] If bacterial overgrowth becomes a problem, the antibiotic sensitivity of the contaminant(s) should be investigated, and the appropriate antibiotic added.

[d] This procedure gradually removes the contaminants from the culture.

3.2 *Cryptosporidium parvum*

3.2.1 Life cycle and morphology

Cryptosporidium spp. (Greek: hidden spore) have a world-wide distribution. Evidence based on morphological analyses and on cross-transmission studies indicate that there are at least four valid species, namely; *C. parvum* and *C. muris* found in mammals, and *C. baileyi* and *C. mealagridis* found in birds (18). In addition, two further species have been documented, namely *C. crotali* in reptiles, and *C. nasorum* in fish. *C. parvum* is the major species responsible for clinical disease in man and domestic animals (18). Humans acquire the disease following the ingestion of infective oocysts, and sporozoites released from excysted oocysts infect the epthelial cells lining the gastro-intestinal tract. The developmental stages can colonize the gastro-intestinal tract from pharynx to rectum, with the jejunum the most frequently affected site (19).

Cryptosporidium completes its life cycle (*Figure 4*) within a single host and transmission is via the thick-walled, environmentally robust oocyst excreted in the faeces of the infected host. Unlike *E. histolytica* and *G. intestinalis*, endogenous re-infection (auto-infection) occurs which, together with the recycling of the asexual stage, allows the build-up of parasite numbers to a high level. In addition, external maturation of oocysts is not required, and some oocysts (the thin-walled oocysts which account for up to 20% of the total) excyst during passage through the intestine releasing infective sporozoites which can further augment the infection. Up to 10^{10} oocysts/gram have been reported in human faeces, and infected calves can excrete up to 10^{10} oocysts daily for up to 14 days (20).

Oocysts of *C. parvum* are smooth, thick walled, colourless, spherical or slightly ovoid bodies containing, when fully developed (sporulated), four elongated, naked (i.e. not within a sporocyst(s)) sporozoites and a cytoplasmic residual body. The modal size measurement of *C. parvum* oocysts is 4.5×5.0 μm (range 4–6 μm).

3.2.2 Transmission

In the last decade, *Cryptosporidium* sp. have been recognized as a common cause of acute self-limiting gastro-enteritis, transmitted by the faecal-oral route. Transmission via the venereal route and from pets has been reported. Secondary cases and possibly asymptomatic excretors may be a source of infection for other susceptible persons. Initial cases of human infection were believed to have been acquired from animals (zooanthroponosis). Both the broad host range exemplified by *C. parvum*, and the high output of infective oocysts from numerous mammalian hosts ensure a high level of environmental contamination. Cryptosporidiosis has been reported in a variety of domesticated animals, livestock, and wildlife, including companion animals which may be reservoirs of human infection (21). In common with

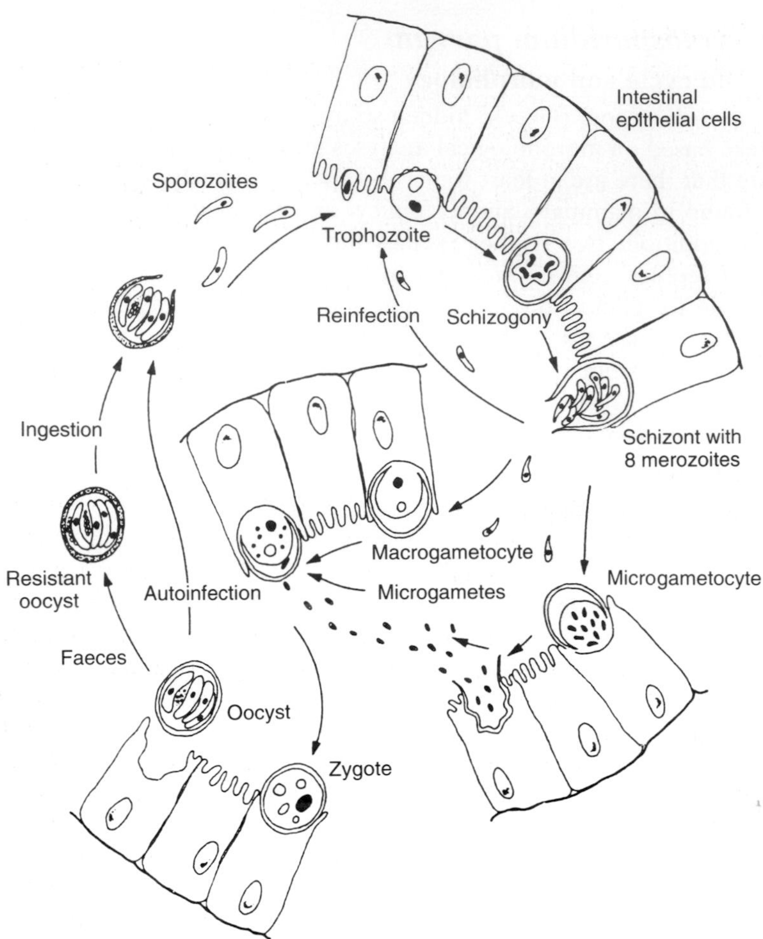

Figure 4. The life cycle of *Cryptosporidium* sp.

other infectious disease agents which contaminate the environment, and can be transmitted to human beings via potable water, the waterborne route of transmission has also been documented for oocysts of *Cryptosporidium* spp. In addition to epidemic cryptosporidiosis from drinking water supplies, there have been two outbreaks reported from the accidental ingestion of swimming pool water. Foodborne and airborne routes have also been documented, but further evidence is required to clarify the significance of both these routes of transmission.

As few as ten oocysts can produce infection in non-human primate infants (22). In humans the ID_{50} is 214 oocysts, although 62% of volunteers ingesting 30 oocysts or more became infected (23).

3.2.3 Symptoms

The incubation period averages three to six days post-infection and oocyst excretion generally occurs from less than three to 30 days (mean: 12 days) and coincides with the presence of symptoms (24, 25). Oocyst shedding can be intermittent and can continue for up to 50 days after the cessation of symptoms (25). The clinical symptoms include a flu-like illness, diarrhoea, malaise, abdominal pain, anorexia, nausea, flatulence, malabsorption, vomiting, mild fever, and weight loss (25).

In the immunocompromised, such as those with acquired immune deficiency syndrome (AIDS), cryptosporidiosis is a common life-threatening condition causing profuse intractable diarrhoea with severe dehydration and fluid losses of up to 10–17 litres per day (19). The spread of parasites to other organs can also occur (26).

3.2.4 Diagnosis

Optimal laboratory diagnosis of cryptosporidiosis is based on the demonstration of oocysts in stools. Auramine–phenol counterstained with strong carbol fuchsin (*Protocol 7*), cold Ziehl–Neelsen (*Protocol 8*), and a monoclonal antibody which recognizes epitopes on the oocyst wall (*Protocol 9*) have all been used to detect oocysts in faeces. Stool samples from most symptomatic individuals with cryptosporidiosis will contain large numbers of oocysts, but increased sensitivity can be achieved by employing a concentration method such as formol ether (*Protocol 2*). In some laboratories, the formol ether concentration technique is used routinely, and the sample used for this examination can be reused for the examination for oocysts by removing the coverslip and allowing the fluid remaining on the slide to dry. Difficulties in discriminating between *Cryptosporidium* sp. oocysts and other spherical objects of similar size (e.g. fungal spores are stained by acid fast methods) do arise, which can make positive diagnosis difficult when only a few oocysts are present (*Plate 2c*).

Protocol 7. Detection of *Cryptosporidium* sp. oocysts in faecal smears by auramine–phenol staining

Equipment and reagents

- Microscope slides (76 × 26 mm)
- Coplin jars or similar, methanol (94%)
- Fluorescence microscope equipped with FITC filters and ×20 and ×40 objective lenses
- Auramine–phenol (Lempert) solution
- Strong carbol fuchsin stain (Paramount Reagents Ltd.)

Method

1. Fix an air dried direct or concentrate smear[a] in methanol for 3 min.
2. Immerse in auramine–phenol stain for 5 min.

Protocol 7. *Continued*

3. Rinse slide in tap-water to remove excess stain.
4. Counterstain in cold strong carbol fuchsin for 10 sec.
5. Rinse in tap-water to remove excess stain.
6. Air dry the slide and examine for the presence of oocysts using a fluorescence microscope equipped with FITC filters. Scan the slide using the ×20 objective lens and confirm the presence of oocysts under the ×40 objective lens.[b]
7. Measure the size and shape of the fluorescent bodies.

[a] For best results, smears of moderate thickness are recommended for this technique and the modified Ziehl–Neelsen staining procedures. Fluid stools should be mixed thoroughly and a sample removed with a pipette or a swab on to a microscope slide, and made into a smear. Formed stools should be emulsified in 150 mM saline to produce a more liquid emulsion before the smear is made and air dried.

[b] *Cryptosporidium* sp. oocysts appear ring-shaped (4–6 μm diameter) and exhibit a characteristically bright fluorescence against a dark red background.

Protocol 8. Detection of *Cryptosporidium* sp. oocysts using modified cold Ziehl–Neelsen stain

Equipment and reagents

- Microscope slides (76 × 26mm)
- Coplin jars or similar
- Light microscope with ×40 and ×100 (oil) objective lenses.
- Methanol (94%)
- Strong carbol fuchsin (Paramount Reagents Ltd).
- 0.4% malachite green (w/v) in distilled water
- 1% HCl (v/v) in methanol (94%)

Method

1. Fix the air dried direct or concentrate smear[a] in methanol for 3 min.
2. Immerse the slide in cold carbol fuchsin and stain for 15 min.
3. Rinse the slide thoroughly in tap-water.
4. Decolorize in 1% HCl (v/v) in methanol for 10–15 sec.
5. Rinse the slide in tap-water.
6. Counterstain with 0.4% malachite green for 30 sec.
7. Rinse the slide in tap-water.
8. Air dry the slide and scan the slide using the ×40 objective lens. Confirm the presence of oocysts[b,c] under the oil immersion objective lens.

9. Measure the size and shape of the red stained bodies.

[a] Moderately thick smear.

[b] *Cryptosporidium* sp. oocysts stain red and appear as spherules (4–6 μm diameter) on a pale green background (*Plate 2c*). The degree and proportion of staining varies with individual oocysts. In addition, the internal structures take up the stain to varying degrees. Some may appear amorphous whilst others may contain the characteristic crescentic forms of the sporozoites.

[c] *Isospora belli* oocysts stain red and appear as large elongated ovoid bodies (20–30 × 10–19 μm), tapered at the end and containing either a granular zygote or two sporoblasts (*Plate 2d*).

3.2.5 Identification of *Cryptosporidium* by immunofluorescence

There is no currently, commercially available antibody preparation which is specific for the epitopes on *C. parvum* oocysts.

The three criteria recommended for the identification of *Cryptosporidium* sp. oocysts by immunofluorescence are:

- characteristic apple-green fluorescence delineating the oocyst wall
- shape (spherical)
- size (4–6 μm diameter)

Direct (*Protocol 9*) or indirect immunofluorescence can be used and although more time-consuming, the use of a second antibody in the indirect method can increase the assay sensitivity.

Protocol 9. Detection of *Cryptosporidium* sp. oocysts by immunofluorescence

Equipment and reagents

- Multispot microscope slides (4 well, Henley, Essex) and coverslips (22 × 64 mm)
- Adjustable automatic pipette (5–50 μl), and disposable tips
- Humidified chamber
- Fluorescence microscope with FITC filters and × 20 or 25 × 40, and × 100 objective lens suitable for fluorescence
- 37 °C incubator
- Acetone
- FITC labelled anti-*Cryptosporidium* Mab (diluted optimally)
- Oocyst positive and negative controls
- Glycerol-based mounting medium (e.g. 50% glycerol: 50% 150 mM PBS pH 7.2)
- Photobleaching inhibitor such as Citifluor (City University, Department of Chemistry)

Method

1. Pipette 25 μl of emulsified stool or formol ether concentrate on to and spread over a well of the multispot slide.[a]
2. Air dry the slide at room temperature.
3. Fix the slide for 1–5 min in acetone and air dry.

Protocol 9. *Continued*

4. Place 25 μl of the FITC labelled monoclonal antibody (at the predetermined working dilution) on to the fixed air dried specimen and the oocyst positive and negative controls.
5. Incubate the slide(s) horizontally in the dark in a humidified chamber for 30 min at 37 °C.
6. Rinse the slide in a gentle stream of water (e.g. with a wash bottle).
7. Drain the excess moisture from the slide and add two or three drops of the mounting medium supplied.
8. Apply a coverslip[b] to the slide ensuring that no air bubbles are trapped over the specimen.
9. Examine the negative and positive controls and record your findings.
10. Examine the test well for fluorescing oocysts[c] using the × 20 (or × 25) objective lens. Cover the whole area of the spot with either vertical or horizontal sweeps. Ensure that the whole area is viewed. Note any oocysts present.
11. Assess the numbers of oocysts present.[d]

[a] Always include known negative and positive samples in each test.

[b] Do not press down on the coverslip, but allow its weight to displace the mounting medium. Inverting the slide on an absorbent tissue will remove the excess mounting medium.

[c] Specific fluorescence localized on the oocyst wall, on circular objects measuring 4–6 μm diameter, should be demonstrable in the positive control only. Specific fluorescence is apple-green in colour, background fluorescence is red (due to the presence of Evans blue which reduces non-specific fluorescence). Non-specific fluorescence is yellow. Always refer to the positive control to ensure that the size, shape, and colour of the putative oocyst are consistent with those of the positive control.

[d] Numbers can be recorded as scanty, moderate, or numerous.

3.3 *Isospora belli*

Isospora spp. are coccidian parasites of mammals, birds, and amphibians. The species responsible for disease in man is *Isospora belli*, and man is the only known host. *I. belli* has a world-wide distribution, and is found more commonly in tropical and subtropical climates than in temperate climates, however, its prevalence remains unknown. It has been implicated in various outbreaks of diarrhoea in institutions in the USA. In immunocompromised individuals it is an opportunistic pathogen (27), being found in 15% of AIDS patients in Haiti (28).

3.3.1 Life cycle and morphology

Humans acquire the infection following the ingestion of infective oocysts from either symptomatic or asymptomatic excretors. The mature oocyst contains two sporocysts, each of which contains four sporozoites. Sporozoites are released and infect the epithelial cells lining the intestinal tract. *I. belli* completes its life cycle within a single host and transmission is via the oocyst excreted in the faeces of the infected host or via rectal intercourse in homosexuals. Both asexual (schizogony) and sexual (sporogony) developmental cycles occur in the epithelial mucosa. Unlike *Cryptosporidium* sp., immature oocysts are excreted in faeces and an external maturation period is required before the oocysts become infective.

3.3.2 Clinical features

The incubation period is about a week. Whilst most infections are asymptomatic, a self-limiting illness characterized by an acute onset, fever, malaise, abdominal pain, and weight loss, lasting for two to three weeks may occur in the immunocompetent host. More rarely, a protracted illness with malabsorption may occur. Oocysts can be detected in faeces for varying time periods (range nine to 122 days) after infection. In the immunocompromised host, symptoms may be severe and prolonged (27).

3.3.3 Diagnostic features of *Isospora belli* oocysts

Immature oocysts are elongated with tapering extremities and measure 20–33 μm × 10–19 μm (median 29 × 13 μm). The thin oocyst wall is smooth, clear, and colourless and is composed of two layers. Within the oocyst wall, in freshly voided faeces, is the unsegmented granular zygote. More rarely, oocysts containing two sporoblasts are seen in freshly voided faeces. The mature oocyst contains two sporocysts, each of which contains four uninucleate, long, slender crescentic sporozoites and a granular mass known as the sporocystic residue.

Oocysts can be stored, and will remain viable, in either 0.5% formaldehyde for seven months, or 2% $K_2Cr_2O_7$ for over two months at 4 °C.

3.3.4 Diagnosis

The examination of both stools and intestinal fluid or mucus for immature oocysts can help establish the diagnosis. When present in stools, immature oocysts are sufficiently large not to be missed on direct faecal examination, however, as they can occur infrequently and in small numbers concentration of the sample is recommended. The formol ether technique (see *Protocol 2*) is recommended.

The immature oocyst (containing a granular zygote) is more likely to be seen in intestinal and faecal specimens, however, the immature oocyst (containing two sporoblasts) may also be encountered. Depending upon the age of the stool, the mature oocyst (containing two sporocysts, with four sporozoites within each sporocyst) may be seen.

Oocysts are transparent and are best seen with reduced illumination. The use of the modified Ziehl–Neelsen stain (*Protocol 8*) has been advocated for the demonstration of oocysts in direct smears, intestinal fluid, and mucus (*Plate 2d*).

3.4 Coccidial enteritis caused by other coccidia

Whilst *Sarcocystis* spp. are coccidian parasites of many vertebrates, they differ from *Cryptosporidium* sp. and *I. belli*, in that they require two hosts to complete their life cycle (heteroxenous). The transmissive stage (the muscle sarcocyst) in the intermediate (prey) host is ingested by the definitive (predator) host where it undergoes sporogony in the intestinal mucosa to produce thin-walled oocysts which contain two sporocysts in the lumen. Oocysts rupture in the lumen releasing the infective sporocysts which are voided in the faeces. Transmission to the intermediate host occurs following the ingestion of sporocysts. These excyst in the intestine and sporozoites undergo schizogony, and eventually remain dormant as sarcocysts in muscle cells. Man is the definitive host for *Sarcocystis bovihominis* and *Sarcocystis suihominis* formerly known as *Isospora hominis*, which have bovine and porcine intermediate hosts respectively. Transmission to man is by eating undercooked beef or pork containing sarcocysts. The deep-freezing of infected meat destroys sarcocysts.

Most infections are thought to be asymptomatic, although some symptomatic cases have been described. Symptoms include abdominal pain, anorexia, nausea, bloating, and diarrhoea associated with the passage of sporocysts. Mature sporocysts can be demonstrated in faeces from nine days post-infection.

3.4.1 Diagnosis

Sporocysts are sparse in faeces and require concentration techniques for their demonstration, as for *I. belli* formol ether concentration is favoured. Sporocysts of *S. bovihominis* and *S. suihominis* are larger than those of *I. belli*, occur singly or in pairs, and contain four sporozoites and a polar residual body. The oocysts of *S. bovihominis* (13.1–17μm × 7.7–10.8 μm) are slightly larger than those of *S. suihominis* (12.6 × 9.3 μm).

3.5 *Balantidium coli*

B. coli is a ciliate parasite of numerous mammals including man and pigs which is found throughout the world. Human infection is prevalent in some areas of the tropics and subtropics and is sporadic in temperate climates. It exists in two distinct forms, namely the trophozoite which infects the caecal and sigmoidorectal regions of the large intestine, and the cyst which is the transmissive stage. Cysts excyst in the small intestine and the trophozoites pass into the large intestine where they can burrow into the mucosal surface and forms colonies. Reproduction is by transverse binary fission. Trophozoites are oval or spheroid in shape, and can measure 30–200 μm in length by

40–60 μm in width. The surface is covered by spiral longitudinal rows of cilia, and at the anterior end is a narrow triangular peristome, ventral to the midline, which leads into the mouth (cytosome).

The cyst is spheroid or ovoid measuring 40–60 μm in diameter, and contains the macronucleus and the contractile vacuoles. Recently encysted organisms retain their cilia and are motile within the cyst, but subsequently lose their cilia and become quiescent. The unstained trophozoite and cyst appear yellowish green.

Person to person, foodborne, and waterborne routes of transmission have been implicated, as has zoonotic transmission from pigs. Asymptomatic excretors may be a source of infection for other susceptible persons. Trophozoites can encyst after being passed in the stool, and may survive for up to ten days in moist conditions outside the body.

3.5.1 Symptoms

A wide spectrum of disease exists ranging from recurrent diarrhoea to mild or fulminating dysentery. Most infections are asymptomatic or chronic and may last for years. Trophozoites can be found in large numbers in superficial colonic exudates, follicles and embedded in the tissues at the base of ulcers. In advanced cases a mass of ulcers, resembling those of amoebic dysentery, may be present. Rarely, trophozoites invade into the submucosa, penetrate the muscular coat, and migrate into the liver and lymph nodes. Liver abscesses containing trophozoites, vaginitis, and urinary tract infections have been reported.

3.5.2 Diagnosis

Diagnosis depends upon the demonstration of either trophozoites or cysts in stools. The methods employed to demonstrate trophozoites are similar to those used for the intestinal amoebae (Chapter 6, section 1.1). Trophozoites can be found in 90% of mucoid and bloody stools by direct examination of faeces or following fixation and staining with iron haematoxylin. Cysts are found less frequently, but can be demonstrated in semi-formed or formed stools, following formol ether concentration of the sample.

3.6 *Chilomastix mesnili*

Trophozoites of *Chilomastix mesnili* reside in the large intestine, and infections are persistent.

3.6.1 Diagnostic morphology

The pear-shaped trophozoite is rounded at its anterior end and tapers posteriorly. The body is asymmetrical as a result of a spiral groove which runs obliquely across the ventral surface. The cleft-shaped cytosome is anterior, extending backwards half the length of the body and has a median constriction. Within the cytosome lies a delicate flagellum. Anteriorly, there are three flagella (two short, one long). Flagella arise from small basal bodies situated anteriorly to the nucleus. The spherical nucleus (3–4 μm in diameter) is medial and situated near the anterior pole. The cytoplasm contains numerous vacuoles and bacteria. The trophozoite plasma membrane is pliable. Reproduction is by longitudinal binary fission. Unfixed trophozoites measure 6–20 μm × 3–10 μm (length × breadth), whereas fixed specimens measure 10–15 μm × 5–6 μm.

The cysts, which appear in formed stools, are thick walled, characteristically lemon-shaped, broadly round at one end, and bluntly conical at the other, and measure 7–10 μm in length and 4.5–6 μm in breadth. The cyst wall is thickened at the conical end and the dense cytoplasm is often separated from this narrower end of the cyst. Occasionally, two nuclei will be present in the cyst.

Trophozoites are seen only in liquid stools, trophozoites and cysts are seen in semi-solid stools, and only cysts are seen in formed stools. Encystation may occur in unformed stools or during centrifugation.

Iodine neither demonstrates nuclear detail nor cytostomal fibrils, however, its inclusion into the cyst highlights the characteristic shape making identification straightforward.

4. Testing of water for intestinal protozoa

Protozoan cysts and oocysts occur in low numbers in the aquatic environment, and therefore large volumes (between 100–1000 litres) of water need to be analysed. Confirmation of organism identity, however, can still only be made on the basis of morphology and recognition of at least two internal features. Some cysts and oocysts may not be viable, and as only viable cysts and oocysts can cause infection, it is important to be able to distinguish between them. There is no standard method for assessing the viability of individual cysts and oocysts, however, the method outlined for *Giardia* cysts, and based on the inclusion or exclusion of fluorogenic dyes, has been used successfully in the author's laboratory for the last three years. Its advantage is that it can be used in conjunction with the identification method, therefore, both the identification and viability of individual cysts can be determined simultaneously.

The following method (*Protocols 10* and *11*) can be used to detect the presence of both *Giardia* spp. cysts and *Cryptosporidium* spp. oocysts in water-related samples.

The current procedure is documented in a HMSO booklet (29) and can be divided into three sections, namely:

- sampling
- elution, clarification, and concentration
- identification

Protocol 10. The filtration of water for *Giardia* spp. cysts and *Cryptosporidium* spp. oocysts

Equipment

- Cartridge filter (AMF Cuno Microwynd 11 DPPPY, polypropylene filters, 1 μm nominal pore size)
- Filter holder (AMF Cuno 1N1); polyethylene tubing and clips to attach on the inlet and outlet of the filter holder housing[a]
- Water meter and flow valve (*Figure 5*)
- Submersible pump and petrol generator
- Polythene bags and seals (to contain individual filters)
- Labels
- Indelible pen
- Cool-box for carrying used cartridges

Method

1. Ensure filtration equipment is clean.
2. Connect the equipment correctly ensuring that a seal is formed between the outlet pipe within the filter holder cap and the plastic filter core. Screw the holder tightly on to the body assembly. Place the water meter downstream of the filter (*Figure 5*). Record the meter reading.
3. Dependent on the water sample to be taken (e.g. raw or treated) connect the inlet pipe to the submersible pump (for raw water) or to a sampling tap (for treated water).
4. Commence sampling. Adjust the flow rate with the flow valve to the desired level (about 1.5 litre/min) and collect a volume of 100–500 litres.
5. Disconnect the filter assembly, remove the filter, and place it in a clean, thick-gauge polythene bag. Seal the bag and mark it with the location, type of water, and date. Store it in a cool box until returned to the laboratory. If the filters cannot be processed on return to the laboratory, store them either in a refrigerator or in a cool-box. Process the filter(s) the next working day.
6. Where multiple sampling with the same filter assembly is necessary, wash the complete assembly, excluding the new filter, thoroughly with water from the new sampling point and then place the new filter in the assembly. Ensure that the assembly is watertight. Continue from step **2**.

[a] Use separate filtration assemblies for raw and treated water.

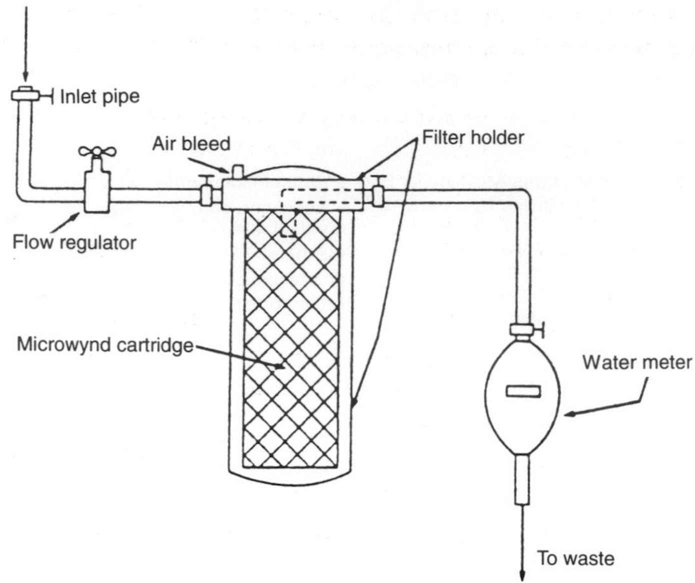

Figure 5. Layout of apparatus for *Protocol 10*.

Protocol 11. Elution, clarification, and concentration of a filter

Equipment and reagents

- Large forceps
- Polyethylene beakers (5 litre capacity)
- Centrifuge bottles (4 × 750 ml), graduated polyethylene screw-capped centrifuge tubes (250 ml capacity [Cat. No. 25330–50, Corning]) (centrifuge tubes should not be reused for sequential analyses)
- 'Stanley' knife and blades
- Stainless steel tray to accommodate a cartridge filter
- Gloves (both disposable and protective)
- Polythene bags (to contain shredded filter)
- Scissors
- Vortex mixer
- Wash bottle
- Vacuum pump (e.g. Buchner pump)
- 10 ml and 50 ml syringes
- Stainless steel cannulae (15 gauge, 10 cm long)
- Microcentrifuge (capable of 10 000 *g*)
- Centrifuge(s) with swing-out buckets for 1 litre, 250 ml, and 50 ml tubes capable of speeds of 1500 *g* for 10 min.
- Stomacher or hand agitate
- Tween-80 (polyoxyethylene sorbitan monooleate) solutions: 0.1% and 2% (v/v) in distilled water
- 'Antifoam'
- Sucrose solution (1.18 S.G.): dissolve 256 g sucrose (Analar) in 300 ml of distilled water, and make up to 500 ml; check the specific gravity at 4 °C with a hydrometer and adjust if necessary (store in a screw-capped bottle at 4 °C)

Method

1. Wearing protective gloves, cut the filter lengthways with a Stanley knife on a stainless steel tray.

2. Separate the cut filter from its plastic core and divide it into three equal sections. Tease the sections apart with forceps on the stainless steel tray.
3. Place the teased inner section into a 5 litre beaker and add 750 ml of 0.1% Tween-80. Hand agitate for 5 min (wear protective gloves), or place in stomacher for 5 min, and agitate for 5 min.
4. Drain the washings into a clean 5 litre beaker and add a further 750 ml of 0.1% Tween-80 to the teased inner section. Wash for 5 min.
5. Remove the inner section from the beaker with forceps, and place it into a polythene bag. Seal the polythene bag and cut the bottom corner of the bag with scissors. Express the fluid through the cut hole into the washings beaker. Discard the wrung inner section of the filter, but retain the polythene bag.
6. Place the teased middle section of the filter into the 750 ml washings contained in the washing beaker. Wash for 5 min.
7. Drain the washings into the same 5 litre beaker used for step **4**, and repeat remainder of step **4**.
8. Remove the middle section (as for the inner section) and repeat step **5**.
9. Place the teased outer section into the 750 ml washings left from step **8**. Repeat as for steps **6–8**.
10. If the outer section still appears dirty, repeat the washing procedure with a further 750 ml of 0.1% Tween-80. Squeeze the residual fluid from the filter as in step **5**. Collect and pool the washings into the same beaker used at step **10**.
11. The total volume of the washings should be approximately 3–4 litres. Pour an equal volume of the washings into each of four 1 litre centrifuge buckets and centrifuge at 1500 *g* for 10 min. Discard the supernatants without disrupting the pellets, resuspend the pellets, and pool them in a final volume of about 200 ml. Pour the suspension into a 250 ml conical centrifuge tube.
12. Centrifuge at 1500 *g* for 10 min.
13. Carefully aspirate the supernatant with a Buchner pump, by sucking at the meniscus only, leaving behind about 3 cm of fluid above the pellet.
14. Cap the tube and resuspend the pellet on a vortex mixer. Transfer the suspension to a 50 ml centrifuge tube, and centrifuge at 1500 *g* for 10 min. Repeat step **13** and reduce the sample volume to 20 ml. Resuspend the pellet by vortexing.
15. Split the sample into two 10 ml aliquots and store one 10 ml sample in a sterile Universal container at 4°C for submission to an independent expert, or collaborating laboratory for cross-checking.

Protocol 11. *Continued*

16. To the other 10 ml sample in the 50 ml centrifuge tube, add 10 ml of 2% Tween-80 and vortex for 30 sec. Frothing can be reduced by the addition of one or two drops of an anti-frothing agent (e.g. antifoam). Centrifuge at 1500 *g* for 10 min.

17. Carefully aspirate the supernatant with a Buchner pump by sucking at the meniscus only to leave 10 ml of fluid in the centrifuge tube. Vortex to resuspend the pellet.

18. Suck up 10 ml of cold sucrose solution (1.18 S.G.) into a 10 ml syringe through the cannula. Carefully, underlay the suspension with the sucrose solution by inserting the tip of the cannula into the bottom of the centrifuge tube. Squeeze the syringe plunger slowly to expel the sucrose solution.[a]

19. Centrifuge at 1000 *g* for 5 min.

20. Insert the cannula into the supernatant and recover all the fluid including the interface into a 50 ml syringe. Do not disturb the pellet. About 15 ml of fluid should be recoverable.

21. Expel the fluid from the syringe into a clean 50 ml centrifuge tube, and centrifuge at 1500 *g* for 10 min.

22. Aspirate the supernatant carefully by sucking at the meniscus only and resuspending the pellet by vortexing.

23. Add sufficient distilled water to fill the centrifuge tube and centrifuge at 1500 *g* for 10 min.

24. Repeat steps **22** and **23** to remove traces of sucrose.

25. Reduce the fluid to the desired volume by aspirating without disturbing the pellet. Note this volume.[b] (This is important.) Resuspend the pellet and retain it for the identification procedure. For final waters the fluid volume can be reduced to 1 ml as described below.

26. Reduce the volume of the suspension by further centrifuging in the same tube (1500 *g* for 10 min).

27. Transfer the suspension into two 1.5 ml polyethylene microcentrifuge tubes placing equal volumes in each tube. Wash the 50 ml centrifuge tube with 500 μl of distilled water. Transfer this to the microcentrifuge tubes. Cap the tubes.

28. Centrifuge at 10 000 *g* for 1 min in a microcentrifuge. Aspirate 50% of the fluid from each tube, resuspend the pellets, and pool them into one tube.

29. Centrifuge at 10 000 *g* for 1 min and aspirate down to the 1 ml mark. Resuspend the pellet and retain it for the identification procedure.

[a] The sediment will float on the sucrose layer. Do not inject air in with the sucrose solution as this disrupts the interface.

[b] This volume is dependent upon the amount of sediment present in the sample.

There are two methods available for the identification of cysts and oocysts which differ only in the solid phase on to which cysts or oocysts are attached. In one method they are stained on a 13 mm membrane in an enclosed system, whereas in the method outlined below, they are stained on microscope slides (*Protocol 12*). In both methods identification is by fluorescence microscopy (*Protocol 13*).

It is important to test a representative aliquot of the concentrated suspension. For final waters, at least 10%–20% of the concentrated sample should be tested for the presence of cysts and/or oocysts. Always include known positive and negative controls in each analysis.

The positive control consists of a suspension of cleaned cysts or oocysts air dried on the multispot slides. The negative control consists of the fluid used to suspend the cysts or oocysts (distilled water), or a known negative water concentrate, air dried on to multispot slides. Both positive and negative control can be slides stored at −20 °C in polythene bags containing silica gel until used.

The working strength of the Mabs and second antibody (if used) should be assessed initially and thence periodically, dependent upon the frequency of use, by diluting the antibody in PBS and preparing a series of twofold dilutions, and testing each sample in this series of dilutions against an individual well of the positive slide. The dilution which highlights 50% of cysts or oocysts by fluorescence is the end-point of the antibody and the working dilution is one or two dilutions below the end-point.

Protocol 12. Immunofluorescence staining of *Giardia* spp. cysts and *Cryptosporidium* spp. oocysts

Equipment and reagents

- Multispot microscope slides, 4 × 10 mm diameter multispot slides (Henley)
- Coverslips (22 × 64 mm)
- Humidified chamber
- Single channel adjustable automatic pipette (5–50 µl) and disposable tips
- Coplin jars or similar
- Fan heater
- 37 °C incubator
- Epifluorescence and brightfield microscope fitted with differential interference contrast (DIC) optics and FITC filters and × 20 (or × 25), × 40, × 100 (oil) objective lenses, eyepiece graticule, and calibration slide
- Phosphate-buffered saline (PBS) 150 mM pH 7.2
- *Giardia* and/or *Cryptosporidium* spp. specific monoclonal antibody kits together with diluent and glycerol-based mountant, Meridan diagnostics and Cellabs Diagnostics Pty Ltd. (Giardia only)
- Fluorescence mounting medium: 50% glycerol, 50% PBS (if not provided with the kit).

Method

1. Mark each slide with the sample number. Apply aliquots of only one sample per slide.
2. Dispense four 25 µl replicates from *Protocol 11*, step 29, one per spot

Protocol 12. *Continued*

on to each slide with an automatic micropipette.[a] Ensure even coverage of the spot, air dry the samples.

3. Fix the air dried samples by placing the slide horizontally and covering the wells for 5 min with a few drops of absolute methanol.
4. Air dry the slide and apply 25 μl of the Mab at its working dilution on to each spot. Ensure the complete coverage of each well with the Mab. Incubate, in a humidified chamber in the dark at 37 °C for 30 min. Rinse each slide individually with a gentle stream of PBS to remove the residual Mab. Immerse the slide in a Coplin jar or similar containing PBS. Wash in three changes of PBS, with 5 min for each change. Drain off the excess moisture.
5. Remove any residual PBS on the wells of the multispot slides by placing the slide in a warm current of air from a fan heater. Do NOT allow the samples to dry out completely.
6. If the assay is based on direct immunofluorescence apply one drop of mounting medium on to each sample and cover with a coverslip,[b] ensuring that no air bubbles are trapped over the specimen.
7. If the assay is based on indirect immunofluorescence, apply 25 μl of FITC labelled second antibody at its working dilution on to each spot. Ensure the complete coverage of each well with the antibody. Incubate, wash, and mount as in steps **4–6**.

[a] In general adhere to the manufacturer's instructions when applying the Mab.

[b] Do not press down on the coverslip, but allow its weight to displace the mounting medium. Inverting the slide on an absorbent tissue will remove the excess mounting medium.

Protocol 13. Examination and identification of fluorescent stained cysts and oocysts

1. Examine the positive control. *Giardia* cysts appear as apple-green ovoid objects 8–12 μm in length and 7–10 μm in width. *Cryptosporidium* oocysts appear as apple-green circular objects 4–6 μm in diameter. If difficulty arises in measuring fluorescent objects (dark-field), increase the bright-field illumination slowly until the fluorescent intensity is reduced. Relate the fluorescent image to the bright-field image and measure it with the eye-piece graticule. Note the background fluorescence, if any, and autofluorescence (yellow green).
2. Examine the negative control. No apple-green fluorescence should be noted.
3. Examine each well of a multispot slide using the × 20 (or × 25) object-

ive lens. Cover the whole area of the spot with either vertical or horizontal sweeps. Ensure that the whole area is viewed. Note any cysts or oocysts present. For *Giardia* assess the presence of internal organelles in cysts by Differential Interference Contrast (DIC) with the × 40 objective lens.

4. Add up the number of cysts or oocysts present in each of the four replicates. This gives the number present in 100 μl of the measured concentrated suspension (*Protocol 11*, step 25 or 29).
5. If the sample underwent step 29, multiply the sum of the four replicates by ten. This is the number of cysts or oocysts present in the 10 ml concentrated suspension. Multiply this figure by two. This is the number of cysts and oocysts present in the 20 ml concentrate which is equivalent to the volume filtered.

   As the filtration and concentration efficiencies can vary from sample to sample, at present the numbers of cysts or oocysts detected in the concentrated suspension are reported as the same numbers occurring in the original sample.
6. Calculate the number of cysts or oocysts per litre from the following formula, if using step **5**.

$$\frac{N \times 10 \times 2}{V}$$

where N = sum of cyst or oocyst numbers in four replicates
10 = dilution factor effective at *Protocol 11*, step 29
2 = dilution factor effective at *Protocol 11*, step 15
V = volume of water sample filtered

Reaction of the stain results in apple-green fluorescence located on the cyst or oocyst wall, thus defining the size and shape of the object. A limitation of the commercially available anti-*Giardia* Mabs is that they recognize epitopes on *G. duodenalis*-type cysts excreted by humans, cats, dogs, and sheep. At present there is uncertainty as to whether cysts from non-human sources are infective to humans, thus the detection of cysts which may not be infective to man can lead to confusion. Until further information becomes available, all viable cysts recovered from environmental waters should be considered potentially infective to human beings.

Similarly, the commercially available anti-*Cryptosporidium* Mabs also have their limitations, as neither is specific for *C. parvum* epitopes. Thus, all oocysts of the correct size and shape must be documented, immaterial of whether they are infective to man.

Autofluorescence, Mab cross-reactivity, or non-specific Mab binding may result in certain organisms/artefacts exhibiting similar fluorescence to *Giardia*

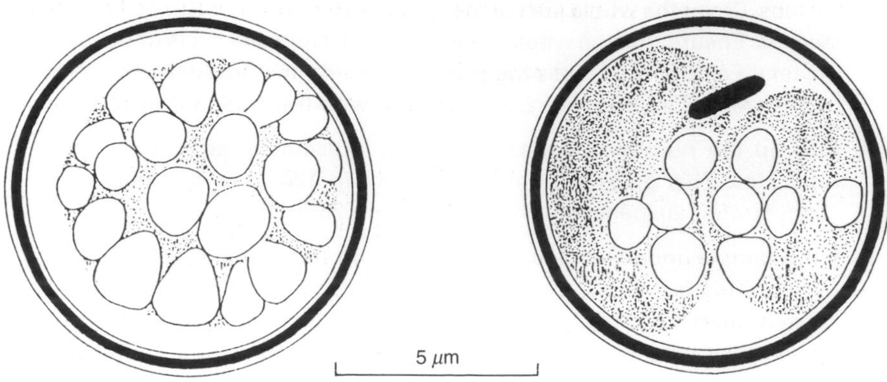

Figure 6. Semi-diagrammatic drawings of coccidian oocysts from human stool, unsporulated and sporulated.

cysts or *Cryptosporidium* oocysts, and when they are of similar size and shape to *Giardia* cysts or *Cryptosporidium* oocysts false positives may result.

For *Giardia*, confirmation of the identity of fluorescent objects can be made following bright-field or DIC microscopy as long as the sample is not too opaque: cysts should be the correct size and shape and at least two internal organelles (e.g. 2–4 nuclei, median body, axonemes) should be discernible, specimens with equivocable results should be referred to an expert.

For *Cryptosporidium*, confirmation of the identity of fluorescent objects is more difficult because of the size of the oocyst. Size and shape are the only criteria which can be used on a regular basis. Surface folds can be seen in up to 60% of samples. Occasionally, when the specimen is sufficiently transparent to observe sporozoites within the putative oocyst, DIC microscopy can be used for confirmation. Difficult specimens should be sent to a reference laboratory.

Unlike cysts or oocysts detected in faeces, cysts or oocysts detected in water-related samples may have been in such an environment for a long time and therefore their morphology and their potential for taking up stains can vary. In such instances, possible cysts or oocysts should be referred to a reference laboratory.

5. Microsporidia

Microsporidia are eukaryotic, obligate intracellular parasites. They are sufficiently unique to be classified into a separate phylum, Microspora (31). Classification is based upon the size, nuclear arrangement (mono or diplokaryotic), mode of division (32, 33), and association of proliferative forms within the host cell (i.e. whether the development of the organism occurs within a parasitophorous vacuole or in direct association with the host cytoplasm).

In excess of 100 genera and nearly 1000 species are currently known, with the majority of species occurring in invertebrates (insects) and lower vertebrates (fish).

The species of Microsporidia infective to mammals are unicellular, Gram-positive organisms, with the mature spore size ranging from 0.5–2 × 1–4 μm in diameter. At present only five genera, namely *Encephalitozoon, Nosema, Pleistophora*, *Septata*, and *Enterocytozoon* have been recognized in humans, with only the genus *Enterocytozoon* being unique to man (34).

The sources of human infection are not clearly defined. Postulated routes of transmission include, person to person contact, spread to humans from animals, birds, lower vertebrates, or invertebrates. In some animals (foxes, dogs, squirrel, monkeys) transplacental transmission of *E. cuniculi* takes place, whereas in other (mice, rabbits) the most important source of infection is via contaminated urine.

The first reported human infection caused by Microsporidia occurred in a nine-year-old Japanese boy (35). This individual suffered from a severe neurological illness, with convulsions, vomiting, headaches, fever, and periods of unconsciousness. Light microscopy of urine and cerebrospinal fluid of this child resulted in identification of oval bodies, which were suspected to be *Encephlitozoon* sp. The second reported case of human microsporidial infection was in a two-year-old child in Colombia (36). Again, the child was afflicted with similar symptoms to those described above. Spores of Microsporidia were recognized in urine samples from this child on two occasions.

More recently, with the increasing occurrence of the human immunodeficiency virus (HIV), organisms which had previously been regarded as opportunistic, have become important medically. Diarrhoea is commonly observed in HIV sufferers, leading to weight loss and cachexia. Despite the evidence for the human immunodeficiency virus itself being capable of colonizing the intestinal tract, thus inducing diarrhoea, in 50% of the patients, the cause remains unidentified.

In a study (37), HIV sufferers with unexplained diarrhoea were examined for prevalence and clinical and biological features of intestinal Microsporidia. Spores were detected in 9 of 18 patients by examination of stools, with Microsporidia being the sole pathogen in eight individuals. Furthermore, Microsporidia (*E. bieunsi*) were found in all of these patients following duodenal and jejunal biopsies.

5.1 Examination of faeces for Microsporidia

Unformed liquid faeces are fixed by adding three volumes of 10% formalin to one volume of faeces. Formed faeces are diluted in distilled water until liquid, and fixed in 10% formalin. The spores of Microsporidia may be detected in faeces by staining with optical brighteners (*Protocol 14*), Giemsa stain (*Protocol 15*), or Trichrome stain (*Protocol 16*).

Protocol 14. Detection of Microsporidia spores in faecal smears using calcoflour white M2R

Equipment and reagents

- Microscope slides (76 × 26 mm)
- Coverslips (22 × 64 mm)
- Adjustable automatic pipette (5–25 μl) and disposable tips
- Coplin jars or similar
- Absolute methanol
- Fluorescence microscope equipped with a UV filter block (excitation 350 nm, emission 450 nm) and × 40 and × 100 objective lenses
- Diamond marker
- 0.5% aqueous calcofluor white M2R (Sigma Chemical Company)
- 0.5% aqueous Evans blue
- 150 mM phosphate-buffered saline (PBS) pH 7.2
- Glycerol-based mounting medium (e.g. 50% glycerol, 50% 150 mM PBS pH 7.2)[a]

Method

1. Score the reference number of the specimen on a microscope slide with a diamond marker, and use separate microscope slides for each stool specimen. Place two drops (about 20 μl) of the faeces–formalin slurry on to the microscope slide and make a smear with a wooden applicator stick.[b]
2. Fix the slide by immersion in absolute methanol for 1–5 min and air dry.
3. Immerse the slide in 0.5% calcofluor white for 5 min.
4. Rinse the slide in PBS.
5. Dip the slide momentarily into 0.5% aqueous Evans blue and rinse in PBS.
6. Remove the excess moisture from the slide, place two or three drops of mounting medium across the slide, position the coverslip on the slide without forming air bubbles, and a view under the × 40 and × 100 objective lenses of a fluorescence microscope equipped with a UV filter block.
7. Measure the size and shape of the sky blue-fluorescing bodies under the × 100 objective lens. Calcofluor white M2R binds to chitin in the endospore layer of the spore wall causing the spore to fluoresce sky blue. Immature spores, containing little chitin, fluoresce less brightly than mature spores. Calcofluor white M2R is not specific for spores of Microsporidia. Other organisms which contain chitin, e.g. fungal spores, will also fluoresce sky blue. The spores of Microsporidia reported to

infect human beings range from 1.0–1.6 × 0.9 μm to 4.0–4.5 × 2.0–2.5 μm (see Table 1).

[a] A photobleaching inhibitor such as Citifluor, City University, Department of Chemistry, London, UK can be used.
[b] As for the conventional demonstration of other protozoan parasites, the best results are obtained when smears are of an optimal thickness. They should be neither too thick, nor too thin.

Table 1. Dimensions of the spores of Microsporidia infecting humans

Species	Spore size
Encephalitozoon cuniculi	2.5–3.2 × 1.2–1.6 μm
Encephalitozoon hellem	2.0–2.5 × 1.0–1.5 μm
Encephalitozoon sp.	1.7–1.8 × 0.8 μm
Nosema connori	4.0–4.5 × 2.0–2.5 μm
Nosema corneum	3.7 × 1.0 μm
Nosema ocularum	3.0 × 5.0 μm
Microsporidium ceylonensis	3.5 × 1.5 μm
Microsporidum africanum	4.5–5.0 × 2.5–3.0 μm
Enterocytozoon bieneusi	1.0–1.6 × 0.9 μm
Pleistophora sp.	2.8 × 3.2–3.4 μm
Septata intestinales	1.2–1.5 × 2.5–3.0 μm

Protocol 15. Detection of Microsporidia spores in faecal smears using Giemsa stain

Method

1. Score the reference number of the specimen on a microscope slide with a diamond marker, and use separate microscope slides for each stool specimen. Place two drops (about 20 μl) of the faeces–formalin slurry on to the microscope slide and make a smear with a wooden applicator stick.[a]
2. Fix the slide by immersion in absolute methanol for 1–2 min and air dry.
3. Immerse slide in Giemsa stain for 35 min.
4. Rinse slide in distilled water (pH 7.2) to remove excess stain and air dry.
5. Confirm the presence of spores under the × 100 oil immersion objective lens.

Protocol 15. *Continued*

6. Measure the size and shape of the pale blue stained bodies under the × 100 objective lens.[b]

[a] As for the conventional demonstration of other protozoan parasites, the best results are obtained when smears are of an optimal thickness. They should be neither too thick, nor too thin.

[b] Spores and pre-spores stain pale blue with reddish nuclei. The spores of Microsporidia reported to infect human beings range from 1.0–1.6 × 0.9 μm to 4.0–4.5 × 2.0–2.5 μm (see Table 1).

Protocol 16. Detection of Microsporidia spores in faecal smears using Trichrome stain

Equipment and reagents

- Microscope slides (76 × 26 mm)
- Coplin jars or similar
- Absolute methanol
- Bright-field microscope with × 100 oil immersion objective lens
- Diamond marker
- Trichrome stain: Chromotrope 2R (Gurr) 6 g, fast green 0.15 g, phosphotungstic acid 0.7 g; add the reagents to 3 ml glacial acetic acid, mix, and allow to stand for 30 min; add 100 ml distilled water
- Acid alcohol: add 4.5 ml acetic acid to 995.5 ml of 90% ethanol and stir
- 95% ethanol
- 100% ethanol
- Xylene

Method

1. Score the reference number of the specimen on a microscope slide with a diamond marker, and use separate microscope slides for each stool specimen. Place two drops (about 20 μl) of the faeces–formalin slurry on to the microscope slide and make a smear with a wooden applicator stick.[a]
2. Fix the slide by immersion in absolute methanol for 5 min and air dry.
3. Immerse slide in Trichrome stain for 90 min.
4. Rinse in acid alcohol.
5. Rinse in 95% ethanol.
6. Dehydrate in 95% ethanol for 5 min.
7. Measure the size and shape of the pinkish-red stained bodies under the × 100 objective lens.[b]

[a] As for the conventional demonstration of other protozoan parasites, the best results are obtained when smears are of an optimal thickness. They should be neither too thick nor too thin.

[b] Spores stain pinkish-red. The spores of microsporidia reported to infect human beings range from 1.0–1.6 × 0.9 μm to 4.0–4.5 × 2.0–2.5 μm (see Table 1).

5.2 Examination of urine for Microsporidia

Urine should be centrifuged at 1250 *g* for 10 min or at 6500 *g* for 5 min in a microcentrifuge to pellet any spores that might be present. The supernatant is aspirated to waste and the pellet resuspended and washed in distilled water. The suspension is centrifuged (1250 *g* for 10 min or at 6500 *g* for 5 min in a microcentrifuge), the supernatant aspirated to waste, and the pellet resuspended in 150 μl of distilled water. Approximately 10 μl of suspension is smeared on to a microscope slide, and one of *Protocols 14–16* followed, depending on the stain of choice.

6. Cyclospora

Named previously as both cyanobacterium-like body and coccida-like body (CLB) (38) and found in the stools of patients presenting with prolonged water diarrhoea, *Cyclospora* sp. is a recently described coccidian parasite of human beings (39) which infects enterocytes of the small bowel and can produce disease (40). Endogenous stages are intra-cytoplasmic and contained within a vacuole (40), and the transmissive stage, the oocyst, is excreted in the stool. CLBs have been isolated from the stools of children, immunocompetent and immunocompromised adults. CLBs have been described in the stools of residents in, and travellers returning from, developing nations, and in association with diarrhoeal illness in individuals from North, Central and South America, the Caribbean, the Indian sub-continent, Southeast Asia, Australia and Europe.

Symptoms include explosive, watery diarrhoea, fatigue, anorexia, weight loss and nausea. In immunocompetent individuals, the symptoms are self-limiting and oocyst excretion is associated with clinical illness (41), whereas in immunocompromised individuals, diarrhoea may be prolonged. The sources of human infection are not clearly defined. Postulated routes of transmission include person to person contact and waterborne transmission (42).

Identification of the parasite is based upon the appearance of the oocyst either in direct or concentrated wet films. Concentration either by the formalin-ether method (*Protocol 2*) or sucrose flotation (*Protocol 3*) is effective. In two cases, oocysts have also been reported from jejunal aspirates (40). The oocyst wall auto-fluoresces under UV illumination. Organisms do not stain with Lugol's iodine. Staining of air dried smears with acid fast stains can aid identification, and according to Wurtz (42), the rapid dimethyl sulphoxide-modified acid fast staining method reported by Brondson (43) is more effective than either the Kinyouin or the modified Ziehl–Neelsen method.

6.1 Diagnostic features of *Cyclospora* sp. oocysts

In wet mounts, oocyst walls appear as well-defined non-refractile spheres measuring 8–10 μm in diameter, and within an oocyst is a central morula-like structure containing a variable number of inclusions (*Figure 6*). At higher (× 400) magnification, the inclusions appear refractile, exhibiting a greenish tinge. Oocysts are remarkably uniform in size (39). Occasionally, oocysts which either have collapsed into crescents or are empty are encountered. Under UV illumination (330–380 nm) the oocyst wall is fluorescent causing the organisms to appear as blue circles. Oocysts stain variably with acid fast stains ranging from deep red to unstained. Organisms seen in stool samples are normally the unsporulated oocysts of *Cyclospora* sp., and excreted oocysts sporulate in the environment.

Organisms of the genus *Cyclospora* have an oocyst with two sporocysts, each of which contain two sporozoites. A proportion (10–20%) of purified oocysts incubated in 2.5% potassium dichromate at 25 °C and 32 °C, for up to two weeks will sporulate completely to produce two sporocysts, each containing two crescentic sporozoites. In instances where excystation *in vitro* have been successful, exposure of oocyst/sporocysts to an excystation medium at 37 °C for up to 4 min, causes the emergence of two crescentic sporozoites from each sporocyst (44, personal communication Y. Ortega, C. R. Sterling & M. M. Marshall).

The number of species of *Cyclospora* infective to human beings is unknown. Ortega *et al.* (44) have proposed that CLB should be designated *Cyclospora cayetanensis* on the basis of the development of the oocyst *in vitro*. However, Bendall *et al.* (40) prefer the use of the term CLB (denoting cyclospora-like body) until further information is forthcoming regarding the biology of this coccidian parasite.

6.2 Treatment

Clinical disease can resolve without treatment (45). Co-trimoxazole has been used successfully to treat the symptoms of diarrhoea in a small group of patients, reducing the mean duration of oocyst excretion as compared to untreated controls (46).

Acknowledgements

I am grateful to Drs R. W. A. Girdwood and M. J. Colloff, SPDL, and Department of Zoology, University of Glasgow, and to Professor K. Vickerman, FRS, Department of Zoology, University of Glasgow for stimulating and productive discussions. Thanks are due to Dr J Vara for permission to quote the calcofluor white M2R method cited in the training manual ‘Diagnosis of Microsporidia’. I am grateful to Professor E. U. Canning, Department of Zoology, Imperial College at Silwood Park, Berks, SL5 7PY for allowing me to use data from the training manual entitled ‘Diagnosis of Microsporidia’.

References

1. Allen, A. V. H. and Ridley, D. S. (1970). *J. Clin. Pathol.*, **23**, 545.
2. Craun, G. F. (1988). *J. Am. Water Works Assoc.*, **80**, 40.
3. Rendtorff, R. C. (1979). In *Waterborne transmission of Giardiasis* (ed. W. Jakubowski and J. C. Hoff), pp. 64–81. U.S. Environmental Protection Agency. Office of Research and Development, Environmental Research Centre, Cincinnati, Ohio 45268, USA, EPA-600/9–79–001.
4. Wolfe, M. S. (1979). *Pediatr. Clin. North Am.*, **26(2)**, 295.
5. Wolfe, M. S. (1984). In *Giardia and Giardiasis. Biology, pathogenensis, and epidemiology* (ed. S. L. Erlandsen and E. A. Meyer), pp. 147–61. Plenum Press, New York and London.
6. Lopez, C. E., Dykes, A. C., Juranck, D. D., Sinclair, S. P., Cann, J. M., Christie, R. W., *et al.* (1980). *Am. J. Epidemiol.*, **112**, 495.
7. Danciger, M. and Lopez, M. (1975). *Am. J. Trop. Med. Hyg.*, **24**, 237.
8. Faubert, G. M., Bemrick, W. J. and Erlandsen, S. L. (1988). *Parasitology Today*, **4**, 66.
9. Saveitz, W. G. and Faust, E. C. (1942). *Am. J. Trop. Med.*, **22**, 130.
10. Lin Shun Dar. (1985). *J. Am. Water Works Assoc.*, **77**, 40.
11. Green, E. L., Miles, M. A., and Warhurst, D. C. (1985). *Lancet*, **(ii)**, 691.
12. Rosoff, J. D., Sanders, C. A., Sonnad, S. S., De Lay, P. R., Hadley, W. K., Vincenzi, F. F., *et al.* (1989). *J. Clin. Microbiol.*, **27**, 1997.
13. Butcher, P. D. and Farthing, M. J. G. (1989). *Biochem. Soc. Trans.*, **17**, 363.
14. Lewis, D. J. M., Green, E. L., and Ashall, F. (1990). *Lancet*, **336**, 257.
15. Mahbubani, M. H., Bej, A. K., Perlin, M. M., Schaefer, F. W., Jakubowski, W., and Atlas, R. M. (1992). *J. Clin. Microbiol.*, **30**, 74.
16. Keister, D. B. (1983). *Trans. R. Soc. Trop. Med. Hyg.*, **77**, 487.
17. Gillin, F. D. (1984). In *Giardia and Giardiasis. Biology, pathogenensis, and epidemiology* (ed. S. L. Erlandsen and E. A. Meyer), pp. 11–30. Plenum Press, New York and London.
18. Current, W. L. (1988). *Am. Soc. Microbiol. News*, **54**, 605.
19. Current, W. L. (1989). In *Cryptosporidiosis. Proceedings of the first international workshop* (ed. K. W. Angus and D. A. Blewett), pp. 1–17. The Animal Diseases Research Association, 408 Gilmerton Rd, Edinburgh EH17 7JJ, UK.
20. Blewett, D. A. (1989). In *Cryptosporidiosis. Proceedings of the first international workshop* (ed. K. W. Angus and D. A. Blewett), pp. 85–105. The Animal Diseases Research Association, 408 Gilmerton Rd, Edinburgh EH17 7JJ, UK.
21. Casemore, D. P. (1990). *Epidemiol. Inf.*, **101**, 1.
22. Miller, R. A., Brondson, M. A., and Morton, W. R. (1990). *J. Infect. Dis.*, **161**, 312.
23. Dupont, H. L., Chappell, C. L., Sterling, C. R., Okhuysen, P. C., Rose, J. B., and Jakubowski, W. (1994). Infectivity of *Cryptosporidium parvum*. Presented at the Clinical Research Meeting of the American Association of Physicians, Baltimore, Maryland, 1994.
24. Fayer, R. and Ungar, B. L. P. (1986). *Microbiol. Rev.*, **50**, 458.
25. Jokipii, L. and Jokipii, A. M. M. (1986). *N. Engl. J. Med.*, **315**, 1643.
26. Soave, R. and Armstrong, D. (1986). *Rev. Infect. Dis.*, **8(6)**, 1012.
27. Soave, R. and Johnson, W. D. (1988). *J. Infect Dis.*, **157**, 225.

28. de Hovits, J. A., Pape, J. W., Boncy, M., and Johnson, W. D. (1986). *N. Engl. J. Med.*, **315**, 87.
29. Anon. (1990). Isolation and identification of *Giardia* cysts, *Cryptosporidium* oocysts, and free living pathogenic amoebae in water etc., 1989, HMSO, London.
30. Sprague, V. (1977). In *Comparative pathobiology* (ed. L. A. Bulla, and T. C. Cheng), vol. 2. Plenum Publishing, New York.
31. Curgy, J. J., Vavra, J., and Vivares C. (1980). *Biol. Cell*, **38**, 49.
32. Canning, E. U. and Hollister, W. S. (1987). *Parasitol. Today*, **3**, 267.
33. Canning, E. U and Lom, J. (1986). *The microsporidia of vertebrates*. Academic Press, New York.
34. Matsubayashi, H., Koike, T., Mikata, T., and Hagiwara, S. (1959). *Arch. Pathol.*, **67**, 181.
35. Bergquist, N. R., Stintzing, G., Smedman, L., Waller, T., and Anderson T. (1984). *Br. Med. J.*, **288**, 902.
36. Molina, J. M., Sarfati, C., Beauvais, B., Lemann, M., Lesourd, A., Ferchal, F. *et al.* (1993). *J. Infect. Dis.*, **167**, 217.
37. Weber, R., Bryan, R. T., Owen, R. L., Wilcox, C. M., Gorelkin, L., and Visvesvara, G. S. (1992). *N. Engl. J. Med.*, **326**, 161.
38. Long, E. G., Ebrahimzadch, A., White, E. H., Swisher, B., and Calloway, C. S. (1990). *J. Clin. Microbiol.*, **28**, 1101.
39. Ashford, R. W. (1979). *Annal. Trop. Med. Parasitol.*, **73**, 497.
40. Bendall, R. P., Lucas, S., Moody, A., Tovey, G., and Chiodini, P. L. (1993). *Lancet*, **341**, 590.
41. Shlim, D. R., Cohen, M. T., Eaton, M., Rajah, R., Long, E. G., and Ungar, B. L. P. (1991). *Amer. J. Trop. Med. Hyg.*, **45**, 383.
42. Wurtz, R. M. (1994). *Clin. Infect. Dis.*, **18**, 620.
43. Brondson, M. A. (1984). *J. Clin. Microbiol.*, **19**, 953.
44. Ortega, Y. R., Sterling, C. R., Gilman, R. H., Cama, V. A. and Diaz, R. (1993). *N. Engl. J. Med.*, **328**, 1308.
45. Berlin, P. G. W., Novak, S. M., Porschen, R. K., Long., E. G., Stelma, G. N. and Schaeffer, F. W. III. (1994). *Clin. Infect. Dis.*, **18**, 606.
46. Madico, G., Gilma, R. H., Miranda, E., Cabrera, L., and Sterling, C. R. (1993). *Lancet*, **342**, 122.

6

Diagnosis of amoebic infection

D. C. WARHURST

1. Introduction

During the life cycle of the intestinal amoebae of man, the trophozoite or feeding stage multiplies by simple binary fission in the large intestine. It subsequently rounds up and develops a wall, to give the resistant infective form or cyst which withstands the conditions outside the body when it is excreted with the faeces. Nuclear division may or may not take place within the cyst. The infection is acquired by direct ingestion of faeces, or by ingestion of faecally contaminated food or water. When the cysts pass through the stomach acid they are unharmed and, after exposure to the secretions of the small intestine and bile, hatch in the large intestine to give rise to multiplying generations of trophozoites.

1.1 Examination of faecal material

Faecal material is the most important specimen for the detection and identification of intestinal amoebae. It should be examined as fresh as possible, and this particularly applies to unformed liquid faeces, where the active trophozoites may be detected on direct microscopical examination if the material is still warm.

It is possible to cultivate trophozoites from fresh material and to hatch and cultivate trophozoite cysts in stools which are several days or more old. For detection of the cysts in formed faeces, concentration techniques are recommended as being much more sensitive than direct examination (Chapter 5, *Protocol 2*). The preparation of smears of faeces, followed by fixation (*Protocols 1* and *2*) and staining with trichrome (*Protocol 3*) or iron haematoxylin is also used to enable the detection and identification of faecal protozoal infections.

2. Identification of amoebae of the human gut

Seven species of amoebae inhabit the human digestive tract but only one, *E. histolytica*, is recognized as a pathogen. It is vital to be able to distinguish the pathogenic species from the non-pathogens. The identification of these species rests largely on morphology under the light microscope, reaction to stains, and measurement of the cyst forms.

2.1 *Entamoeba*

Intestinal infection with *Entamoeba histolytica* is an important cause of diarrhoea world-wide, especially where sanitary conditions are poor. Infection mainly affects the colon resulting in a dysenteric syndrome. It differs clinically from bacterial dysentery in that the onset is less acute, developing over several days. The patient may experience 6–12 stools per day which are faecal and may be blood stained. Abdominal cramps are less severe than in bacterial dysentery. Clinical symptoms increase in the first few days and will persist for one to two weeks if untreated, and diminish in severity over the next four weeks. Episodic relapses may continue to develop over a number of years and most patients eliminate the infection even in the absence of treatment.

The commonest and clinically most threatening complication is amoebic liver abscess. Infection is carried to the liver via the portal vein and is more likely to develop in the right lobe. The abscess expands and will, if untreated, rupture through the skin or more rarely through the diaphragm into the chest. Patients complain of right upper quadrant pain and there is local tenderness. An enlarged tender liver can sometimes be palpated. Swelling and redness of the skin indicate an abscess which may soon rupture resulting in a cutaneous infection. Amoebic liver abscess (ALA) usually does not present in the acute phase of intestinal infection but arises months or years after initial exposure. There is often no history of amoebic dysentery.

Other complications of amoebic infection are less common. An amoebic ulcer can erode into a colonic vessel giving rise to a catastrophic haemorrhage. Ulcers placed in the rectum can give rise to intense tenesmus. Metastatic abscesses can be located in any organ of the body including the lungs, brain, or peritoneal cavity. Cutaneous infection is difficult to treat and a destructive variant of this infection, penile amoebiasis, has been found in male homosexuals.

2.2 Diagnosis

The diagnosis of amoebic dysentery is made by finding stages of *E. histolytica* in stools. In patients with acute diarrhoea and fluid stools it is valuable to look for the presence of motile trophozoites. Specimens of rectal ulcer scrapings may also be collected at sigmoidoscopy, the diagnosis is made by finding trophozoites. The trophozoites of *E. histolytica* can be differentiated from non-pathogenic species by the presence of ingested red cells (*Plate 6a*). In patients with formed stools motile trophozoites are rarely seen and the cyst form should be sought. Serology has little role to play in the diagnosis of intestinal amoebiasis as fewer than 50% of patients with intestinal amoebiasis develop an antibody response.

The recent description of an ELISA test for the detection of galactose-inhibitable adherence protein of *E. histolytica* (necessary for amoebic adherence) in serum and faeces may prove to be of use (1), since it detects invasive *E. histolytica*.

Faecal microscopy is not always helpful in the diagnosis of amoebic liver abscess as the majority of patients will not have amoebic cysts in their stools. In countries where amoebiasis is endemic carriage rates may be high and the significance of cysts can not be inferred with certainty. The diagnosis of amoebic liver abscess depends on three types of evidence: non-specific, imaging, and serology.

Patients with amoebic liver abscess are febrile and have a leucocytosis, predominantly a neutrophilia. The diagnosis of amoebic liver abscess has been transformed by the availability of effective imaging techniques for the liver: ultrasound and CT scanning. These techniques are highly sensitive and have good specificity. Unfortunately, CT and ultrasound scanning are often not available where this disease is most common. Up to 95% of patients with amoebic abscess will have positive serology and rapid diagnosis can be achieved using the cellulose acetate precipitin test (see *Protocol 7*). This test is positive early in the course of the infection and becomes negative approximately three months after treatment. Antibodies may also be detected using the indirect fluorescent antibody test. This test is positive in up to 50% of patients with intestinal amoebiasis and in almost all patients with ALA. Antibody concentrations remain elevated for an extended period.

Four of the species of amoebae found in the human alimentary tract belong to the genus *Entamoeba* and have a characteristic nuclear structure when stained with iodine- or haematoxylin. Material ('chromatin') lining the nuclear membrane and a small central staining dot can be seen.

2.2.1 *Entamoeba* spp.

E. gingivalis is the only member of the genus which lives in the buccal cavity, around the roots of the teeth, and has no cyst form, being transmitted by mouth to mouth contact. It may be detected by direct examination of material from between the teeth, or by culture, a more sensitive method. The other three species live in the large intestine and only *E. histolytica* has the capacity to cause ulceration, dysentery, and colitis. The spherical cysts of these species are distinctive, that of *E. coli* having the largest average diameter, 18 μm, ranging from 15–30 μm (*Figure 1*). During maturation of the cyst in the intestine, nuclear division takes place three times, to give a maximum of eight daughter nuclei. The cyst of *E. histolytica* has a mean diameter of 12 μm (10–15 μm) and nuclear division takes place twice only, giving four nuclei in the mature form. *E. hartmanni* is morphologically similar to *E. histolytica* but the cyst rarely reaches 10 μm in diameter, averaging 6–7 μm. Inclusions in

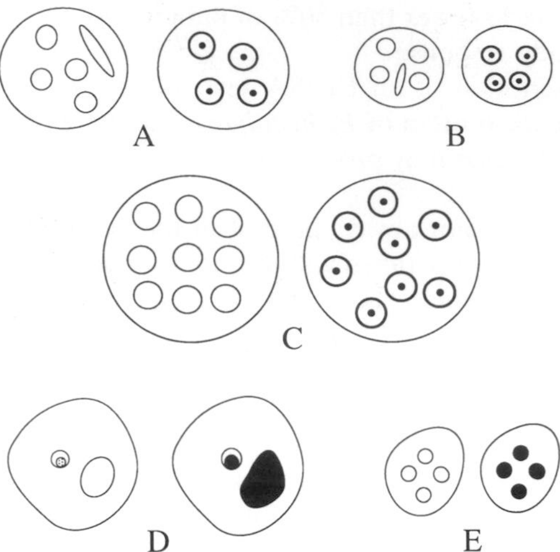

Figure 1. Identification of amoebic cysts in faeces (the right-hand drawing shows the appearance using iodine containing stains). A, *Entamoeba histolytica* (10–14 μm); B, *Entamoeba hartmanni* (7–9 μm); C, *Entamoeba coli* (15–30 μm); D, *Iodamoeba butschlii* (9–15 μm); E, *Endolimax nana* (7–9 μm).

addition to nuclei in the cysts are of value in diagnosis. In all the immature cysts of *Entamoeba* spp., some storage carbohydrate in the form of glycogen is present. This is very marked in *E. coli* and gives a reddish-brown tinge to a large area of the cyst when stained with iodine. Less obvious glycogen is seen in the cysts of *E. histolytica* and *E. hartmanni*. As the nuclear divisions progress, the amount of glycogen present lessens. It is often possible to see in the unstained *E. histolytica* or *E. hartmanni* cyst, blunt-ended refractile inclusion bodies termed 'chromidial bars' or 'chromatoids' which are composed of ribonucleoprotein (in fact, ribosomes in a crystalline form). These stain with thionine-based stains such as Burrow's or Sargeaunt's stain, but tend to be obscured by iodine staining. They are clearly seen, stained reddish or black, in fixed material stained with trichrome or iron haematoxylin.

The trophozoites or actively feeding and dividing forms are, in *E. histolytica*, characterized by their ability to ingest and digest erythrocytes (*Figure 2*). Whilst still warm, they tend to move actively in a directional manner, by means of a lobose pseudopodium, but as conditions in the specimen deteriorate they will round up and push out occasional 'explosively extruded' pseudopodia, without necessarily covering any distance. *E. histolytica* trophozoites from asymptomatic amoebiasis are not, in my experience, generally found to contain ingested erythrocytes. *E. dispar* is a recently described species which is morphologically identical to *E. histolytica*. It can be differentiated on the basis of zymodeme pattern, monoclonal antibody and lectin binding (2).

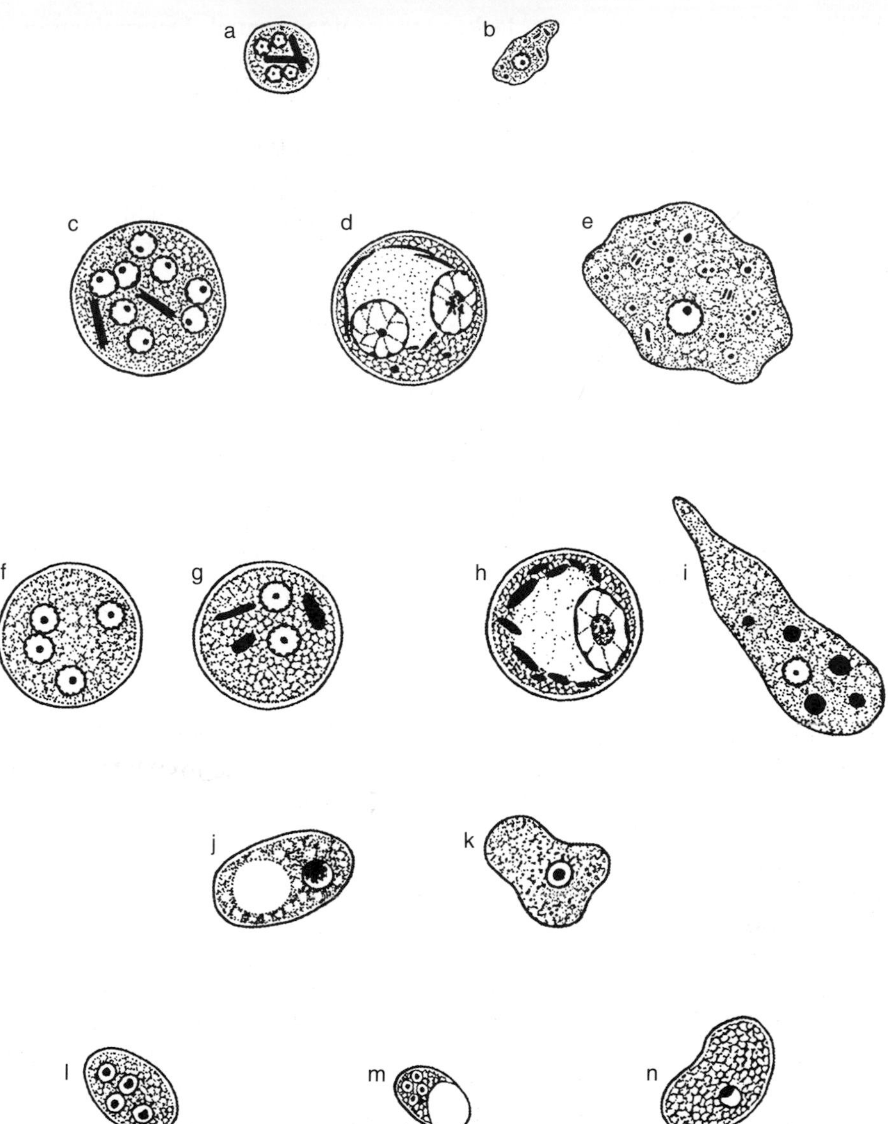

Figure 2. Trophozoites and cysts of amoebae. *E. hartmanni* (a) cyst, (b) trophozoite; *E. coli* (c) cyst, (d) early cyst, (e) trophozoite; *E. histolytica* (f) and (g) cyst, (h) early cyst, (i) trophozoite; *Iodamoeba butschlii* (j) cyst, (k) trophozoite; *Endolimax nana* (l) and (m) cysts, (n) trophozoite (stained with trichrome or iron-haematoxylin).

Unlike *E. histolytica, E. dispar* lacks pathogenic potential. Determination of the species cannot be achieved by methods available to routine laboratories.

2.2.2 *Endolimax, Iodamoeba,* and *Dientamoeba*

The nuclei of these three remaining species have little staining material on the nuclear membrane but possess a large staining karyosome which takes up 1/2–2/3 or more of the space inside the nucleus. These belong to three different genera and species:

(a) *Iodamoeba bütschlii* is the largest of these amoebae and the cysts are often similar to those of *E. histolytica* in size, though usually irregularly oval in shape and having only a single large nucleus. There is a marked, dense, and well-defined glycogen vacuole, staining strongly with iodine. This, as with other glycogen vacuoles, disappears in permanent preparations stained with haematoxylin or trichrome (*Figure 1*).

(b) *Dientamoeba fragilis* has no cyst stage, and the trophozoite, when seen in fresh preparations, moves rapidly on a broad front, and, on staining can often be seen to have two nuclei. This organism is not detected by the concentration procedures.

(c) *Endolimax nana* is the smallest of the intestinal amoebae. Its cysts are oval or spherical and average 6 μm in diameter. The mature cyst has four nuclei and a characteristic larger karyosome. The cyst of *E. nana* tends to stain in iodine with a greenish rather than a yellow to brown tinge as in the case of the other cysts (*Figure 1* and *2*).

Protocol 1. PVA fixative technique

Reagents

- Mercuric chloride
- 95% alcohol
- Distilled water
- Polyvinyl alcohol, must be *c.*40 000 M_r (Fluka)
- Glacial acetic acid
- Glycerol

Method

1. Dissolve 7 g mercuric chloride in 100 ml distilled water at 75 °C, cool.
2. Add 33 ml 95% alcohol to 66 ml of the $HgCl_2$ solution, then take 93.5 ml of the $HgCl_2$/alcohol mixture and add:
   - 5 ml glacial acetic acid
   - 1.5 ml glycerol
   - 5 g polyvinyl alcohol
3. Heat on a water-bath at 75 °C until the powder dissolves.
4. Cool to room temperature. This may be stored stoppered on the bench.

5. Emulsify one part faeces in three parts PVA mixture. Larvae, ova, and trophozoites will be preserved well, cysts may show a variable degree of distortion. When required, smears are made from the mixture on slides and allowed to dry. Before staining they must be treated with 70% alcohol containing iodine. This removes mercury residues which interfere with staining.
6. Stain with iron haematoxylin or trichrome (*Protocol 3*).

Protocol 2. Preparation and use of fixatives and stains

A. *Schaudinn's fixative*

1. Dissolve 110 g mercuric chloride in one litre warm, distilled water and allow to cool, when crystals should form at the bottom of the container.
2. Add 600 ml of saturated $HgCl_2$ solution to 300 ml 90% (v/v) ethanol to prepare the stock solution.
3. Add 5 ml glacial acetic acid to 95 ml stock solution to give fixative.
4. Smear the fresh faeces and allow to dry only at the edge of the smear before placing in the fixative.
5. Leave for 1 h and then transfer to 70% ethanol in which the film can be stored until iodine treatment can be carried out (see above).

B. *Double strength Lugols iodine*

1. Dissolve 1.0 g iodine and 2.0 g potassium iodide in about 10 ml of distilled water by shaking in a stoppered tube, and make up to 50 ml.
2. Add one drop of the iodine solution to one drop of faecal concentrate or to a small volume of fresh faeces.

C. *Bayer's solution*

1. Add 7 g of $CuCl_2$ and 70 ml of glacial acetic acid to one litre of 20% formalin to make a stock solution.
2. The stock solution is diluted 1:10 with distilled water and the faecal sample is emulsified in an equal volume. This method has been found useful for preserving the staining qualities of cysts and avoids shrinkage often seen on storage.

D. *Burrow's stain*

1. Add 20 mg Thionin (Sigma) to 24 ml distilled water, 3 ml ethanol, and 3 ml glacial acetic acid.

Protocol 2. *Continued*

2. Leave an equal volume of the stain and formalinized faecal concentrate overnight. Chromidial bars will stain blue.

E. *Sargeaunt's stain*

1. Add 200 mg malachite green (Sigma) to 3 ml 95% (v/v) ethanol, 3 ml glacial acetic acid, and make up to 100 ml with distilled water.
2. Use only following formol ether concentration. Mix one drop of faecal concentrate with one drop of stain and examine under a coverslip.
3. Chromidial bars stain as solid green blocks, and other nuclear and cytoplasmic detail is visible to a greater or lesser extent.

Protocol 3. Preparation and use of trichrome stain

1. Dissolve the dry stains in the glacial acetic acid first (leave 30 min), then add the water. May be stored indefinitely in sealed bottles.
2. Smears to be stained should have been fixed in Schaudinn's fluid (1 h), or in PVA, and must be iodine treated (see *Protocol 1*) before staining, and then washed briefly in two changes of 70% ethanol.
3. Stain in trichrome stain for 10 min and then rinse in 70% ethanol.
4. Expose all the slides individually to acid alcohol (99 ml 90% ethanol with 1 ml glacial acetic acid) for about 3 sec (vary if necessary) and then rinse well in tap-water.
5. Dehydrate in absolute ethanol (two changes) and clear in inhibisol or xylene before mounting in DPX.

Entamoeba may be cultured for definitive identification by zymodeme analysis. The method described by Robinson (3) is most frequently used and is described in *Protocol 4*.

Protocol 4. Cultivation of *E. histolytica* from faeces in Robinson's medium

Reagents

- Saline agar slopes: make 1.5% plain agar (Oxoid L28) in 0.7% (w/v) saline and aliquot in 2.5 ml quantities into bijou glass bottles —after autoclaving, allow the agar to solidify on a slope
- Erythromycin solution: make a 20% solution in 70% ethanol as a stock, then dilute in sterile distilled water to 0.5% (store at 4 °C)
- 20% sterile Bacto peptone in 5 ml volumes
- Rice starch (sterilize by dry heat for 1 h at 160 °C)
- Phthalate buffer: dissolve 204 g potassium phthalate in 100 ml, 40% NaOH and make up to 2 litres with distilled water, pH should be adjusted to 6.3 and the solution aliquoted in 5 ml volumes and autoclaved—a working solution is prepared by diluting the stock by 1:10

- 'R' medium for *Escherichia coli*: the concentrated stock is sodium chloride 125 g, citric acid monohydrate 50 g, potassium dihydrogen phosphate 12.5 g, ammonium sulfate 25 g, magnesium sulfate heptahydrate 1.25 g, lactic acid 100 ml, distilled water 2.5 litres. The concentrated stock solution is stable at room temperature. For use, 100 ml of this solution is mixed with 7.5 ml of 40% (w/v) NaOH and 2.5 ml of 0.04% bromothymol blue in ethanol made up to 1 litre. Adjust the pH to 7.0 and then autoclave. Store at room temperature for one month before using.
- 'BR' medium: inoculate a faecal strain of *E. coli* into shallow layers of 'R' medium in sealed medical flat bottles, and incubate at 37 °C for 48 h. The resultant suspension of bacteria may be kept on the bench for up to two months. Check the pH does not rise above 7.3 by noting the colour of the indicator.
- 'BRS' medium: mix equal volumes of horse or sheep serum and 'BR' medium and incubate for 48 h in a shallow layer in a medical flat bottle. The resultant medium will retain its usefulness for one month at room temperature.

Method

1. Add a large loopful of faeces to an agar slope. Then put in four drops of erythromycin solution (0.5%), a knife-point of starch, and fill up with 1.5 ml of 'BR' medium.
2. Incubate (37 °C) overnight, remove the supernatant with a Pasteur pipette, and replace with fresh supernatant composed of equal parts of 'BRS' medium and phthalate solution. Add two drops each of erythromycin and phthalate solution.
3. Incubate a further 24 h and then examine a small drop of the starchy sediment for amoebic trophozoites, with and without the addition of Lugol's iodine. If no growth has occurred, even after a further 24 h, the culture is deemed negative. The amoebae which grow in the culture may be cultivated continuously in the BRS/phthalate mixture as above, taking care to add some starch when subcultures are made (at three day intervals).

3. Serological diagnosis of invasive amoebiasis

The detection of extraintestinal amoebic invasion by *E. histolytica* relies to a great extent on identification of specific serum antibody, because in approximately 50% of such cases, an intestinal infection may not be detectable. However serological tests are not sufficiently sensitive for reliable routine diagnosis of intestinal amoebiasis, especially dysentery. Chronic invasive infections and amoeboma are more likely to be accompanied by seropositivity. In laboratories with a low work-load for serological diagnosis of amoebiasis the IFAT (3) (see *Protocol 5*) and CAP tests (4) see (*Protocol 6*) are the most useful. EWSA tests (1) may be introduced into wider usage in the future, but will not be described in this chapter. Amoebic liver abscess (ALA) is a medical emergency for which definitive diagnosis by serology is required.

3.1 Indirect immunofluorescence (IFA) against *E. histolytica* (4)

Protocol 5. Indirect fluorescent test for *Entamoeba histolytica* antibody

Equipment and reagents

- *Entamoeba histolytica* culture (HK9, NIH200 or HM1)
- Teflon-coated small-welled slides
- Fluorescein labelled anit-immunoglobulin
- Evan's blue
- UV microscope
- Benchtop centrifuge
- Humidified chamber

Method

A. *Preparation of sample*

1. Take an axenic culture of *Entamoeba histolytica* in the logarithmic phase, remove the supernatant and add chilled PBS to remove the amoeba. Wash the amoebae twice in PBS by centrifugation at 700 g. Resuspend the amoeba in PBS to give 100 organisms in 3 μl.
2. Put 3 μl of the suspension on each well of the teflon coated slide and dry in a current of warm air. Fix in methanol[a].
3. Dilute patient sera from 1/80 to 1)640 and add 20 μl of each addition to wells and leave in a moist chamber for 30 min.
4. Wash twice for 20 min with two charges of PBS.
5. Add 20 μl fluorescin labelled anti-immunoglobulin diluted 1/50 in PBS to each well. Leave in a moist box for 30 min. Wash twice for 20 min with three changes of PBS.
6. Counterstain with 1/30 000 Evan's blue (in PBS) for 5 min and wash in PBS for 5 min. Allow slides to dry and place one drop of commercial mountant or buffered glycerol, pH 7.6 on each well and add a coverslip.
7. Examine under UV illumination (490 nm). The end point is defined as the well in which half of the amoebae are fluorescing.[b]
8. Any serum which gives a positive reaction at 1/80 diluation is considered antibody positive.[c]

[a] Slides prepared in this way can be stored at −20°C to −70°C wrapped individually in absorbent tissue.

[b] The strongest reaction is seen at the membrane.

[c] In sera from persons returning from overseas 20% of 1/80 titres will be false positives. Higher specificity will be found at titres of 1/160 and 1/320. More than 95% of amoebic liver abscess patients will show a positive serological test in the IFAT. Only 50% of intestinal amoebiasis cases will show detectable antibody.

3.2 Cellulose acetate precipitin test

This test is carried out on all sera with a reciprocal titre of 80 or higher in the IFAT. The test was described by Stamm and Phillips (5). It is useful for the rapid diagnosis of amoebic liver abscess, and confirmation of sera with a titre greater than 80 in the IFAT.

Protocol 6. CAP test for *E. histolytica* antibody

Equipment and reagents

- Cellulose acetate membrane (Gelman Sciences Inc.)
- Perspex template (*Figure 3*)
- Nigrosin (Sigma)

Method

1. Cut a 40 mm × 40 mm square of cellulose acetate membrane ('Sepraphore III' (62092), Gelman Sciences Inc.).
2. Label the membrane on each edge, +, −, test 1, and test 2, as in *Figure 3*.
3. Float on PBS pH 7.2 without wetting top surface for 5 min.
4. Blot very lightly.
5. Make 4 + 1 wells using an indented perspex template as shown in *Figure 3* and rounded metal rod (diameter approximately 4 mm). Care must be taken not to cut the cellulose acetate membrane at the edges.
6. Place in PBS pre-wetted moist chamber with edges in contact with damp foam. The membrane should be placed symmetrically over a 30 mm square hole cut in the foam and placed in a suitable plastic box with a piece of foam glued to the lid to humidify the air above the membrane.
7. Add 3 μl of antigen (6 μl/ml crude amoebic soluble protein) to central well, and 5 μl of each of 4 sera (undiluted) to peripheral wells.
8. Incubate with lid closed at room temperature for 4 h.
9. Wash in normal saline for 30 min.
10. Fix 10 min in 3% acetic acid.
11. Stain for 7 min in nigrosin in methanol/acetic acid/water.
12. Wash in 3% acetic acid.
13. Observe in bright light for precipitin lines.

4. Diagnosis of infection caused by *Blastocystis hominis*

This organism is commonly found in the stools of healthy people. It has previously been classified as a trichomonas, as a yeast, and later placed

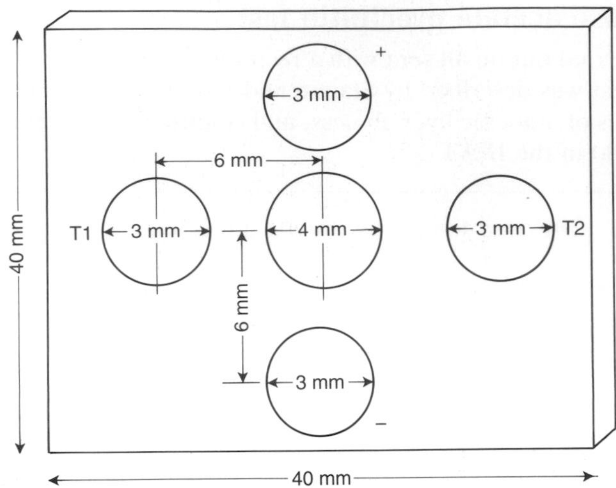

Figure 3. Perspex template for CAP test. All holes have bevelled edges; hole diameters are to the edge of holes. Positions for control sera (+, −) and two test sera (T1, T2) are shown.

among the algae, and lastly the protozoa. It was first classified with the Sporozoa, but latterly with the Amoebida based on its motility in culture and its ability to phagocytose. The role of this organism in human disease is uncertain. The prevalence is between 10% and 20% of the population and a large proportion of these infections are asymptomatic. It is widely accepted that small numbers of Blastocystis in the stool are unlikely to be responsible for clinical symptoms. Some authors, however, consider that when larger numbers are present (more than five per high power field) clinical disease may follow. Reported symptoms include anorexia, flatus, and diarrhoea. Fever, nausea, and vomiting are less common.

4.1 Diagnosis

This organism is readily demonstrated in stool specimens using unstained smears or by staining with Giemsa or Gram's stain. In a stool a vacuolated spherical structure is seen varying in size from 5–30 μm in diameter (*Figure 4*). An amoebic form is only rarely seen in patient specimens but is more common in artificial culture. This is irregular in shape and 10–15 μm in diameter. A larger granular form is even less rarely found in stools (10–60 μm in diameter) but is found in culture in media containing 20% human serum. Blastocystis has been shown to be susceptible to a number of agents *in vitro* including metronidazole, furazolidine, and trimethoprim-sulfamethoxazole. The role of these in the management of human infection can not be interpreted in view of the difficulties of assigning pathogenicity in any individual patient.

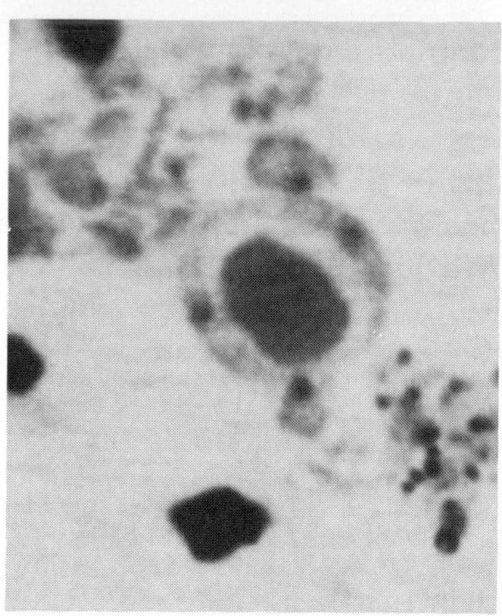

Figure 4. *Blastocystis hominis* in human faeces stained with Giemsa. Reproduced by kind permission of R. S. Jackson, Department of Microbiology, University of Leeds.

5. Infections caused by free-living amoebae

5.1 *Naegleria fowleri*

N. fowleri is a free-living environmental organism which is responsible for a rare and usually fatal form of meningitis (6). The amoeboid trophozoite invades tissues during acute infection. The flagellate form is highly motile by virtue of two flagella and is found in fresh water. A highly resistant non-motile cyst is also formed. This is capable of surviving for prolonged periods in the environment. Pathogenic *Naegleria* tolerate temperatures of up to 46°C and salinity of up to 0.85%.

Infections are usually associated with swimming in rivers or swimming pools with high ambient temperatures (which may have been chlorinated). Infections have also been reported after bathing in thermal springs and some have acquired infection following snuffing water as part of religious rituals.

The organisms gain access to the body through the nose. The clinical syndrome associated with *N. fowleri* infection is primary 'amoebic' meningo encephalitis (PAM). This is a rapidly progressive meningitis with all of the clinical features of acute pyogenic meningitis. The main lesions are found in the olfactory bulb and the maxillary and sphenoid sinus can be filled with the products of infection.

The application of specific therapy after early diagnosis of the condition has led to recovery in only four of more than 144 (7) recorded cases. Although relatively few cases of PAM are recorded, the disease is significant among those associated with recreational water use, particularly because of its almost invariably fatal outcome. In the two year period 1989 and 1990, three cases of PAM were reported among 1062 cases of illness associated with recreational water use in the USA (8).

5.1.1 Diagnosis

The diagnosis is usually made when a history of swimming in stagnant water is obtained in a patient with severe meningitis. The organisms in CSF are difficult to differentiate from inflammatory cells when stained by Gram's method but are readily identified using Wright's stain. When *Naegleria* are suspected they can be identified by their motility in wet preparations. A method for cultivation has been described using 1.5% non-nutrient agar seeded with *E. coli*.

The major problem in diagnosis of PAM is to distinguish between it and other encephalitides of rapid onset such as meningococcal, acute tubercular, and viral meningitis. Distinction from all but non-tubercular bacterial meningitis is relatively straightforward since on CSF examination there is a markedly raised cell count, mainly polymorphonuclear cells. In tubercular or viral meningitis the cellular increase when present is composed of mainly mononuclear cells. CSF protein is generally above 1 g/litre and may be up to 10 g/litre, and this contrasts with viral meningitis where low values are usually found. Glucose may be lower than normal, as in bacterial meningitis, but this is not a useful diagnostic feature.

5.2 *Acanthamoeba*

Acanthamoeba spp. have previously been classified as *Hartmannella*. Several species have been isolated from human infection of which *A. culbertsoni* is most common. Others include *A. castellanii*, the type species, *A. polyphaga*, and *A. astronyxis*. *Acanthamoeba* have a simple life cycle with an amoeboid trophozoite and a resistant cyst form.

Eye infections can be a precursor to meningitis but in other cases a chronic corneal ulcer is the outcome. Amoebic keratitis has a poor prognosis for vision with some patients requiring corneal transplantation or enucleation.

5.3 Diagnosis and treatment

The diagnosis of *Acanthamoeba* infections depends on the demonstration of amoebae in the CSF or in corneal scrapings. In the case of meningitis the diagnosis is often made at post-mortem examination. Immunoperoxidase techniques can be used to detect the presence of amoebae and to identify them. *Acanthamoeba* spp. vary in anti-microbial sensitivity. Treatment of menigitis is usually unsuccessful.

5.3.1 Granulomatous amoebic encephalitis (GAE)

Acanthamoeba spp. which cause GAE and chronic acanthamoeba keratitis (CAK) are found world-wide and also feed on bacteria, but they are not necessarily associated with warm water, and can also multiply in brackish conditions. The life cycle consists only of the trophozoite and cyst forms, and either of these can be a source of infection for man. Several species of the genus have been isolated from human tissue, and the ubiquitous distribution of these organisms means that human exposure is widespread. For example, it is estimated that humans inhale one of the resistant cysts every day (9). As a corollary of this wide exposure, the organism finds it difficult to colonize man, and infections are generally restricted to the immunodeficient or to immunoprivileged sites, the most common of which is the cornea. Infections are generally of a chronic type and there is marked granulomatous tissue reaction. Successful treatment by medical or surgical means is so far restricted to the ocular infection. It is estimated that more than 200 cases of CAK have been recorded since 1974.

Several species of *Acanthamoeba* have now been identified in cases of human granulomatous amoebic encephalitis (GAE). The organism produces infections in various tissues in the immunocompromised or debilitated, including those with AIDS (10).

Clinical

The incubation period is generally prolonged. The signs and symptoms are typical of a variety of conditions resulting from space-occupying lesions in the brain and include hemiparesis, seizures and, in about 70%, altered mental ability (stupor or lethargy through disorientation to irritability and combativeness). The predisposing factors include use of steroids (42%), antibiotics, chemotherapy, alcoholism, AIDS, diabetes, and immunocompromised states. Acute *Acanthamoeba* meningoencephalitis was seen associated with *Acanthamoeba* keratitis and uveitis in a child (11).

The characteristics of GAE mimic a deep mycosis with systemic dissemination. In the five cases reviewed by Jager and Stamm (12) there was a frontal headache, fluctuating coma, with or without significant history of a predisposing disease. The route of infection of the brain in the Hodgkin's lymphoma case they reviewed is thought to have been intranasal, since there were basal cortical changes in the brain, with the olfactory lobes affected. Presence of amoebae in the vessel walls gives rise to a vasculitis of an allergic type. Dead and dying organisms are found, and there is evidence of a foreign body giant cell reaction. It is noteworthy that amoebic cysts are seen in the tissues in GAE and CAK, unlike the situation in *Naegleria* PAM.

Diagnosis

The CSF cell count was raised in all patients, lymphocytes being markedly elevated, composing 19% to 100% of the cells present. Glucose concentrations, where measured, were not appreciably lowered, as would be found in bacterial meningitis or PAM.

Although amoebic trophozoites have been reported in CSF in a few cases of GAE, there is no doubt that this is an extremely unusual finding.

In view of the chronic nature of the infection and the invasive character of attempts to obtain biopsy specimens, the ideal initial investigation would seem to be serological (13).

Cerebral biopsy is not an uncommon procedure, and specific polyclonal antibody has been used on wax-embedded sections in immunofluorescence (14) or immunoperoxidase techniques. *Acanthamoeba*-specific monoclonal antibodies have been developed which are likely to prove valuable in diagnosis.

Treatment

As yet there has been no successful treatment of systemic *Acanthamoeba* infection in man. There are reports of the successful use of rifampin and of paromomycin in treatment of infections in mice.

5.3.2 Chronic *Acanthamoeba* keratitis (CAK)

Acanthamoeba is present in all types of environments throughout the world. Since its cysts are resistant to drying the chance of cyst inoculation on a mucous surface is high. The cornea is an immunoprivileged site, since there is no direct contact with the blood, and it is possible for cysts or trophozoites of this organism to infect corneal stroma.

Acanthamoeba keratitis or kerato-uveitis presents a serious diagnostic and treatment problem to ophthalmologists. Since the first reports from UK and USA in the early 70s (15, 16) many further cases have been seen in Europe, the USA, and other countries. The major part of the increase in developed countries is probably related to contact lens use and is related to direct inoculation of the amoebic trophozoites or cysts into the cornea during insertion of the contaminated lens.

The first ocular infections (15, 16) were thought to be associated with trauma to the cornea, leading to invasion of the amoebae, and were not linked to contact lens use. However, 85% of *Acanthamoeba* eye infections in a recent USA survey were in hard or soft contact lens wearers (17). Symptoms characteristically mimic those of herpes keratitis, although the condition is generally more painful than viral disease. Retrospective studies of keratitis material prior to 1973 in London failed to reveal any earlier cases (18).

The disease runs a slow relapsing course, often a ring abscess is persistent, epithelial breakdown is recurrent with varying degrees of hypopyon.

5.3.3 Diagnosis of acanthamoebic keratitis (19)

Clinical signs have been confused not only with other infective entities but also topical anaesthetic abuse (20).

Diagnosis may be made by observation of characteristic cysts in wet mounts

(10% KOH wet mount is reported satisfactory (21)) of corneal ulcer scrapings, and subsequent culture. Cultures made from superficial scrapings of the cornea, or from punch biopsies (22), are valuable. Suggestive but not con clusive evidence for the infection is obtained when the amoeba is isolated from contact lenses themselves, the cases or the washing fluid. The fluorescent dye calcofluor has been used to stain the cysts in smears.

The temperature of the eye is lower than that of the rest of the human body. Therefore *Acanthamoeba* strains that grow at lower temperatures may also contribute to infection. Recent evidence indicates that perhaps only a limited number of species cause ocular disease. Delineation of the exact species of *Acanthamoeba* that cause keratitis is a prerequisite for the study of the ecology of the keratitis-producing amoebas (23).

5.3.4 Treatment of acanthamoebic keratitis

The most effective therapeutic drugs so far examined have been the diamidines propamidine and dibromopropamidine (24). It is important to remember that *Acanthamoeba*, unlike *Naegleria*, encysts in infected tissues. Clinical cure generally utilizes medications in combination with surgical procedures such as keratoplasty or, sometimes, debridement (25). Anti-inflammatory steroids are thought to increase the susceptibility of the eye to *Acanthamoeba* infection, but the judicious use of steroids in conjunction with drug treatment has been valuable in many cases. This problem is discussed with respect to several eye infections by Stern and Buttross (26).

References

1. Abd-Alla, M. D., Jackson, T. F. H. G., Gathiram, V., El-Haweg, A. M., and Ravdin, J. I. (1993). *J. Clin. Microbiol.*, **31**, 2845.
2. Sargeant, P. G. and Williams, J. E. (1978). *Trans. R. Soc. Trop. Med. Hyg.*, **72**, 164.
3. Robinson, G. L. (1968). *Trans. R. Soc. Trop. Med. Hyg.*, **62**, 285.
4. Gonzalez-Ruiz, *et al.* (1992). *J. Clin. Microbiol.*, **30**, 2807.
5. Stamm, W. P. and Phillips, E. A. (1977). *Trans. R. Soc. Trop. Med. Hyg.*, **71**, 49.
6. Warhurst, D. C. (1985). *Parasitol. Today*, **1**, 24.
7. Ma, P., Visvesvara, G. S., Martinez, A. J., Theodore, F. H., Daggett, P. M., and Sawyer, T. K. (1990). *Rev. Infect. Dis.*, **12**, 490.
8. Herwaldt, B. L., Craun, G. F., Stokes, S. L., and Juranek, D. D. (1991). *MMWR. CDC. Surveill. Summ.*, **40**, 1.
9. Kingston, D. and Warhurst, D. C. (1969). *J. Med. Microbiol.*, **2**, 27.
10. Kilrrington, S. and White, D. G. (1994). *Rev. Med. Microbiol.*, **5**, 12.
11. Jones, D. B., Visvesvara, G. S., and Robinson, N. M. (1975). *Trans. Ophthalmol. Soc. UK*, **95**, 221.
12. Jager, B. V. and Stamm, W. P. (1972). *Lancet*, **ii**, 1343.
13. Kenney, M. (1971). *Hlth. Bab. Sci.*, **8**, 5.
14. Warhurst, D. C. (1982). In *Immunofluoresence techniques in diagnostic micro-*

biology (ed. J. M. B. Edwards, C. E. D. Taylor, and A. H. Tomlinson), pp. 46–8. London, HMSO.

15. Nagington, J., Watson, P. G., Playfair, T. J., McGill, J., Jones, B. R., and Steele, A. D. McG. (1974). *Lancet*, **ii**, 1537.
16. Visvesvara, G. S., Jones, D. B., and Robinson, N. M. (1975). *Am. J. Trop. Med. Hyg.*, **24**, 784.
17. Stehr-Green, J. K., Bailey, T. M., and Visvesvara, G. S. (1989). *Am. J. Ophthalmol.*, **107** 331.
18. Ashton, N. and Stamm, W. P. (1975). *Trans. Ophthalmol. Soc. UK*, **95**, 214.
19. Visvesvara, G. S. (1988). In *Laboratory diagnosis of infectious disease* (ed. A. Balows, W. J. Hausler, M. Ohashi, and A. Turano), pp. 723–30. Springer, New York.
20. Rosenwasser, G. O., Holland, S., Pflugfelder, S. C., Lugo, M., Heidmann, D. G., Culbertson, W. W., *et al.* (1990). *Ophthalmology*, **97**, 967.
21. Sharma, S., Srinivasan, M., and George, C. (1990). *Indian J. Ophthalmol.*, **38**, 50.
22. Lee, P. and Green, W. R. (1990). *Ophthalmology*, **97**, 718.
23. De-Jonckheere, J. F. (1991). *Rev. Infect. Dis.*, **13**, S385.
24. Wright, P., Warhurst, D. C., and Jones, B. R. (1985). *Br. J. Ophthalmol.*, **69**, 778.
25. Osato, M. S., Robinson, N. M., Wilhelmus, K. R., and Jones, D. B. (1991). *Rev. Infect. Dis.*, **13**, S431.
26. Stern, G. A. and Buttross, M. (1991). *Ophthalmology*, **98**, 847.

7

Trichomonads

J. P. ACKERS

1. Introduction

Trichomonas vaginalis and *Pentatrichomonas hominis* (previously classified as *Trichomonas hominis*) are two of the three trichomonad parasites infecting humans, the third being the uncommon and little studied oral parasite *Trichomonas tenax*. All three are closely related flagellate protozoa with simple life cycles which do not include a resistant cyst stage. *T. vaginalis* is sexually transmitted, and the most common protozoan infection in Europe and North America, but with an even higher prevalence in many developing countries. *P. hominis* inhabits the large bowel and is much less common; it is usually regarded as a non-pathogen although it can probably cause mild gastro-intestinal symptoms when present in large numbers. It is transmitted by the ingestion of trophozoites derived from the faeces of infected patients, and is unusual in being sufficiently resistant to gastric acid despite the absence of a cyst. Because of their very different epidemiology and clinical presentation, these two organisms will be dealt with separately.

2. *Trichomonas vaginalis*

2.1 Introduction

It is now generally accepted that the majority of cases of human trichomoniasis are sexually transmitted; nevertheless symptomatic infections are much more common in women than in men, and it is also much easier to recover the organism from the former than the latter.

2.1.1 Trichomoniasis in women

T. vaginalis is a parasite of the urogenital system, being most commonly found in the vagina. The organism has a predilection for squamous epithelial cells, and is thus rarely found in the endocervix. In up to 90% of cases the organism may be recovered from the urethra and Skene's glands, but it is not clear whether true bladder infection occurs. Further dissemination, to the ureter, kidney, or more distant sites has only very occasionally been reported, and parasitaemia is not believed to occur. Up to half of infected women may be asymptomatic; in the remainder symptoms include discharge (frequently irritating or pruritic but by no means always frothy or malodorous), dyspareunia, and dysuria. On examination diffuse vulval erythema, excessive discharge, and vaginal wall inflammation may be found, but it is important to note that no combination of signs and symptoms is diagnostic (1) (for a clinical review see ref. 2).

2.1.2 Trichomoniasis in men

Trichomoniasis in males is frequently regarded as either non-existent or unimportant; however not only is there good epidemiological evidence that infected men are the source of most infections in women, but male trichomoniasis is not as invariably asymptomatic as is frequently supposed (3). As with women, this is a disease of the urogenital tract, but there is also limited evidence that the organism penetrates into the tissues such as the prostate.

2.2 Specimen collection

If serodiagnosis is being considered then blood will need to be collected. Otherwise the organism is sought in samples taken from the genito-urinary tract.

2.2.1 Women

Material for wet film and culture is collected from the posterior fornix of the vagina using a cotton wool tipped swab, but considerably more material (and thus greater sensitivity) may be obtained by using an absorbent polyester swab (4), and for certain diagnostic kits the manufacturer's own swab must be used. Urine or urethral smears may also be examined, but the urinary tract is seldom the only site of infection.

2.2.2 Men

The organism is difficult to detect in males and therefore several different specimens should be examined if possible. Freshly produced semen is probably the best, but urethral exudate collected on an absorbent swab (4), urine sediment, and prostatic secretions can also be used.

2.3 Diagnostic methods

The methods which are available for the diagnosis of *T. vaginalis* infections in both men and women may be summarized as follows:

- wet film examination
- stained films
- direct detection with labelled antibodies
- culture
- antibody detection
- antigen detection

2.4 Wet film examination

This is the most widely used method, despite its poor sensitivity, found to be between 38% and 82% (5) but it retains its popularity because it is quick, cheap, and specific. Specimens should be mixed with a little isotonic saline and examined immediately. Trichomonads survive well in Stuart's transport medium for up to 24 hours, but after that viability begins to decline (5). A well stopped-down bright-field, dark-field, or phase-contrast illumination may be used, and there are no studies showing significantly better results with any one of the three. Trichomoniasis is diagnosed by finding living trichomonads, with characteristic morphology: a pear-shaped organism about 13 μm × 10 μm (*Figure 1*), with four anterior flagellae clearly visible, or alternatively beating so rapidly that only the disturbance which they produce in the surrounding debris can be seen. The undulating membrane beats more slowly and is also diagnostic, but may be hidden depending on the orientation of the organism. The projecting axostyle may or may not be clearly seen; it sometimes appears much longer than as usually illustrated. In our experience, trichomonads which are seen almost always grow—i.e. if culture is the standard, the specificity approaches 100%. The importance of looking at fresh or well handled specimens can not be overstated; in a wet preparation dead or dying trichomonads will become an inert and unrecognizable blob.

2.5 Stained films

Several attempts have been made to improve the sensitivity of wet film examination by staining the organisms. The only method to have received even limited acceptance is the use of acridine-orange. Although the sensitivity is usually reported as better than wet film examination the specificity may be rather lower, immediacy is lost, and an expensive fluorescence microscope is required (6). Conventional microscopical stains, although excellent for showing detail in cultured organisms (*Figure 2*) have found little application in routine diagnosis (5). One important but controversial diagnostic tool is the Papanicolaou stained smear. There is no doubt that perfectly fixed and stained smears can clearly show the presence of *T. vaginalis*; and this should be particularly valuable since infection may produce changes in the nucleus of cells which make the detection of pre-malignant states unreliable. However, serious doubts have been cast on the specificity of this method (7, 8) and it is probably not suitable for routine use. For the one method of preparing demonstration slides from culture, see section 3.5(b).

2.6 Direct detection with labelled antibodies

There are many attractions in the idea of preparing films from clinical specimens and then staining them with specific, labelled antibody, the chief ones being that the procedures are basically familiar and that, providing that the

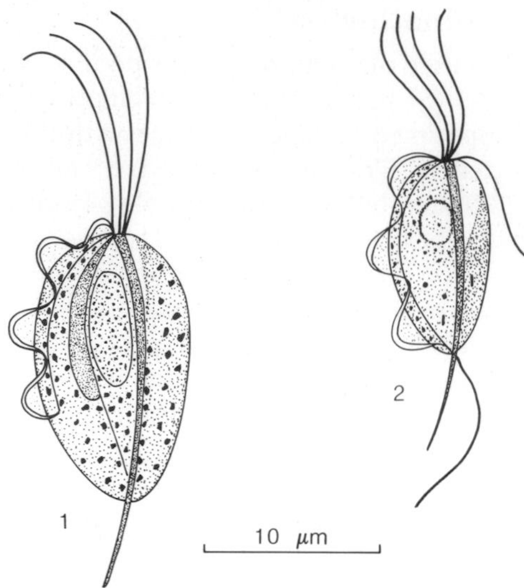

Figure 1. Trichomonads of man: 1. *Trichomonas vaginalis,* 2. *Pentatrichomonas hominis* (× 2500).

antibody is completely specific, any labelled body, however unrecognizable, must be the organism sought. In principle, no parasitological experience should be needed, and dead or fragmentary organisms should be detectable. In practice background staining can seldom be completely prevented and it is impossible to give reliable guidance on how to manage a patient whose specimen is culture negative but clearly shows fluorescent but not recognizable bodies. The most successful examples of this technique have employed monoclonal antibodies. Krieger *et al.* (9) and Chang *et al.* (10) both described methods, and antibody-based detection kits are now commercially available. In a recent comparison (11) such a kit (Integrated Diagnostics Inc. Berkeley, California, USA) was judged to be almost as sensitive as culture and clearly superior to both wet films and acridine-orange stained films. Enzyme labelled antibodies have the advantages of not requiring a fluorescence microscope and of producing a permanently stained slide; they have been applied to both tissue sections and cervical cytology smears (12), but the method has not been widely investigated for routine diagnosis.

The method described here was evaluated on 2000 vaginal smears sent to a reference laboratory (Wozniak *et al.* in preparation); 55 specimens were positive by culture, 25 by wet film examination, and 55 by immunofluorescence (sensitivity: 94.5%; specificity: 99.8%; predictive value of positive result 94.5%; predictive value of negative result 98.5%).

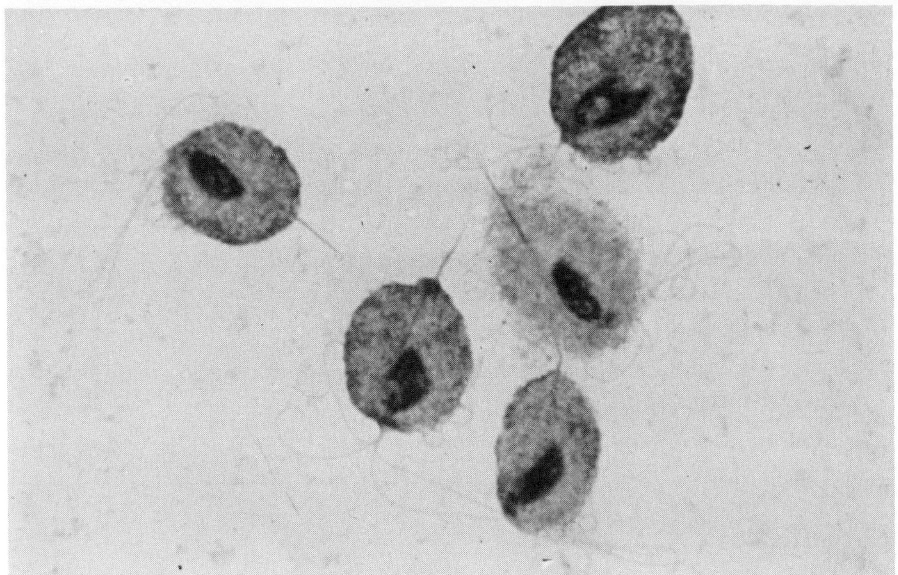

Figure 2. Stained *T. vaginalis* (Geimsa; ×2000)

2.6.1 Selection of monoclonal antibodies and diagnosis using an immunofluorescent method

Monoclonal antibodies are prepared by conventional methods using whole cultured organisms as the antigen. Candidate antibodies are selected from those which fluoresce brightly with all of ten isolates grown in culture (to avoid possible strain-specific antigens); three which give particularly bright fluorescence and clear definition of morphology are then produced as ascitic fluids, mixed in equal proportions, and the optimum working dilution determined by titration using cultured organisms and following *Protocol 1*.

Protocol 1. Immunofluorescent staining of smears

Equipment and reagents

- Optimum dilution of mixed monoclonal antibodies in 0.1 M Hepes buffer containing 1% BSA and 0.1% sodium azide
- Working dilution of fluorescein labelled heterologous anti-mouse immunoglobulin in PBS (either the manufacturer's recommendation or determined by chequerboard titration; we use sheep antibody at 1:50)
- Ten-well Teflon coated slides, with one or more positive control wells—the latter should be spotted with about 5000 cultured *T. vaginalis* organisms and air dried
- 90% glycerol in PBS, or a commercial mountant such as 'Citifluor'
- PBS

Protocol 1. *Continued*

Method

1. Make smears directly from vaginal swabs on to one well of the slide.
2. Air dry and fix in acetone for 10 min.
3. If testing is not to be done immediately, slides may be stored at −20 °C.
4. Place 25 μl of diluted monoclonal antibody on each well, and incubate in a moist chamber for 20 min at room temperature.
5. Rinse with PBS and then soak in PBS for 10 min. Drain and carefully blot off excess.
6. Place 25 μl of fluorescein labelled anti-mouse immunoglobulin on each well; incubate, rinse, and wash as above.
7. Mount and examine under UV illumination.

2.7 Culture

Numerous studies (5, 13) have shown that culture methods are 20–30% more sensitive than wet film microscopy, and they now represent the 'gold standard' against which other diagnostic methods are evaluated. Nevertheless there is no doubt that on occasions genuinely positive specimens do not grow, and the overall sensitivity is probably between 86%–97% (13). Possible causes include using sequential specimens (one of which may be better than the other) for culture and wet film examination, poor quality medium, the presence of inhibitory substances in the collecting equipment, or inaccurate identification; the most controversial is the postulated, but not widely accepted, existence of infectious but non-cultivable organisms. It is also clear that while there are many perfectly satisfactory media available, others are less able to grow organisms from small innocula than the best (14–16).

2.7.1 Choice of media

Because so many excellent media exist, we shall give instructions (*Protocol 2*) for the preparation and use of only one—modified Diamond's medium (MDM)(17–20). This medium is widely used, is always as good as any other in comparative trials, and is available commercially in many countries of the world.

Protocol 2. Preparation of modified Diamond's medium (MDM)

Equipment and reagents

- The ingredients listed below
- Sterile, heat inactivated mycoplasma-free horse serum[a]
- Antibiotics (see step **7**)

Method

1. Ingredients:
   - trypticase (BBL) 20.00 g
   - yeast extract (Difco) 10.00 g
   - maltose 5.00 g
   - L-ascorbic acid (analytical grade) 1.00 g
   - KCl 1.00 g
   - $KHCO_3$ 1.00 g
   - KH_2PO_4 1.00 g
   - K_2HPO_4 1.00 g
   - $FeSO_4.7H_2O$ 0.18 g
   - Glass-distilled water 900 ml
2. Dissolve all the dry ingredients in the water, by stirring and warming if necessary. Cool, filter, check the pH (which should be about 6.8[b]), and adjust if necessary.
3. Dispense in appropriate volumes and autoclave at 15 p.s.i. for 15 min.
4. Medium may be stored at 4 °C for up to one month, or at −20 °C indefinitely.
5. Immediately before use add the serum to 10% (v/v) final concentration, together with antibiotics chosen from step **7**.
6. Dispense into small bottles or tubes (glass or tissue culture grade plastic). *T. vaginalis* is inhibited by oxygen, therefore while strict anaerobiosis is not required, tubes should be completely filled to exclude as much air as possible.
7. Antibiotics. The following list is recommended by Linstead (20) and agrees with our experience. Amounts recommended are **final concentrations per millilitre** of complete medium. If isolates are being maintained in long-term axenic culture, routine addition of antibiotics seems unnecessary and undesirable.
   (a) For routine use, add benzyl penicillin (1000 IU), streptomycin sulfate (100 μg), and nystatin (50 U).
   (b) If resistant bacteria are a problem, try gentamicin (up to 200 μg), flucloxacillin (500 μg), neomycin (500 μg), or chloramphenicol (250 μg).
   (c) If fungal overgrowth occurs, try Amphotericin B (15 μg) or miconazole nitrate (50–100 μg).
   (d) It is not usually necessary to eliminate mycoplasma unless isolates are to be maintained for research purposes, but if required try kanamycin (100 μg) or tylosin (60–120 μg).

[a] Horse serum is traditional, but probably many others are suitable.

[b] Linstead (20) suggests that the medium should be adjusted to a lower pH (about 6.2) if difficulty is experienced in growing organisms from very small innocula.

2.7.2 Use of culture medium in diagnosis

Vaginal and other specimens should be inoculated into tubes or small bottles containing 5–15 ml of medium and incubated at 37 °C; sterile swabs may be broken off inside the tube. Cultures should be examined daily for motile organisms, either by removing a loopful of medium and making a temporary wet preparation, or as follows. Plastic tissue culture tubes filled with 15 ml of medium are used; the technique is expensive in medium and in disposable plasticware, but the tubes may be checked very rapidly, conveniently, and sensitively by examining the flat face with an inverted microscope. Some strains grow in suspension while others adhere to the plastic. The ability to examine cultures repeatedly without opening them is a great advantage. Most culture will show visible growth within 48 hours, but all should be kept for at least 96 hours before being discarded as negative; in rare cases we have had specimens from male patients which were not clearly positive for seven to ten days.

2.8 Antibody detection

A very great deal of effort over the years has been put into trying to diagnose *T. vaginalis* infections by serological means, since many patients would much prefer to have a blood sample taken rather than a speculum examination. The final conclusion of this work, however, has to be that while antibodies can be detected in the majority of infected women, there are too many cases where they can not be found for the method to be useful in patient management. Other problems include pre-existing natural antibodies, the possible existence of different serotypes, and very poor sensitivity in males. A recent review (21) discusses the whole subject in much greater detail.

2.9 Antigen detection

The detection of antigen rather than antibody has certain inherent advantages, of which the most important are that there is no interference from previous infections; recent infections, when an antibody response may not yet have occurred, can be detected, as can those (see above) who never respond adequately. Strictly speaking, antigen detection includes both the immunological staining of whole organisms (described in section 2.6) as well as the detection of parasite-specific molecules in clinical specimens; it is the latter which is discussed here. The original descriptions were of microplate ELISA techniques utilizing antibodies to capture antigen from clinical specimens, followed by separate detection using an enzyme-linked second antibody (22, 23); subsequently a more rapid sandwich ELISA utilizing an anti-*T. vaginalis* monoclonal antibody was described (24), and a very rapid latex agglutination test (now available commercially in kit form from Mercia Diagnostics, Guilford, Surrey, UK) (25). These new techniques promise to provide the speed of wet film examination with the sensitivity of culture, but since they are still research methods and the optimum procedures have not yet been established, the interested reader should consult the original papers for detailed instructions.

2.10 Anti-microbial sensitivity testing

T. vaginalis infections are usually treated with metronidazole or one of the other 5-nitroimidazoles, for there are no other effective or approved chemotherapeutic agents. Introduced in the early 1960s, this class of compound usually provides a rapid and complete cure. Treatment failures are now well recognized, and a proportion of them are due to resistant isolates of the parasite. The need may, therefore, arise to determine anti-microbial sensitivity. The biochemical basis of 5-nitroimidazole resistance, and procedures for managing such infections are discussed in recent reviews (26–29). It was only slowly appreciated that the sensitivity of *T. vaginalis* to metronidazole is greatly affected by the oxygen tension in the medium during the assay; the geometric mean minimum lethal concentration (MLC) of 199 isolates from patients successfully treated with a single 2 g dose was found to be 1.6 μg/ml under anaerobic conditions compared with 24.1 μg/ml under aerobic conditions (30). The corresponding figures for 53 treatment-resistant isolates were 5.5 μg/ml and 195.5 μg/ml respectively; since plasma levels following this dose of drug usually peak at about 40 μg/ml and remain above 16 μg/ml for 16 hours (31) this and other evidence suggests that aerobic MLCs should be appropriate predictors of treatment failure. However such failures appear to occur almost at random, and only become likely when the MLC exceeds 3.1 μg/ml (anaerobic) or 100 μg/ml (aerobic) (30).

Protocol 3. Metronidazole sensitivity testing (30)

Equipment and reagents

- Culture medium for sensitivity testing
- Sterile round-bottom 96-well microtitre plates and lids
- Solutions containing 8 and 80 μg/ml metronidazole in DMSO
- 50 μl eight-row multipipettes
- 150 μl pipette
- Anaerobic jar(s)
- Moist chamber(s)
- Well-grown cultures of the strains to be tested—these should not yet be in stationary phases and contain few if any non-motile organisms

Method

1. The recommended medium contains:
   - trypticase (BBL) 20.00 g
   - yeast extract (BBL) 10.00 g
   - maltose 5.00 g
   - L-ascorbic acid (analytical grade) 0.20 g

Protocol 3. *Continued*

- L-cysteine hydrochloride.H_2O 1.00 g
- KH_2PO_4 0.80 g
- K_2HPO_4 0.80 g
- glass-distilled water 900 ml

2. The medium is prepared as in *Protocol 2*, except that:
   - the pH is adjusted to 5.9
   - newborn calf serum is recommended
   - penicillin (1000 IU/ml) and streptomycin (1 μg/ml) alone are added (note the very low concentration of streptomycin)
3. It will be noted that the medium is very similar to the MDM medium described in *Protocol 2*. It is however known that the concentrations of both iron and reducing agents are critical, and that in general small changes in composition can have a significant effect on the results (32).
4. Count the cells in the culture of *T. vaginalis* (haemocytometer or Coulter counter) and dilute with medium to 66 600 cells/ml.
5. Orientate the plate with eight horizontal rows of 12 wells; four rows are used for each strain so that each plate may be used to test two strains. If anaerobic and aerobic testing are to be done simultaneously, duplicate plates must be prepared for each pair of strains.
6. Dilute the standard metronidazole solutions, and pure DMSO, 1:10 with medium. Thus diluted, the 8 μg/ml standard will give a maximum final concentration of 100 μg/ml (suitable for sensitive strains); the 80 μg/ml will give 1000 μg/ml.
7. Place 50 μl medium in every well.
8. Place 50 μl diluted DMSO in the first well of the first and fifth row.
9. Place 50 μl diluted standard metronidazole in the first wells of the other six rows.
10. Using an eight-channel pipette set to 50 μl, make doubling dilutions across the plate, finally discarding 50 μl from the last wells.
11. Using four of the eight channels, add 150 μl (10^4 cells) of the first strain to all the wells in the top four rows. Add cells of the second strain to the lower four rows.
12. Cover with a sterile cover and incubate at 37 °C, either in a moist box (aerobic) or in an anaerobic jar.
13. After 48 h examine each well with an inverted microscope; the end-point is the minimum concentration at which no motile cells are seen.

14. Notes:

(a) If at all possible standard resistant and sensitive strains should be included in each assay; suitable strains are available from the American Type Culture Collection (30).

(b) Mason (33) has proposed adding 0.003% bromocresol purple to the medium; growth of the *T. vaginalis* produces acid causing the colour to change to deep yellow.

3. *Pentatrichomonas hominis*

3.1 Specimen collection

P. hominis is found only in faeces, and only there in the form of a fragile trophozoite, which must be detected either by microscopy or culture. It is therefore necessary that a fresh, preferably warm specimen be obtained and examined as quickly as possible; concentration techniques which are widely applicable when searching for faecal cysts or eggs are not appropriate here, since they destroy the trophozoite. Several specimens should be obtained and examined before infection may be excluded.

3.2 Diagnostic methods

Since *P. hominis* is one of the rarer human large bowel parasites, and since it is widely (but not exclusively) regarded as a non-pathogen, relatively very little work has been devoted to developing diagnostic methods, and virtually no quantitative data on specificity and sensitivity has been published.

3.3 Wet film examination

Temporary preparations should be made, either directly from liquid stools, or after mixing with a little isotonic saline, and a coverslip applied; they are then examined as for *T. vaginalis* (see section 2.4). In the presence of so much faecal debris it is even more important to find the characteristically motile organisms. The features which distinguish *P. hominis* from *T. vaginalis*, a fifth anterior flagellum and a longer recurrent flagellum (*Figure 1*), will not be visible, but each of the three human trichomonads has been shown to be site-specific (34), and any found in faeces may be assumed to be *P. hominis*.

3.4 Stained preparations

Little work has been done on the use of fixed and stained films for the diagnosis of *P. hominis*, but it is likely that, as with *T. vaginalis*, immediacy is lost without any real gain in sensitivity or specificity.

3.5 Culture

Culturing faecal specimens will certainly reveal infections missed on direct examination, but whether the sensitivity is as high as with *T. vaginalis* is simply not known, nor have different media been systematically compared. Nevertheless it is a useful technique which should be more widely applied. A valuable medium, and the only one with which we have personal experience, is Robinson's (35). This old-fashioned, biphasic medium is still one of the best for establishing faecal protozoa in culture; a great advantage is that it will grow *Entamoeba histolytica* as well as other amoeba. The preparation and use of this medium is described in Chapter 6, *Protocol 4*; a drop of medium should be withdrawn daily for several days and a wet preparation made and examined for motile flagellates. Since Robinson's medium is so good at growing many faecal protozoa, an attempt should be made to see the undulating membrane which is characteristic of all trichomonads. If this proves difficult, try:

(a) Placing a drop of culture on a slide and then exposing to acetic acid vapour (by inverting the slide over the mouth of a small bottle containing glacial acetic acid) for a few seconds. This immobilizes the organisms and makes flagellae and the undulating membrane much easier to see.

(b) Staining. Make a smear from culture and fix **without** allowing to dry by exposing to osmium tetroxide vapour. (This is highly toxic and corrosive; seek appropriate advice.) Allow the film to dry, re-fix in methanol, and stain with highly diluted Giemsa (try 1:40 in buffered water pH 7.2 for 20 min). Many organisms will be overstained or badly orientated, but some should be very clear. This method may also be used for cultured *T. vaginalis*.

If desired, *P. hominis* may be axenized and grown without bacteria, but not as easily as *T. vaginalis*. A brief discussion of the most suitable media to use is given by Linstead (20) and elsewhere (36).

3.6 Other techniques

Little, if any work has been done on the immunological diagnosis of *P. hominis* infections; by analogy with asymptomatic passers of *E. histolytica* cysts, it seems unlikely that serum antibodies will often be present; no doubt a faecal antigen detection test could be developed if anyone felt that it was worthwhile. If treatment is needed, 5-nitroimidazoles are regarded as effective, but we know of no determinations of *in vitro* sensitivity.

References

1. Schaaf, V. M., Perez-Stable, E. J., and Borchardt, K. (1990). *Arch. Intern. Med.*, **150**, 1929.

2. Rein, M. F. (1989). In *Trichomonads parasitic in humans* (ed. B. M. Honigberg), pp. 225–34. Springer-Verlag, New York.
3. Krieger, J. N. (1989). In *Trichomonads parasitic in humans* (ed. B. M. Honigberg), pp. 235–45. Springer-Verlag, New York.
4. Oates, J. K, Selwyn, S., and Breach, M. R. (1971). *Br. J. Vener. Dis.*, **47**, 289.
5. McMillan, A. (1989). In *Trichomonads parasitic in humans* (ed. B. M. Honigberg), pp. 297–310. Springer-Verlag, New York.
6. Fripp, P. J., Mason, P. R., and Super, H. (1975). *J. Parasitol.*, **61**, 966.
7. Mason, P. R., Super, H., and Fripp, P. J. (1976). *J. Clin. Pathol.*, **29**, 154.
8. Perl, G. (1972). *Obstet. Gynecol.*, **39**, 7.
9. Krieger, J. N., Holmes, K. K., Spence, M. R., Rein, M. P., McCormack, W. M., and Tam, M. R. (1985). *J. Infect. Dis.*, **152**, 979.
10. Chang, T. H., Tsing, S. Y., and Tzeng, S. (1986). *Hybridoma*, **5**, 43.
11. Bickley, L. S., Krisher, K. K., Punsalang, A. Jr., Trupei, M. A., Reichman, R. C., and Menegus, M. A. (1989). *Sex. Trans. Dis.*, **16**, 127.
12. O'Hara, C. M., Gardener, W. A., and Bennett, B. D. (1980). *Acta Cytol.*, **24**, 448.
13. Lossick, J. G. (1988). *J. Am. Med. Assoc.*, **259**, 1230.
14. Clay, J. C., Veeravahu, M., and Smyth, R. W. (1988). *Genitourin. Med.*, **64**, 115.
15. Thomason, J. L., Gelbart, S. M., Sobun, J. F., Schulien, M. M. B., and Hamilton, P. R. (1988). *J. Clin. Microbiol.*, **26**, 1869.
16. Gelbart, S. M., Thomason, J. L., Osypowski, P. J., James, J. A., and Hamilton, P. R. (1989). *J. Clin. Microbiol.*, **27**, 1095.
17. Diamond, L. S. (1957). *J. Parasitol.*, **43**, 488.
18. Hollander, D. H. (1976). *J. Parasitol.*, **62**, 826.
19. Kulda, J., Honigberg, B. M., Frost, J. K., and Hollander, D. H. (1970). *Am. J. Obstet. Gynecol.*, **108**, 908.
20. Linstead, D. (1989). In *Trichomonads parasitic in humans* (ed. B. M. Honigberg), pp. 91–111. Springer-Verlag, New York.
21. Ackers, J. P. and Yule, A. (1988). In *Immunological diagnosis of sexually-transmitted diseases* (ed. H. Young and A. McMillan), pp. 275–302. Marcel Dekker, New York.
22. Watt, R. M., Philip, A., Wos, S. M., and Sam, G. J. (1988). *J. Clin. Microbiol.*, **24**, 551.
23. Yule, A., Gellan, M. C. A., Oriel, J. D., and Ackers, J. P. (1987). *J. Clin. Pathol.*, **40**, 566.
24. Lisi, P. J., Dondero, R. S., Kwiatkoski, D., Spence, M. R., Rein, M. R., and Alderete, J. F. (1988). *J. Clin. Microbiol.*, **26**, 1684.
25. Carney, J. A., Unadkat, P., Yule, A., Rajakumar, R., Lacey, C. J. N., and Ackers, J. P. (1988). *J. Clin. Pathol.*, **41**, 806.
26. Müller, M. and Gorrell, T. E. (1983). *Antimicrob. Agents Chemother.*, **24**, 667.
27. Lossick, J. G., Müller, M., and Gorrell, T. E. (1986). *J. Infect. Dis.*, **153**, 948.
28. Lossick, J. G. (1989). In *Trichomonads parasitic in humans* (ed. B. M. Honigberg), pp. 324–41. Springer-Verlag, New York.
29. Grossman, J. H. and Galask, R. P. (1990). *Obstet. Gynecol.*, **76**, 521.
30. Müller, M., Lossick, J. G., and Gorrell, T. E. (1988). *Sex. Trans. Dis.*, **15**, 17.
31. Monro, A. M. (1974). *Curr. Med. Res. Opin.*, **2**, 130.
32. Meingassner, J. G. and Heyworth, P. G. (1982). *J. Parasitol.*, **68**, 1163.

33. Mason, P. R. (1985). *J. Parasitol.*, **71**, 128.
34. Honigberg, B. M. (1989). In *Trichomonads parasitic in humans* (ed. B. M. Honigberg), pp. 342–93. Springer-Verlag, New York.
35. Robinson, G. L. (1968). *Trans. R. Soc. Trop. Med. Hyg.*, **62**, 285.
36. Fukushima, T., Mochuzuki, K., Yamazaki, H., Watanabe, Y., Yamada, S., Aoyama, T. *et al.* (1990). *Jikken Dobutsu.*, **39**, 187.

8

Leishmania and *Trypanosoma*

J. E. WILLIAMS

1. Introduction

The genera *Leishmania* and *Trypanosoma* belong to the family Trypanosomatidae of the order Kinetoplastida. All members of this family are parasitic and possess a single locomotory flagellum, which arises from a flagellar pocket. All members of the Kinetoplastida have a DNA-containing organelle, the kinetoplast, which is part of a simple mitochondrion and is located adjacent to the flagellar basal body. Only the *Leishmania* and *Trypanosoma* have species which infect and cause disease in man. Two genera of sandfly act as vectors, *Phlebotomus* in the Old World and *Lutzomya* in the New World.

1.1 Life cycles and morphology

All the Trypanosomatidae undergo replication by simple binary fission and use an invertebrate host as a vector for transmission. They also all undergo morphological changes during their life cycle, either during their development in one host, or during the transition from one host to the other. Not all of the eight morphological forms are found in the two genera discussed here; the ones that are of significance are the amastigotes (*Plate 2e*), promastigotes (*Figure 1*), epimastigotes (*Figure 2*), and trypomastigotes (*Plates 3a*). These terms relate to the position of the kinetoplast to the nucleus, the course of the flagellum along the body, and its point of exit from the body. *Figure 3* is a diagrammatic representation of the four morphological forms and the species they appear in.

2. Leishmaniasis

Leishmaniasis is the disease caused by parasites of the genus *Leishmania*. They form a large group of organisms, infecting diverse vertebrate hosts in many areas of the world. All species are intracellular parasites (amastigotes) within macrophages of mammalian hosts and flagellated extracellular forms (promastigotes) within insect vectors. Two genera of sandfly, *Phlebotomus*

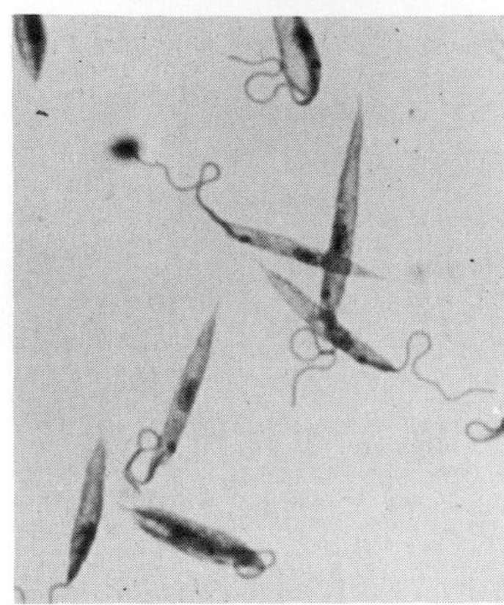

Figure 1. Cultured promastigotes of *L. donovani* (Giemsa stain).

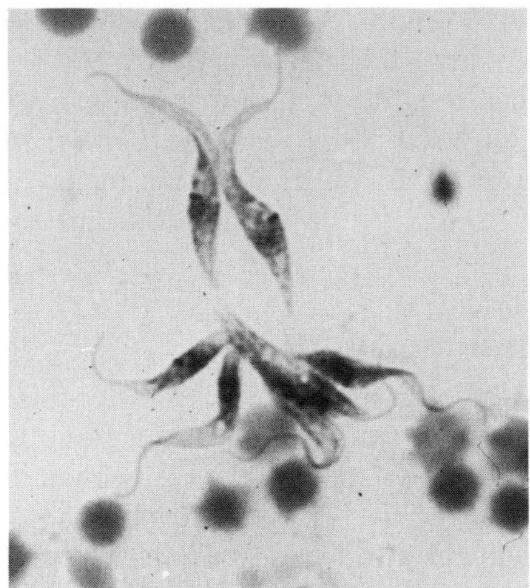

Figure 2. Cultured epimastigotes of *T. cruzi* (Giemsa stain).

and *Lutzomya*, act as vectors in differing areas of the world. The disease in man can be categorized into three main clinical forms: visceral, cutaneous, and muco-cutaneous.

2.1 Visceral leishmaniasis (Kala-azar)

Kala-azar is distributed throughout the tropics and sub-tropics, occurring in most of Asia, China, India, Africa, the Mediterranean area, South and Central America. *Leishmania donovani*, the causative parasite, is a complex of three subspecies:

- *L.(L.) donovani* in East Africa, India, and China

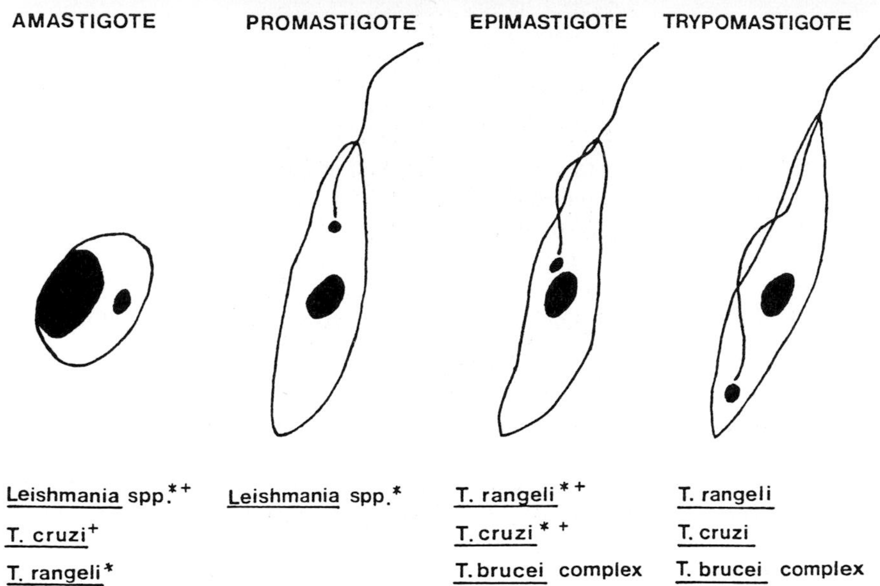

Figure 3. Diagram to show the significant morphological forms of the genera *Leishmania* and *Trypanosoma* and their distribution in man and their vectors.

- *L. (L.) infantum* in West and Central Africa, the Middle East, the Mediterranean area, and China
- *L. (L.) chagasi* in Central and South America

Visceral leishmaniasis is not confined to macrophages at the site of infection, but is a systemic infection of the reticulo-endothelial system and may be found in macrophages associated with all parts of this system. Although skin lesions do not usually occur, it has been recently shown that cutaneous infections with *L. donovani* are possible and number of cases have been associated with HIV infection. Several of these infections have been in patients who have only lived in, or travelled to, countries in the Mediterranean region (1).

2.1.1 Diagnosis

Diagnostic methods can be divided into three categories:

(a) Parasitological diagnosis by demonstration of the parasites using biopsy methods followed by staining and/or culture techniques.
(b) Serological methods.
(c) Molecular techniques using specific kinetoplast DNA (kDNA) or complementary DNA (cDNA) probes.

2.1.2 Parasitological diagnosis

Parasites can be found in samples obtained by marrow aspirate, splenic aspiration, lymph node biopsy and, less commonly, blood. In HIV infected patients with suspected diffuse cutaneous infection, then punch biopsy specimens are best taken and processed as described in *Protocol 6*. Ideally, stained smears (*Protocol 1*) and cultures (*Protocol 2*) should be made from any material obtained by these methods.

i. Splenic aspiration

Although spleen puncture has always been controversial because of the risk of complications, it provides the most accurate method of demonstrating parasites from an infected person. The use of a syringe and fine-bore needle (21G) guided into the anterior surface of the spleen (2), minimizes the danger from tearing of the tissue and subsequent haemorrhage. Part of the contents of the biopsy needle should be expelled on to a clean slide and smeared for staining (*Protocol 1*) and the rest put into NNN culture medium (*Protocol 2*).

ii. Marrow puncture

This method is safer to carry out, but yields far fewer parasites than samples from the spleen. It is not uncommon to fail to demonstrate parasites in stained films from marrow samples, whereas cultures of the marrow, as for splenic specimens, will usually be positive. Smears of the marrow should be made as for normal haematological purposes and stained by *Protocol 1*.

iii. Lymph gland puncture

This has some use in cases exhibiting lymphadenopathy, but as in marrow specimens it is not always possible to demonstrate parasites from these specimens. Culture and stained smears should both be carried out to give the best chance of diagnosis.

iv. Blood buffy coat

It is sometimes possible to isolate parasites from blood, usually from patients with Kala-azar from Kenya and Eastern India. Blood in anticoagulant (type not critical) should be centrifuged (aseptically) at 2000 *g* for 10 min and the cells from the buffy coat removed and used to prepare smears and inoculate cultures.

Amastigotes can be found in the cytoplasm of macrophage cells, or lying free around them. They may be in groups or single and are round ovoid bodies 2–3 μm in size. A definitive diagnosis can only be made if both the nucleus and kinetoplast are seen in the parasite, see *Plate 2e*. There are many other bodies, both artefacts and other organisms, which have a superficial resemblance to amastigotes. Particular care should be taken in immunocompromised patients not to misidentify intracellular *Histoplasma capsulatum* for amastigotes. They are of a similar size, but more solid in appearance and lack the obvious nucleus and kinetoplast, although they often have a number of chromatin-like inclusions, see *Plate 2f*.

Protocol 1. Staining method for biopsy smears

Equipment and reagents

- 10 ml disposable syringe with a 1½″ × 19G dropping needle
- Staining dish or rods
- Methanol (Analar grade)
- Giemsa stain, (BDH) 'R66 improved'
- Buffered distilled water pH 7.2: 3.0 g Na_2HPO_4 anhydrous, 1.2 g $NaH_2PO_4.2H_2O$, made up to 1 litre (or buffer tablets from BDH)

Method

This method can also be used for staining blood smears, gland fluid, and cerebrospinal fluid for the identification of trypanosomes.

1. Ensure smears are completely dry, flood with methanol, and allow to fix for 1–3 min.
2. Draw up 1 ml of Giemsa stain into the syringe, followed by 9 ml of buffered water to give a final dilution of 1:10. Mix, by drawing a small amount of air into the syringe and inverting several times.
3. Shake off excess methanol, no need to dry, and either stain face down in a dish[a] or face up on staining rods for 20 min.[b] Do not overstain else the amastigote morphology will be obscured.
4. Wash the slide briefly in buffered water and drain dry, do not blot.
5. Examine slide using an oil immersion lens (× 50 or × 63 is ideal, if unavailable then × 100). Search the whole of the smear, as only small numbers of parasites may be present.

[a] Staining face down gives better results, as stain precipitate falls away from the specimen and makes subsequent scanning for amastigotes easier.

[b] If staining for trypomastigotes in blood or other samples, then increase time to 30 min. Promastigotes from culture require 15 to 20 min.

Protocol 2. Isolation of *L. donovani* using NNN medium

Equipment and reagents

- Purified agar, e.g. Oxoid purified agar 1.4 g
- Sodium chloride 0.6 g
- Distilled water 90 ml
- 1/4 oz narrow neck McCartney bottles (bijou bottles) or 20 ml Gibco, narrow neck, screw-cap culture tubes
- 250 ml conical flask

Protocol 2. *Continued*

Method

1. Add the ingredients to the conical flask and heat with continuous mixing to prevent the agar from burning.
2. Add 3 ml of agar to bijou bottles or 5 ml of agar to culture tubes.
3. Sterilize the agar by autoclaving bottles or tube at 121 °C for 15 min and allow to cool to approximately 50 °C.
4. Add sterile rabbit blood [a] to each bottle or tube (defibrinated or citrated) to give a final concentration of about 15%. Mix gently and leave to cool in a sloped position. As soon as slope is firm, transfer to refrigerator or ice-bath to produce water of condensation at the bottom of the slope. [b] If not to be used immediately, store at 4 °C.
5. Samples of marrow or other material are inoculated into the condensate at the bottom of the slope. Do not add too much sample to the culture, as this will inhibit growth. Two or three drops only are sufficient and this should be added aseptically.
6. Check cultures for promastigotes after five, seven, and ten days. If no growth is observed, leave for 15 days and subculture into fresh medium and check as before.

[a] If rabbit blood is unavailable, washed cells from other species, supplemented with fetal calf serum, can be used.

[b] Visceral organisms grow much better in a minimal medium than a rich one and NNN, without an enriched overlay, has been shown to be the best one for these organisms.

2.1.3 Serological diagnosis

Specific humoral antibodies are found in cases of visceral leishmaniasis and these allow diagnosis using a variety of methods. The indirect fluorescent antibody test (IFAT) and enzyme-linked immunosorbent assay (ELISA) have been most useful, but recently the direct agglutination test (DAT) has given very good results. The Leishmanin test (a skin test described in *Protocol 3*) is usually negative in active visceral leishmaniasis.

i. IFAT

This test (*Protocol 4*) has the advantage that there is a short-lived antibody response which becomes negative after six to nine months after the patient is cured; also, antibodies are demonstrable very early in the infection and these features make this a useful test for detection of relapses of infection. Titres above 1/20 are significant and above 1/128 are diagnostic. A disadvantage of the test is the difficulty in deciding end-point titres and the possibility of cross-reaction with trypanosomiasis. The use of amastigotes as the antigen, instead of promastigotes prevents this problem.

ii. ELISA

The ELISA test (3) is highly specific (100%) with a sensitivity in excess of 98.0%. The antigen is a preparation of *L. donovani* promastigotes and the test can be carried out on serum or plasma, as well as blood spots collected on to filter paper. This makes it a very useful test for field and survey applications, but problems with false positive reactions make it less useful than the IFAT and DAT for laboratory diagnosis.

iii. DAT

The advantage of the DAT is its simplicity, it requires no sophisticated equipment or special skills; also the reagents are stable and inexpensive, which helps both from a field application and in laboratories which may only carry out a few tests each year. Promastigotes of *L. donovani* are used as antigen and the test can be performed on serum, plasma, blood spots, and whole blood and, as titres are very high, a screening serum dilution of 1/3200 is possible. The test has a high specificity and sensitivity. The original test (4) has been improved (5) and is given in *Protocol 5*.

iv. Interpretation

As with all serological methods, interpretation of results need some caution. Care must be taken to ensure that all necessary controls are carried out, serological, reagent, etc. and that any operator bias or inexperience is controlled. The latter two are particularly important in the IFAT, which can often have difficult end-points. If carrying out single screening dilution tests, as in the DAT, any positive samples should be further diluted and 'titred out' to an end-point to determine the antibody concentration.

One problem with all of these tests is the production of the antigen, it is not commonly commercially available, and more importantly, the **standardization** of the prepared antigen. This should always be carried out against reference positive and negative sera of known titres.

Protocol 3. Leishmanin test

Equipment and reagents

- Cultured promastigotes
- Locke's solution: NaCl 8.0 g, $CaCl_2$ 0.2 g, KCl 0.2 g, Na_2HPO_4 1.24 g, $KHPO_4$ 0.17 g glucose 1.0 g, distilled water to 1 litre pH 7.4
- 0.5% phenol in physiological saline
- 1 ml syringe with 26 gauge intradermal needle

Method

1. Harvest promastigotes from culture and wash five times with cold Locke's solution (see *Protocol 2*).
2. Resuspend in 0.5% phenol saline to give a final count of 10^7 promastigotes/ml.

Protocol 3. *Continued*

3. The test is carried out by giving 0.1 ml of suspension (10^6 promastigotes) intradermally. A control solution of phenol saline should be injected at a neighbouring site at the same time.
4. Read test after 48 and 72 h and record diameter of reaction. A positive test is indicated by an induration 5 mm or larger. The result can be graded into four classes, 5–6 mm, 6–8 mm, >8 mm, and >8 mm plus blister (6). Cross-reaction can occur in patients with leprosy, tuberculosis, and some fungal infections, although these are rare. A positive result shows exposure to leishmanial antigen at some time and is not species-specific. It is of limited use in diagnosis of active infection, although a positive result in children under 12 is suggestive of infection.

Protocol 4. Immunofluorescent antibody test (IFAT)

Equipment and reagents

- Teflon coated multispot slides
- Cultured organisms washed four times in PBS pH 7.2[a]
- Fluorescein labelled anti-human globulin (Wellcome MF 01)
- Evans blue (1:50 000 in PBS)
- Glycerol mountant
- Coplin jar

Method

To prepare antigen slides, dilute washed organisms to 10^7/ml and spot on to slides (5 μl). Dry and fix with methanol for 10 min, and store until required at −20 °C.

1. Remove slide from freezer and allow to come to room temperature in a desiccator.
2. Dilute test and control sera (reference negative and positive), at a screening dilution of 1:30.
3. Add 5 μl of sera to appropriate wells, incubate at room temperature in a moist chamber for 30 min.
4. Wash three times in PBS pH 7.2, 15 min per wash, in a Coplin jar.
5. Drain slide and add 20 μl of anti-human globulin (dilution 1:30) to each well, incubate, and wash as in steps **3** and **4**.
6. Stain in Evans blue for 5 min and wash for 10 min in PBS, dry, and mount with glycerol mountant.

7. Examine using a fluorescent microscope, with fluorescein filter block, using a × 20 objective.

[a] This test can be used for *Leishmania*, *T. b. brucei* complex, and *T. cruzi* by using cultured promastigotes, or the appropriate trypomastigote accordingly, to prepare the antigen slides. Method is the same for each.

Protocol 5. Direct agglutination test for visceral leishmaniasis

Equipment and reagents

- Promastigotes of *L. donovani* grown in a suitable medium to late log phase
- Locke's solution pH 7.7
- 0.4% (v/v) Difco 1:250 trypsin in Locke's solution pH 7.7
- 2.0% (v/v) formalin in Locke's solution
- 1.0% (v/v) formalin in 0.9% (w/v) NaCl
- 0.9% (w/v) NaCl
- Coomassie brilliant blue
- Water-bath at 37 °C
- Magnetic stirrer
- 96-well microtitre plates with V-shaped well
- Diluent, 0.9% (w/v) NaCl containing 1% heat inactivated fetal calf serum

A. *Preparation of antigen*

1. Harvest promastigotes by centrifugation at 4000 *g* for 15 min at 4 °C.
2. Wash five times in Locke's solution, centrifuging at 3200 *g* for 10 min each time.
3. Resuspend final pellet in trypsin solution in ratio of 1 vol. promastigotes to 20 vol. trypsin.
4. Mix well and incubate at 37 °C for 45 min.
5. Spin out of trypsin at 3200 *g* for 10 min, and wash five times as in step **2**.
6. Resuspend pellet in cold Locke's solution to give a concentration of 2 × 10^8 cells/ml.
7. Add an equal volume of 2% formalin in cold Locke's solution and leave at 4 °C overnight.
8. Spin formalized cells at 3200 *g* for 10 min at 4 °C. Wash pellet twice with 0.9% NaCl. Resuspend to same volume as in step **7**.
9. Add Coomassie blue to a final concentration of 0.2% (w/v). Stir at medium speed for 90 min.
10. Spin down after 90 min and wash twice with 0.9% NaCl. Resuspend pellet in 1.0% formalin in 0.9% NaCl to the same volume as step **9**, and store at 4 °C. This is the antigen for the test, keep cool (do not freeze), and protect from light.

Protocol 5. *Continued*

B. *Direct agglutination test*

1. Dilute test serum 1/100 with diluent and add 2-mercaptoethanol to a concentration of 0.2 M. Incubate at 37 °C for 60 min.
2. For a 12 row plate, pipette 50 μl of diluent into all wells except well 2. Pipette 10 μl of diluted test serum into well 2.
3. Transfer 50 μl of well 2 into 3, mix, and carry on doubling dilution to well 12. Discard 50 μl from 12 after mixing.
4. Mix antigen gently and add 50 μl to well 1 (control well), and then to each subsequent well, and mix each time.[a]
5. Cover plate with lid or Saran-wrap, place in a moist chamber, and incubate, at room temperature, for a **minimum** of 24 h.
6. Read result over a white background or light box. End-point titre is the last well where agglutination is seen, i.e. the last well with a **diffuse** suspension, unlike control well which should have a discreet blue 'button' of cells.[b]

[a] Pipette tips can be saved if antigen is added to well 12 first and then the same tip can be used for other wells, i.e. increasing serum concentration.

[b] Plate should be read from directly above against a light background. End-point titres of 1/3200 or greater indicates active disease. Negative samples should give titres less than 1/800. Known positive and negative serum samples should be run on every plate. Fresh batches of antigen should also be standardized against sera of known titre.

2.1.4 Molecular methods of diagnosis

Serological diagnosis of Kala-azar is complicated by cross-reactions with related organisms. Specific diagnosis can be achieved using competition ELISAs with monoclonal antibodies, however, this still does not differentiate between current and past infection. There have been significant advances in the use of restriction endonuclease technology to look at minicircle components of kDNA and nDNA of the trypanosomatids. Barker (7) has reviewed DNA probes and their application to the taxonomy and clinical diagnosis of leishmaniasis.

Ideally, DNA probes used for the diagnosis of visceral infections should possess both high sensitivity and specificity. kDNA probes suffer variable sensitivity, due mainly to the diversity of kDNA within the species and it can be difficult to isolate species-specific kDNA sequences (8). Howard *et al.* (9) have recently described a genomic DNA probe, Lmet2, specific to the *L. donovani* complex. They claim that it is of very high sensitivity and specificity and that it has been used to demonstrate human infection from bone marrow samples (Howard, personal communication). As with all DNA probe tests, it is still a lengthy and complex technique, requiring an autoradiography step to visualize the blots. However work is proceeding which may lead to a simplified PCR-based assay, which would be more useful as a routine diagnostic test. The future clinical value of molecular-based tests is undoubtedly great, particularly if they can be developed to give not only a quick and accurate confirmation of infection, but also differentiation of species as well. At this time, although current research in this field is promising, there are no diagnostic tests suitable for use routinely by laboratories.

2.2 Cutaneous leishmaniasis

This disease is caused by a number of different species of leishmania, having the same life cycle as the visceral species, but being confined to the skin in most cases. There are two forms, Old World cutaneous leishmaniasis and New World (American or neotropical) cutaneous leishmaniasis.

2.2.1 Old World cutaneous leishmaniasis

This is distributed throughout the Eastern Mediterranean, Africa, the Middle East, India, and Asia. In the western areas of the Mediterranean, *L. infantum* can cause cutaneous lesions. Three species are responsible for Old World cutaneous leishmaniasis:

- *L. tropica* in Middle East, Afghanistan, Iran, and USSR
- *L. major* in Middle East, Africa, and India
- *L. aethiopica* in East Africa

2.2.2 Lesions

All Old World lesions are confined to the skin and there is no mucosal involvement. They may be single or multiple and localized to the area of the infected sandfly bite. *L. major* tends to be more acute with rapidly healing lesions; local lymph glands may be involved. In contrast, *L. tropica* is a much more chronic infection.

2.2.3 New World cutaneous leishmaniasis

This disease is caused by leishmanial species belonging to two complexes:

i. L. Mexicana complex

- *L. Mexicana* in Mexico, Guatemala, and Belize
- *L. venezuelensis* in Venezuela
- *L. garnhami* in Venezuela (Andes mountains)
- *L. pifanoi* in Venezuela
- *L. amazonensis* in the Amazon basin

ii. L. braziliensis complex

- *L. braziliensis* in Central and South America
- *L. panamensis* in Panama, Columbia, and Costa Rica

- *L. guyanensis* in northern Amazon basin
- *L. peruviana* in Peruvian Andes

2.2.4 Lesions

There is considerable difference between the lesions produced by the parasites of the *L. braziliensis* complex and those of the *L. mexicana* complex or Old World organisms. Lesions produced by the *L. mexicana* complex are similar to those of *L. major*, with parasites usually being plentiful in the lesion. Infections of the ear with *L. mexicana* often involve necrosis of the cartilage with resultant disfiguration. Lesions produced by *L. braziliensis* differ in several ways. Parasites are typically scanty and difficult to demonstrate with mucosal involvement being a serious complication of this disease, it usually following a papule-like lesion elsewhere on the body and symptoms taking up to several years to develop. The nose and nasal septum are usually involved and the septum can become totally destroyed with, ultimately, destruction of the whole front of the face.

The consideration of the types of lesion and their complications is an important aspect of cutaneous leishmaniasis and those interested should consult *Manson's Tropical Diseases* (10) for a full account.

2.2.5 Diagnosis

Diagnosis depends on the isolation of the parasites, as for the visceral form of the disease, and the use of serological tests, or a combination of the two. It is important to try and make a differential diagnosis between infections with *L. mexicana* organisms and *L. braziliensis*, due to the severity of the complications of the latter. This can be done using cultural characteristics, *L. mexicana* grows readily whilst *L. braziliensis* grows poorly, or by biochemical means. Variation in enzyme structure and its demonstration by electrophoresis (zymodeme analysis) is most useful, although not a routine diagnostic method.

2.2.6 Parasitological diagnosis

Demonstration of amastigotes in lesions require some form of biopsy of the lesion and this can be a simple slit skin scrape or larger punch biopsy specimen. In each case, smears or touch preparations should be made, see *Protocol 6*, and these stained with Giemsa as in *Protocol 1*. At the same time, material should be put into culture as it is often very difficult to demonstrate amastigotes from cutaneous lesions, particularly those of the *L. braziliensis* type. Cutaneous organisms are more fastidious than the visceral ones and a richer medium is usually required for successful isolation. The use of a biphasic medium based on 'Difco' blood agar base is recommended, see *Protocol 7*. Many workers use Schneiders Drosophila Medium (Gibco) which is a commercially available insect culture medium. This is supplemented with 10% to 20% fetal calf serum and may be used to isolate and bulk culture all species of *Leishmania*. It can be variable in performance and the World Health Organization Leishmaniasis Reference Laboratory recommend the 'Difco' blood agar base medium for isolation (11).

Protocol 6. Biopsy methods for cutaneous leishmaniasis

Lesions may be either open (ulcerated) or closed (nodular) and in both cases samples must be taken from the inflamed, swollen edge of the lesion. It is here that there is the greatest chance of finding macrophages containing amastigotes.

A. *Preliminary procedures*

Before any biopsy is performed the following preparation of the area of excision must be carried out.

1. Remove any 'crusty' material from the site and cleanse away any pus.
2. Carefully cleanse the edge of the lesion using a swab soaked in 70% isopropanol or ethanol and allow to dry completely. Do not allow alcohol to enter the open part of the lesion.
3. If an open lesion is secondarily infected with bacteria or fungi, swab with 20 vol. hydrogen peroxide.

B. *Skin punch biopsy*

1. Using the dermatological punch (2–4 mm) or scalpel, remove a small core of tissue from the edge of the lesion, e.g. *L. braziliensis*.
2. Place tissue sample on to a sterile dish and with a sterile scalpel blade, cut the tissue to expose a fresh surface.
3. Blot surface on a sterile gauze and using forceps, touch firmly against a clean glass slide. Make two or three further 'impression smears' (touch preparations). Dry, fix, and stain as in *Protocol 1*.[a]
4. Use remainder of tissue to inoculate a suitable culture medium; rub tissue against the side of culture tube to free amastigotes from the tissue, see *Protocol 7*.

C. *Slit skin method*

1. Firmly pinch the skin of the area to be sampled, between finger and thumb,[b] and with a small scalpel blade make a shallow slit in the pinched skin. Maintain firm pressure.
2. Rotate the scalpel through 90° and with the cutting edge of the blade, scrape the cut edges of the slit in an outward direction.
3. Release the pressure and apply a sterile dressing to the cut surface, maintain pressure until bleeding stops.

Protocol 6. *Continued*

4. Make smears and inoculate a suitable culture medium with material collected.

D. *Aspiration method*

1. Inject 0.1–0.2 ml of sterile saline into the edge of the lesion using a 2 ml syringe and short 20 gauge needle.
2. Rotate the needle when in the skin to cut pieces of tissue around the edge of the needle wound.
3. Aspirate the fluid back into the syringe, removing as much as possible. Minimal blood should be obtained, if fluid contains more than a trace, make another aspiration.
4. Make smears and inoculate cultures.

[a] Blot the tissue to remove as much blood as possible from the cut surface, as too much will reduce chances of finding amastigotes in the touch smears.

[b] Firm pressure is required to keep the area as blood-free as possible whilst taking the specimen.

Protocol 7. Blood agar base medium for the culture of cutaneous *Leishmania* spp.

Equipment and reagents

- Difco blood agar base 8 g (Difco Co. 0045–02–5)
- Distilled water 200 ml
- Defibrinated rabbit blood (sterile)
- 500 ml flask
- 20 ml McCartney bottles

Method

1. Dissolve agar in water by gently heating in a boiling water-bath.
2. Dispense in 5 ml amounts in bottles and autoclave at 121 °C for 15 min.
3. Cool to 50 °C and add 0.6 ml of rabbit blood (aseptically),[a] mix gently. Slope and allow to set.
4. Stand at room temperature for 24 h to allow fluid of condensation to form at bottom of slope.
5. To inoculate, add a small sample of specimen to condensate and incubate at 24 °C.
6. Examine every four days for promastigotes using × 40 objective of microscope, see *Protocol 8*. Subculture negative cultures and examine every four days for a further 20 days.

[a] If possible, it is preferable to avoid using antibiotics in the medium, however, if required, add 200 IU penicillin and 200 μg gentamicin per millilitre of blood. An alternative to gentamicin is 2 mg/ml of streptomycin.

2.2.7 Serological diagnosis

In cases of Old World cutaneous leishmaniasis serological diagnosis is of little use, as few antibodies can be demonstrated. The leishmanin skin test, see *Protocol 3*, becomes positive after three months of the lesion forming and remains positive for life. Care is needed in the interpretation of this test, particularly in patients from areas of high endemicity.

In New World cutaneous leishmaniasis serology is of more use and the IFAT test is at present the test of choice, see *Protocol 4*. Unlike the ELISA, which has problems with false positive reactions and which remains positive long after cure is achieved, the IFAT titres fall after the infection is cured and gives valuable information on the efficacy of treatment. An important differential reaction with the IFAT is the negative results obtained with *L. mexicana* infections, unlike those of *L. braziliensis* which give a positive titre (1/16 to 1/512) in every case. The leishmanin test is positive in all cases.

3. Trypanosomiasis

Trypanosomiasis is the disease caused by organisms of the genus *Trypanosoma* and in man this genus can be further subdivided into two subgenera, each being found in different areas of the world. These are the *Trypanozoon*, found in Africa, and *Schizotrypanum* which occurs in the Americas. Both types have a blood sucking insect as the intermediate host and the parasites undergo a developmental stage in this host. Species of *Glossina* (tsetse flies) act as vectors in Africa and various Reduviid bugs (kissing bugs) in the Americas. Although closely related, the species within these two subgenera have very different life cycles and clinical effects in man. The African form gives rise to a disease known as African trypanosomiasis or 'sleeping sickness' whilst the American form causes American trypanosomiasis or 'Chagas' disease

3.1 African trypanosomiasis

There are two subspecies which are capable of infecting and causing disease in man. They belong to the *Trypanosoma brucei* complex and are *T. b. rhodesiense* and *T. b. gambiense*. Recent work has suggested that *T. b. rhodesiense* may not be different to *T. b. brucei*, which is usually regarded as being infective only to animals. All three subspecies are morphologically indistinguishable, although using isoenzyme analysis, *T. b. gambiense* can be differentiated from the other two. They occur in man only in the trypomastigote stage, see *Plate 3a*, and are found in the blood, lymph, and cerebrospinal fluid, where they multiply by binary fission. There is evidence (12) that they may penetrate and divide inside the ependymal cells of the choroid plexus of the brain and that here they may be protected from the action of trypanocidal drugs.

Although, historically, there was a geographical differentiation between *T. b. rhodesiense* (East African) and *T. b. gambiense* (West African), this is artificial and their distribution overlaps as shown below:

- *T. b. rhodesiense* in Tanzania, Kenya, Malawi, Zimbabwe, Uganda, and parts of Zaire and Congo
- *T. b. gambiense* in West Africa, Zaire, Congo, and Uganda

The course of the infection is similar in both forms. At the site of the infected tsetse bite a local lesion (chancre) often occurs, with a variable period of intermittent fever. This is followed by invasion of the central nervous system (CNS) with a progressive meningo-encephalitis resulting in coma and death, usually from intercurrent infection. In *T. b. rhodesiense* this process is usually acute and rapidly fatal (six to nine months), whilst that of *T. b. gambiense* may be much more chronic (two to five years).

3.1.1 Laboratory diagnosis

If travel history is suggestive of possible exposure to tsetse fly bites, then in both cases, diagnosis is best made by demonstration of the trypomastigotes in the blood or tissue fluids. Depending on the duration of the infection this can be done by puncture of the trypanosomal chancre, blood examination, puncture of enlarged lymph glands, and examination of cerebrospinal fluid, where also the presence of a raised cell count, morula cells, see *Plate 3b*, and a raised IgM are all suggestive of possible trypanosome infection. Serological tests are of limited use, although the IFAT gives high titres in the acute stage and an ELISA test is also available.

i. Trypanosomal chancre

It is more common to find trypanosomal chancres in early infections of *T. b. rhodesiense* and when present, trypanosomes can often be demonstrated in serous fluid aspirated from the chancre. This can be done using a small sterile needle to puncture the side of the chancre after cleaning with an alcohol swab. The wound is squeezed to express some serous fluid on to a microscope slide and this is examined as a wet preparation under the microscope, see *Protocol 8*.

ii. Examination of blood

In the acute stage, especially of *T. b. rhodesiense*, it is possible to detect motile trypanosomes in direct wet blood films examined under the microscope. A drop of blood, either from a capillary sample or venous blood taken into heparin, is placed on to a microscope slide and examined as in *Protocol 8*. More commonly, trypanosomes are difficult to find in the blood and a concentration method must be carried out. A number of methods are available of different sensitivities and technical difficulty. Thick blood smears stained with Giemsa or Fields stain should always be made as for the diagnosis of malaria. Trypanosomes can also be found in the buffy coat (13) of blood spun in microhaematocrit tubes, see *Protocol 9*. This method is approximately five to ten times more sensitive than thick blood smears and is simple to perform in any laboratory. The most sensitive of the blood concentration methods is the 'miniature anion exchange column' method (14) which uses the difference in electrical charge on the surface of the trypanosomes from that of the blood cells to effect a separation on an ion exchange chromatography column. This method is extremely sensitive and is able to detect trypanosome concentrations as low as five to ten organisms per millilitre of blood. The method is given in *Protocol 10*.

iii. Lymph gland puncture

In the early stages of gambiense infection, trypanosomes can often be demonstrated in aspirates of swollen lymph glands, see *Protocol 11*. The glands most commonly involved are the cervical glands in the posterior triangle of the neck (Winterbottom's sign). The technique is only possible early in the infection as at this time they are soft and easy to puncture, later they become much harder and difficult to aspirate. Gland puncture should always be carried out in conjunction with other diagnostic methods to maximize the chances of isolating trypanosomes.

iv. Cerebrospinal fluid

In the later stages of disease elevated concentrations of IgM may indicate typanosomiasis. If CSF examination is performed to demonstrate cerebral involvement this procedure should not be undertaken until blood forms have been looked for. In the absence of trypanosomes in the fluid, a raised white blood cells count ($> 5000/ml$), the presence of morula cells, and raised proteins are all indicative of possible trypanosome infection. In later stages of the disease, significantly raised IgM levels are also very significant. CSF should be taken by the normal method and a sample checked immediately for motile trypanosomes using wet smears, see *Protocol 8*, and a cell count performed. Smears, stained with Giemsa should also be made and checked for both trypanosomes and morula cells.

Protocol 8. Preparation of wet smears and microscopical examination

Equipment

- Clean microscope slides
- Coverslips 22 mm × 22 mm
- Compound microscope

Method

1. Place a small drop of fluid to be examined in the centre of the slide and cover with a coverslip. The drop should be large enough to fill the area of the coverslip without leaving air spaces or flowing beyond the edge.

Protocol 8. *Continued*

2. Examine under a compound microscope using a × 40 objective and either bright-field illumination, with the condenser iris closed down to give maximum contrast, or phase-contrast illumination or, if available, dark-field illumination.
3. If looking at a blood specimen, then the trypanosomes may be difficult to see, however, the violent movement of the RBC's surrounding a trypanosome is obvious and with careful searching it is possible to see the actual trypanosome. Samples with few cells, such as CSF, are best viewed under phase-contrast or dark-field illumination.

Protocol 9. Microhaematocrit tube method

Equipment

- Heparinized or plain capillary haematocrit tubes
- Slide for reading spun tubes, see *Figure 4*
- Haematocrit centrifuge

Method

1. Fill two capillary tubes to within a centimetre of the top and seal the clean end using a sealant such as Cristaseal, plasticine, modelling clay, or by rotating the end in a small flame. Heparinized tubes should be used for capillary blood and plain tubes for blood previously taken into anticoagulant.
2. Centrifuge the tubes in the haematocrit centrifuge for 4 min.
3. Examine the tubes using the prepared slide shown in *Figure 4*. This is made using two strips of plasticine (modelling clay) between which the tube is placed. Put a cover glass over the tube and **gently** press on to the plasticine strips. Fill the space under the cover glass with water.[a]
4. Examine the plasma just above the buffy coat layer using a × 10 or × 20 objective, looking for any signs of motile trypanosomes. Ensure the condenser iris is closed sufficiently to give a good contrast. Roll the tube carefully to search the whole area of the interface and focus up and down to ensure all depths are checked. The trypanosomes are seen as small motile organisms in the clear plasma layer. If suspected organisms are seen they should be viewed using the × 40 objective to exclude artefact results such as platelets undergoing Brownian motion.[b]

[a] Examine tubes within a few minutes of centrifugation as the trypanosomes, if present, soon swim away from the buffy coat interface and become less motile, making them difficult to distinguish. CAUTION. It is possible to cut the tube at the region of the buffy coat and expel the contents on to a slide and stain it to help identification of trypanosomes. **This is a hazardous procedure and is not usually necessary or recommended for diagnosis.**

[b] In endemic areas and occasionally in patients who have spent some time in endemic areas, microfilariae may be present in the tubes and these make it impossible to detect trypanosomes by this method.

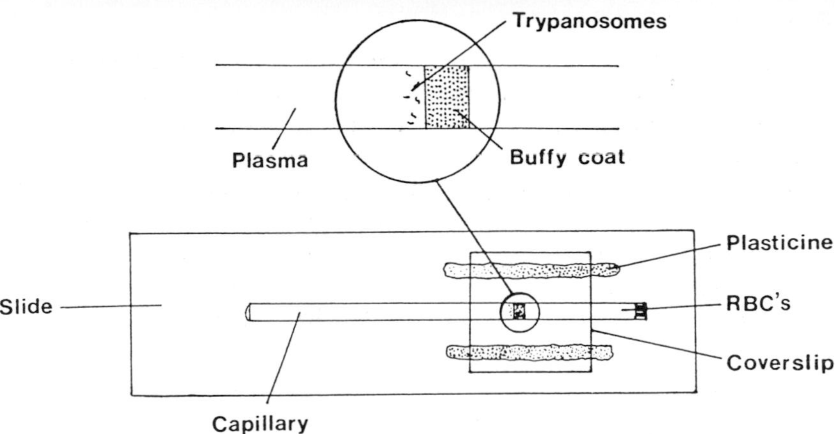

Figure 4. Diagram of a viewing slide for the microhaematocrit tube method of diagnosis of trypanosomes in blood.

Protocol 10. Mini anion exchange column technique

This method (14) relies on the difference in surface charge on the trypanosomes and the host blood cells. Preparation of the cellulose medium must be carried out exactly as described or else the column will fail and either the trypanosomes will be retained on the column and not detected or, red blood cells will be allowed to pass through the column and mask any trypanosomes in the collecting tube.

Equipment and reagents

- 25 g diethylaminoethyl–cellulose (pre-swollen), DEAE 52 (Whatman Ltd. 4057–050)
- PBS-G 4:6, pH 8.0 buffer: Na_2HPO_4 anhyd. 5.4 g, $NaH_2PO_4.2H_2O$ 0.31 g, NaCl 1.7 g, D(+) glucose 26.0 g, made up to 1 litre with distilled water, check pH 8.0 + 0.05
- 1/20 orthophosphoric acid
- 250 ml tall glass beaker
- 25 ml glass Universal bottles (wide-neck McCartney bottles)
- 2 ml plastic syringe
- Cork borer with same diameter as internal diameter of syringe
- Glass Pasteur pipettes
- Collecting pipette made by pulling a fine tip in the end of a glass Pasteur, see *Figure 5*
- Cellulose sponge (type used for dish-washing is ideal)
- Plastic automatic pipette tip (large)
- Bench centrifuge

A. *Preparation of chromedia*

1. Place cellulose in beaker and add 100 ml of PBS-G buffer. Mix well and allow to settle for 20 min, then suck off or decant the supernatant containing any fine particles of cellulose.
2. Repeat washing four times using fresh buffer.
3. After the fifth wash, resuspend in buffer and adjust to pH 8.0, if required,

Protocol 10. *Continued*

using orthophosphoric acid. Do this slowly with constant mixing—**do not overshoot**. Allow to settle.

4. Discard most of the supernatant, leave enough buffer to make a thick slurry that will pour, mix thoroughly, and dispense into approximately 10 ml aliquots in glass 25 ml Universal bottles.
5. Store at −20 °C until required. Thaw in warm water immediately before use and mix well. Store similar aliquots of PBS-G buffer, for running the columns, in the same manner.

B. *Preparation and running of the column*

1. Using a cork borer, cut a piece of sponge so that it is a tight fit inside the barrel of the syringe and push to the bottom of the barrel.
2. Run 1 ml of PBS-G through the sponge to wet it and allow to drain.
3. Shake the cellulose (DE 52) to resuspend it and using a Pasteur pipette load into the barrel up to the 2 ml mark. Allow buffer to drain and cellulose to pack.
4. Run 2 ml of PBS-G through column and when surface is just dry, add 100–150 μl of sample blood (this can be collected by finger prick into a heparinized capillary tube).
5. Allow blood to absorb on to column and then place collecting pipette in position under syringe barrel, see *Figure 5*. Add a few drops of PBS-G to the top of the column.
6. Attach reservoir pipette to the top of the syringe using the rubber plunger taken from the syringe piston, see *Figure 5*, fill with PBS-G, and leave to run.
7. When collecting pipette is full, this should take about 4 min, remove and centrifuge for 10 min at 1600 *g*.
8. Remove plastic tip and place on viewing slide, see *Figure 5*, and examine tip for trypanosomes

Protocol 11. Examination of lymph gland aspirates

Equipment and reagents

- Disposable syringe, 2 ml or 5 ml
- 18 G hypodermic needle
- Sterile 0.9% NaCl
- Alcohol swab
- Slides and coverslips

Method

1. Rinse the syringe with sterile NaCl and draw back the plunger about half-way.

2. Palpate the swollen gland and firmly, without undue pressure, bring it towards the surface of the skin and immobilize.
3. Cleanse the surface with the alcohol swab and allow to dry.
4. Holding the gland firmly, insert the needle, without the syringe attached, into the gland ensuring it penetrates into the centre.
5. Keeping the needle as still as possible, to avoid excessive pain, gently massage the gland to allow fluid to enter the needle. Still holding the gland withdraw the needle.
6. Hold the needle over a slide and attach prepared syringe, then expel the contents of the needle on to the slide and cover with a coverslip.
7. Place a sterile dressing on the wound.
8. Examine the slide immediately for motile trypanosomes, using the × 40 objective of the microscope and phase-contrast illumination or if unavailable, with the condenser iris closed down to give a good contrast.

3.2 American trypanosomiasis (Chagas' disease)

This disease is caused by infection with *Trypanosoma cruzi* and human infection is widespread throughout Central and Southern America, with an estimated 20 million people infected. Although large numbers are infected, many people have little or no symptoms of disease. The highest incidence of severe disease occurs in southern Peru, Bolivia, Paraguay, Uruguay, northern Argentina, and southern Brazil. No Chagas' disease is found in the Amazon basin.

In man *T. cruzi* exists in the blood as the trypomastigote form, and as intracellular amastigotes in the tissues. The trypomastigotes are typically C-shaped with a large kinetoplast and free flagellum, see *Plate 3c*. The amastigotes are similar to those of the leishmanias and are found in pseudocysts in various muscles of the body, particularly heart muscle and the smooth muscle of the gut, see *Plate 3d*. In these sites, *T. cruzi* may cause damage due to humoral and cell-mediated responses to parasites liberated from pseudocysts. This can result in a variety of cardiac symptoms and in some cases damage to the autonomic nerve ganglia of the smooth muscle of the intestine resulting in mega syndrome. The disease runs an acute and chronic course. The majority of infections enter a chronic phase but death can ensue during the early acute phase, particularily in children.

3.2.1 Laboratory diagnosis

When considering a possible infection with *T. cruzi*, history of travel to endemic areas, exposure to Reduviid bugs, or possible blood contamination (e.g. transfusion) should be sought. Laboratory diagnosis of *T. cruzi* by

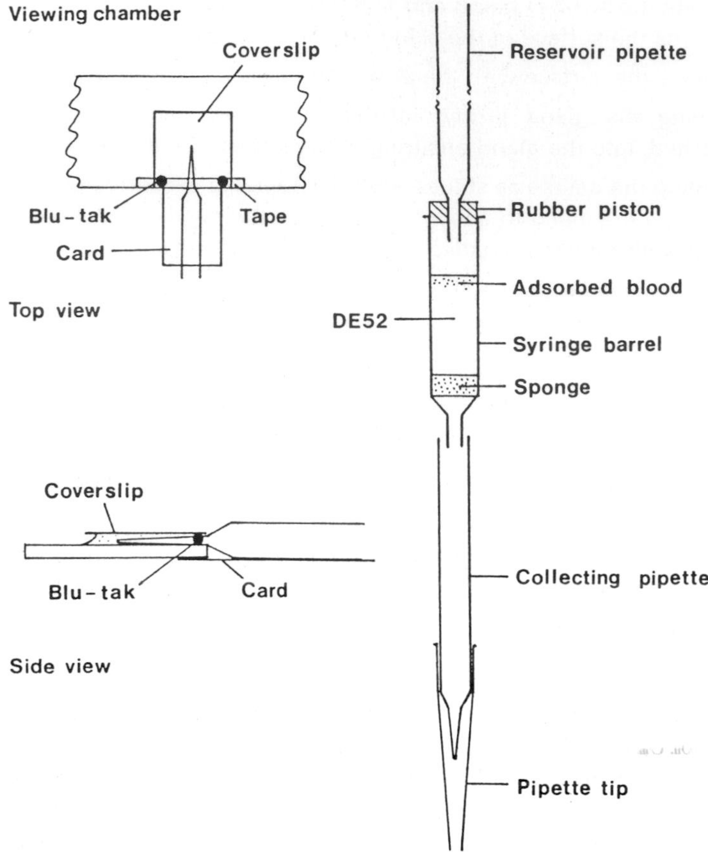

Figure 5. Diagram of the mini anion exchange column and viewing slide.

demonstration of the trypomastigotes in blood can only be made during the early acute phase of the infection as they soon disappear as the parasites enter the tissues. However, blood should always be checked, as during the acute phase it is possible to give effective treatment which may prevent later cardiac damage. Various concentration methods can be employed, including xenodiagnosis and blood culture. Serological methods are important in the confirmation of *T. cruzi* infection.

i. Examination of blood

Trypomastigotes of *T. cruzi* are fragile and thick blood films are not advised. Wet blood films (*Protocol 8*) should be carefully checked for motile trypanosomes and the haematocrit method (*Protocol 9*) is also useful. If motile trypanosomes are found, it is important to make a stained preparation of the sample to exclude the possibility that they may be *T. rangeli*, a non-

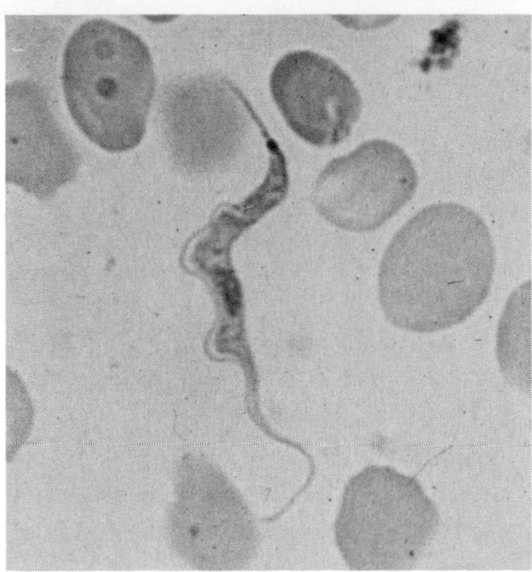

Figure 6. Trypomastigote of *T. rangeli* in human blood (Giemsa stain).

pathogenic trypanosome, transmitted by triatomine bugs and capable of infecting man. They are more slender than *T. cruzi* with a small kinetoplast and an anteriorly placed nucleus, see *Figure 6*.

ii. Xenodiagnosis

This is a good method of detecting trypanosomes during the chronic phase of the infection. Uninfected, triatomine bugs are fed on the patient and the recta examined several weeks later (*Protocol 12*). If trypanosomes had been ingested during the blood meal, epimastigotes and trypomastigotes will be found in the rectal contents. This is a sensitive method of diagnosis, as the bugs are very susceptible to infection, although this does vary from species to species of bug.

iii. Blood culture

When facilities for xenodiagnosis are not available, blood culture (*Protocol 13*), can be used to demonstrate infection during the chronic phase. This method has some disadvantages including the long period often required before cultures become positive, and the need to maintain aseptic conditions to prevent contamination of the cultures. Epimastigotes grow in positive cultures and these may be preceded by immotile amastigote forms.

iv. Serology

When parasites can not be found in blood, serology is a valuable technique for the diagnosis of Chagas' disease. Infection is lifelong, hence antibodies can always be demonstrated. IFAT (*Protocol 4*) and ELISA (*Protocol 14*) are most useful and antibodies can be demonstrated one month after infection. The antigen used in these tests is difficult and hazardous to prepare.

Protocol 12. Xenodiagnosis

Equipment

- Five to ten laboratory reared, uninfected, fifth stage nymphs of *Rhodnius prolixus, Triatoma infestans,* or earlier instars of *Dipetalogaster maxima.* Bugs should be starved for 14 days before use. Bugs can usually be obtained from a local tropical medicine institute or university entomology department.
- Suitable container to put feeding bugs in, covered with a double layer of well secured gauze
- Black cloth to cover container during feeding

Method

1. It is extremely important to explain to the patient what is about to happen and reassure them it will not be painful.
2. Securely strap the container of bugs to the forearm of the patient and cover with the cloth. Leave for 30 min.[a]
3. Remove container and keep in a secure place for 28 days.
4. Examine the rectal contents of each bug for motile epimastigotes or trypomastigotes, using the × 40 objective of a microscope and a wet preparation (*Protocol 8*). This can be done by killing the bug with chloroform and dissecting the gut out, or by gently squeezing the abdomen of the bug with a pair of forceps and expressing the faeces on to a slide with a little saline. For **safety** reasons this operation should be carried out behind a Perspex screen or in a safety cabinet, as the parasites are highly infectious either via a cut or the conjunctiva.
5. If positive, prepare Giemsa stained smears and check that flagellates are those of *T. cruzi* and not *T. rangeli*, which may also be present; epimastigotes of *T. rangeli* are longer and more slender than those of *T. cruzi.*

[a] Try to ensure that the patient does not see the bugs before or during feeding, as this can be very traumatic.

Protocol 13. Blood culture to detect *T. cruzi*

Equipment and reagents

- Culture media: Bacto blood agar base 14.0 g (Difco Co. 00450), Bacto tryptose 5.0 g (Difco. Co. 0124-01), purified agar 3.0 g (Oxoid L28), sodium chloride 6.0 g, distilled water to 1 litre
- 2 litre flask
- Defibrinated rabbit blood, heat inactivated at 56°C for 30 min
- NaCl 0.9 g/litre (sterile) containing 400 IU/ml each of penicillin and streptomycin

Method

1. Dissolve the media components by heating gently in the flask, mix, and dispense in 4 ml amounts in culture tubes (any available type).
2. Autoclave at 121 °C for 20 min, cool to 50 °C, and add 0.3 ml of blood to each tube. Slope and allow to set.
3. Add to each tube 1.0 ml of sterile NaCl containing 400 IU penicillin/ml and 400 IU streptomycin/ml.
4. Test for sterility by incubating at 28 °C for 48 h, store at 4 °C.
5. To use, inoculate 0.2 ml of patient blood into a tube and incubate at 28°C for 14 to 21 days. Examine after 14 days and then every 7 days for 35 days using a microscope, for motile epimastigotes of *T. cruzi*, see *Figure 2*.

Protocol 14. *T. cruzi* ELISA (15)

Equipment and reagents

- ELISA plates (Dynatech Ltd)
- Coating buffer pH 9.6: Na_2CO_3 1.59 g, $NaHCO_3$ 2.93 g, NaN_3 0.2 g, made up to 1 litre with distilled water
- PBS–Tween: PBS + 0.05% Tween-20
- ELISA substrate buffer pH 5.0: 24.3 ml citric acid (19.2 g/100 ml), 25.7 ml phosphate (28.4 g Na_2HPO_4/100 ml), 50 ml distilled water—immediately before use dissolve 40 mg of *ortho*-phenylenediamine (Sigma) in the above, followed by 40 μl 30% H_2O_2
- Skimmed milk powder or bovine serum albumen
- Peroxidase labelled, anti-human globulin
- 2.5 M sulfuric acid, **take care, corrosive**
- ELISA reader

Method

1. Culture *T. cruzi*, harvest and wash in PBS, adjust to 5 × 10^6/ml in coating buffer, freeze-thaw in liquid nitrogen, and sonicate (3 × 30 sec on ice). Put 100 μl of sonicate in each well and incubate at 4 °C overnight.
2. Empty wells, fill with PBS–Tween, leave for 3 min, repeat three times.
3. Block by adding 150 μl of 1% milk powder in PBS–Tween to each well, incubate at 37 °C for 1 h.
4. Wash as in step **2**.
5. Add 100 μl of patient serum and control sera to relevant wells, and incubate for 2 h at room temperature.[a]
6. Wash as in step **2**.
7. Add 100 μl of freshly diluted conjugate and incubate at room temperature for 2 h.
8. Wash as in step **2**.

Protocol 14. *Continued*

9. Add 100 μl of freshly made substrate and incubate for 30 min, at room temperature, in the dark.
10. Stop reaction with 50 μl of 2.5 M H_2SO_4.
11. Read visually or in an ELISA multiscan (Flow laboratories).

[a] Serum samples should be diluted 1:200, as titres can go down to 1:10^6. Positives should be defined at a cut-off of 3 × O.D. of the control, but a standard chequerboard should be carried out with control sera and antigen (16).

References

1. Alvar, J., Blasquez, J., and Najera, R. (1989). *J. Infect. Dis.*, **160**, 560.
2. Kager, P. A., Rees, P. H., Manguyu, F. M., Bhatt, K. M., and Bhatt, S. M. (1983). *J. Geogr. Med.*, **35**, 125.
3. Hommel, M., Peters, W., Ranque, J., Quilici, M., and Lanotte, G. (1978). *Ann. Trop. Med. Parasitol.*, **72**, 213.
4. Harith, A. E., Kolk, A. H. J., Kager, P. A., Leeuwenburg, J., Muigai, R., Kuigu, S., *et al.* (1986). *Trans. R. Soc. Trop. Med. Hyg.*, **80**, 583.
5. Harith, A. E., Kolk, A. H. J., Leeuwenburg, J., Faber, J., Muigai, R., Kuigu, S., *et al.* (1988). *J. Clin. Microbiol.*, **26**, 1321.
6. Pampiglione, S., Manson-Bahr, P. E. C., LaPlaca, M., Borgarth, M. A., and Musumeci, S. (1975). *Trans. R. Soc. Trop. Med. Hyg.*, **69**, 60.
7. Barker, D. C. (1989). *Parasitology*, **99**, 560.
8. Smith, D. F., Searles, S., Ready, P. D., Gramiccia, M., and Ben-Ismail, R. (1989). *Mol. Biochem. Parasitol.*, **37**, 213.
9. Howard, K. M., Kelly, J. M., Lane, R. P., and Miles, M. A. (1991). *Mol. Biochem. Parasitol.*, **12**, 313.
10. Manson-Bahr, P. E. C. and Bell, D. R. (ed.) (1987). *Manson's tropical diseases.* Baillière Tindall, London.
11. Evans, D. A. (ed.) (1989). *Handbook on the isolation, characterisation and cryopreservation of Leishmania.* UNDP/World Bank/WHO Special Programme, Geneva.
12. Ormerod, W. E. (1979). In *Biology of the Kinetoplastida* (ed. W. H. R. Lumsden and D. A. Evans), Vol. 2. London: Academic Press.
13. Woo, P. T. K. (1970). *Acta Trop.*, **27**, 384.
14. Lumsden, W. H. R., Kimber, C. D., Evans, D. A., and Doig, S. J. (1979). *Trans. R. Soc. Trop. Med. Hyg.*, **73**, 312.
15. Voller, A., Bidwell, D. E., and Bartlett, A. (1975). *Lancet*, **1**, (7904) 426.
16. Voller, A., Bidwell, D. E., and Bartlett, A. (1980). In: *Manual of clinical immunology* (ed. R. N. Rose and H. Friedman), pp. 359. Washington DC: American Society of Microbiology.

9

Migrating worms

S. H. GILLESPIE

1. *Toxocara canis*

1.1 Life cycle and morphology

Toxocara canis is an ascarid parasite of canids. In the dog, ingested eggs hatch in the stomach and invade the intestinal wall where larvae are carried to the liver and are distributed to the body via the bloodstream. Lung migration occurs and larvae are coughed up and swallowed, where larvae develop into adult worms in the intestines of the dog. Eggs passed in the faeces may or may not be fertilized (*Plates 3e,f* and *4a*). This life cycle occurs mainly in younger dogs; over the age of six months, larval development is halted at the L_2 stage and larvae migrate in the tissues before becoming dormant. In pregnant bitches, larvae are activated and migrate transplacentally to infect the pups after the 42nd day of gestation. In consequence, almost all pups are infected at the time of whelping (1).

To be infective, eggs must undergo a period of maturation in the soil which takes between 10 and 14 days (*Plate 3f*). *Toxocara* eggs remain viable in the soil for morc than two years. Human infection occurs via the ingestion of embryonated eggs. The eggs hatch normally in the stomach and invade the intestine, but, as in the case of adult dogs and other non-canid hosts, larval development is halted at the L_2 stage, and they continue to migrate in the tissues.

Toxocara larvae produce a complex mixture of glycoprotein antigens, the excretory—secretory antigens (ES). These antigens have complement fixing, anti-cholinesterase, and proteinase activity (2). The inflammatory response is largely directed against ES antigens and this is thought to be responsible for the clinical syndromes associated with *Toxocara* infection.

1.2 Visceral larva migrans

The syndrome of visceral larva migrans occurs when the parasitic larvae, unable to complete their life cycle, migrate within the human host. Although many different genera have been associated with visceral larva migrans, numerically, *T. canis* is the most important pathogen. Current serodiagnostic tests do not distinguish between antibodies to *T. canis* and *T. cati*, however epidemiological data indicates that it is the dog parasite which is most often implicated in human infections (3).

The major clinical syndrome associated with *Toxocara* infection is visceral larva migrans, characterized by fever, malaise, cough, bronchospasm, hepatosplenomegaly, and lymphadenopathy. There is an association between epileptic seizures and seropositivity, although a causal relationship has not been proved.

1.3 Ocular toxocariasis

Single larvae may become trapped in the retina and the subsequent inflammation may result in significant visual loss. This is usually unilateral, but 1%–3% of cases are bilateral. Ocular toxocariasis may present as endophthalmitis, retinal granuloma, retinal detachment caused by fibrotic traction bands, unilateral pars palanitis, and uveitis (4). Infection with *Toxocara* may also be completely asymptomatic, the infection only coming to light as part of the investigation of eosinophilia.

Toxocariasis may also present to the clinician among children who have recently ingested potentially contaminated soil or canine faeces. Patients ingesting canine faeces should be reassured as *Toxocara* eggs require a period of embryonization in the soil before they become infective. In the case of soil ingestion, as infection can be transmitted in this situation, acute and convalescent serum may be taken to demonstrate seroconversion. Should seroconversion occur, the parent should be reassured as most patients who are infected with toxocariasis have mild, transient, or no symptoms.

1.4 Diagnostic tests

Since *T. canis* is unable to complete its life cycle in the human host, the examination of faeces for the presence of eggs is not diagnostic. A definitive diagnosis can be made by examination of tissue biopsy. However, in the case of both ocular toxocariasis and visceral larva migrans, biopsy material rarely becomes available. Moreover, multiple tissue sections are required before evidence of parasitic infection is found, thus this method of diagnosis can not be recommended (5). In consequence, serology forms the mainstay of the diagnosis of toxocariasis. A wide-range of serological techniques and parasite antigens have been used for the serological diagnosis of toxocariasis. Skin testing proved highly specific, but has a low sensitivity and, as toxocariasis principally affects children, it is not the method of choice. Serological techniques using *Toxocara* adult worm extract (6) or *Toxocara* egg antigen, cross-react with antibodies from other ascarid parasites (7). *T. canis* ES antigen is most frequently used as the capture antigen (8). Although there is cross-reaction with *T. cati*, there is minimal cross-reaction with other helminthic parasites. This antigen is also readily obtainable as *T. canis* larvae may be maintained in serum-free medium for periods of more than one year, during which period excretory–secretory antigen is produced. The method for hatching *T. canis* larvae is outlined in *Protocol 1* and the method for purifying *Toxocara* excretory–secretory antigen is detailed in *Protocol 2*. The use of this antigen in an ES antibody capture ELISA is described in *Protocol 3*.

Protocol 1. Hatching of *Toxocara canis* eggs

Equipment and reagents

- RPMI medium with added Hepes buffer (Gibco), Hank's balanced salt solution, 100 IU penicillin/ml, streptomycin 250 μg/ml
- Tissue homogenizer
- Benchtop centrifuge
- Sterilized Baermann apparatus consisting of a cotton wool plug in a tea strainer placed over a sterilized 500 ml beaker
- Sterile Petri dishes
- Microscope
- Sterile Universal containers
- Sodium hypochlorite solution (14% available chlorine)
- Scalpel
- Forceps

Method

1. Identify female *T. canis* adult worms using *Figure 1*.
2. Store the adult females for at least one month in 5% formalin to allow maturation of the eggs (*Figure 1*).
3. Make central incision and express some fluid.
4. Examine using the ×10 and ×40 objective and the stage micrometer (Page 79–81) confirming the identity as *T. canis* on the basis of size and characteristic morphology (*Plates 3 e,f, and 4a*).
5. Homogenize the adult female using a mechanical tissue homogenizer (e.g. Model L2R, Silverson Machines Ltd, Buckinghamshire, UK).
6. Wash by centrifugation in distilled water.
7. Mix the deposit with an equal volume of sodium hypochlorite (14% available chlorine), and incubate for 5 min at room temperature.
8. Add distilled water to make up the volume to 20 ml and centrifuge at 1000 *g* for 8 min. Wash again with distilled water.
9. Transfer the deposit to the Baermann apparatus and incubate overnight in a 37 °C water-bath. Viable larvae migrate through the cotton wool and are collected in the base of the container. Excess RPMI is carefully aspirated and discarded. The larvae are carefully transferred to new culture medium and incubated at 37 °C.
10. Cultures can be maintained for antigen production for more than 18 months. Culture tubes should be examined weekly and passaged providing viability is > 95%. If not, viable larvae can be harvested by following the procedure from step **9**.

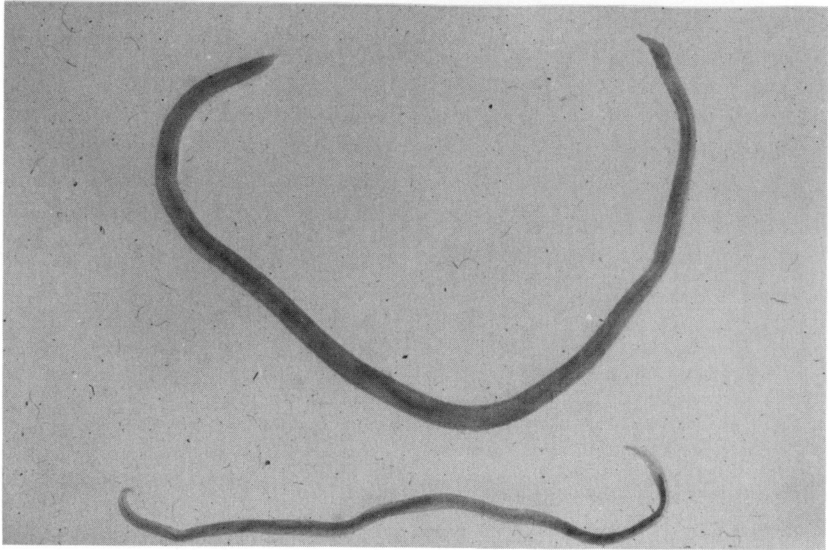

Figure 1. Adult *Toxocara,* the larger worm is the female.

Protocol 2. Purification of excretory–secretory (ES) antigens

Equipment and reagents

- Spent medium from continuous culture of *T. canis*
- Ultrafiltration cell
- Ultrafiltration membrane
- Supply of nitrogen gas
- Beakers, sterile Universals, silicone tubing
- Freeze-dryer
- Benchtop centrifuge
- 0.45 μm filter
- Dialysis tubing

Method

1. 100–200 ml of spent medium from continuous culture of L_2 larvae of *T. canis* is collected. Medium may be stored at −20 °C while an adequate volume is collected.
2. Centrifuge at ~4000 *g* and filter sterilize using 0.45 μm filter.
3. Assemble the ultrafiltration cell (Amicon) using a filter with a molecular exclusion of 10 000 Dalton (YM10).
4. Ultrafilter the spent medium using a nitrogen supply at low pressure sufficient to maintain a steady rate of filtration.
5. Collect the concentrated medium containing ES antigen and dialyse against several changes of distilled water. You will know the dialysis is complete when the concentrate is completely clear.
6. Further concentration is achieved by freeze-drying.

Protocol 3. Anti-toxocara ES IgG antibody ELISA

Equipment and reagents

- Freeze-dried ES antigen concentrate (from *Protocol 2*)
- Microtitre ELISA plates
- Control sera: standardization control, negative control, positive control
- Horse-radish peroxidase-conjugated anti-human IgG monoclonal antibody
- ATBS substrate (2,2′-azino-di-3-ethyl-benzthioazoline sulfonate) (Kirkegaard-Perry)
- Microtitre ELISA reader
- Automatic pipettes, microcentrifuge tubes, plastic tips, etc.
- Humidified chamber
- Phosphate-buffered saline with 0.05% Tween-20
- Phosphate-buffered saline with 0.5% bovine serum albumin
- Bicarbonate buffer 0.06 M, pH 9.6

Method

1. ES antigen solution is made in bicarbonate buffer at a concentration determined previously by chequerboard titration.
2. Plates are coated by adding 100 μl/well of ES antigen solution and incubating overnight at 4°C. Two wells are left uncoated as blocking controls.
3. Wells are washed four times with PBS–Tween.
4. Plates are blocked with PBS plus 1% bovine serum albumin either by incubation overnight at 4°C or for 2 h at room temperature.
5. Wells are washed four times with PBS–Tween.
6. Test and control serum diluted 1:100 is added in 100 μl volumes to wells and incubated in a humidified chamber for 1 h.
7. After washing as before HRP-conjugated anti-human IgG monoclonal antibody is added at the optimum dilution previously defined by chequerboard titration and incubated for 1 h.
8. ATBS substrate is added according to manufacturers' instructions and incubated in the humidified chamber until the positive control reaches on O.D. of 0.75. Optical density is read at 405 nm.
9. Results are calculated as follows: results between plates are adjusted to reduce plate-to-plate variation by multiplying all values obtained by the ratio of the values obtained for the standardization controls. Positive results are defined on the basis of a cut-off equal to three standard deviations above the mean value for a series of control negatives.

1.4.1 Toxocara ES ELISA test

ES antibody capture ELISA is the most widely accepted test for the sero-diagnosis of toxocariasis. The major disadvantage of this method is that it is unable to distinguish old from recent infection. Although a decline in antibody with time after acute infection can be inferred from the difference in the prevalence of toxocariasis in adult and child populations (8, 9), antibody concentration cannot be used to differentiate old and new infection. Ocular infection is, however, associated with lower antibody concentrations and when this diagnosis is likely, a titred assay should be performed (10).

Several attempts have been made to develop a *Toxocara* antigen detection ELISA, and such a system has been successfully applied in the dog (11). Similar systems for use in human diagnosis have failed to live up to their early promise (12, 13).

Clinical laboratories may be requested to perform soil surveys to establish the degree of contamination of public areas with *T. canis* eggs. Soil contamination is related to local veterinary practices with regard to worming and standards of hygiene for domestic dogs. Seroprevalence rates in children are probably broadly related to the level of soil contamination. However, it is impossible to assess the risk of acquiring toxocariasis in a public place on the basis of a single soil survey. Thus, such surveys should only be performed to identify high risk areas or to monitor the effects of control measures. At least 50 g of topsoil should be collected, the specimen numbered, and the position of sample marked on a sampling map. Optimal yield of *Toxocara* eggs can be obtained using a magnesium sulfate flotation technique, which is described in *Protocol 4* (14).

Several reports have been published detailing IgE-specific ES antibody capture ELISAs. Where comparison has been published good agreement has been observed between results in the IgG antibody capture ELISA, and positive results obtained in cases of ocular toxocariasis when IgG concentrations are low.

Protocol 4. Detection of *Toxocara canis* in environmental samples

Equipment and reagents

- Sterile containers
- Site map
- Large sieve pore size 4 mm
- 0.0025% (v/v) Tween-20 solution
- Saturated magnesium sulfate solution
- Tissue homogenizer
- Benchtop centrifuge
- Stage micrometer

Method

1. 25 g of soil is passed through the sieve to remove stones and other solid objects.
2. 100 ml Tween-20 solution is added to each specimen which is then homogenized using a tissue homogenizer for 5 min.
3. The sample is then centrifuged at ~ 2500 *g* for 10 min and the supernatant discarded.
4. The deposit is resuspended in a saturated solution of $MgSO_4$ and this mixture centrifuged at ~ 2500 *g* for 10 min.

5. The centrifuge tube is then topped up with additional $MgSO_4$ and a coverslip placed on top. This is left to stand for at least 5 min, but not more than 15 min.
6. The coverslip is transferred to a microscope slide and examined using the × 10 objective and the stage micrometer. *T. canis* ova are identified on the basis of size and typical morphology (*Plate 3e* and *f*).

2. *Strongyloides stercoralis*

2.1 Life cycle

S. stercoralis is unusual among metazoan parasites in that it is capable of completing its life cycle within the human host and thus, in certain circumstances, capable of causing overwhelming infection. The aetiological agent of strongyloidiasis was first identified by Normand in the intestinal wall of five soldiers who had died of uncontrolled diarrhoea in Cochin-China in 1876. The genus *Strongyloides* has two recognized human pathogenic species: *S. stercoralis* and *S. fuelleborni*.

S. stercoralis is adapted to the moist tropics with a similar distribution to human hookworms and can be found in Africa, Asia, and South America. *S. fuelleborni* is found as an intestinal parasite in chimpanzees and African baboons. Human infections have been reported from the Philippines, Papua New Guinea, and East and Central Africa (15).

Parasitic females are found in the mucosal epithelium of the small intestine where they lay thin-walled eggs which hatch in the intestinal epithelium. The rhabditoid larvae migrate into the lumen and are discharged in the faeces. In soil with an excess of moisture rhabditoid larvae develop in one of two ways: through the rhabditiform L_2 stage into the infective filariform L_3 larvae which are capable of invading intact skin. In tissue it undergoes a heart–lung migration developing to the adult stage in the small intestine and thus completing the life cycle. It may also develop through a free-living cycle where under appropriate conditions transformation into filariform larvae may occur and the parasitic cycle re-entered. *Strongyloides* infection in the human host can be maintained by filariform larvae penetrating intact skin, by the auto-infection cycle where rhabditiform larvae develop into filariform larvae in faecal material on the perianal skin, or where rhabditiform develop into filariform larvae in the intestine and penetrate the gut wall. The auto-infection cycle is probably the mechanism whereby the parasite is able to maintain itself in the host for prolonged periods. Active *Strongyloides* infection has been found in approximately 8% of prisoners of war taken by the Japanese more than 40 years later (16). It is also crucial in the hyperinfection syndrome where uncontrolled auto-infection leads to production of massive numbers of larvae which penetrate every organ of the body.

2.2 Clinical syndromes

Strongyloides is well adapted to the human host, only causing disease under certain circumstances. The initial penetration by filariform larvae is not known to be associated with cutaneous reaction. It may be that with frequent exposure through auto-infection that sensitization occurs leading to the symptoms associated with larva currens. The term larva currens (which means 'running larva') describes the cutaneous reaction to the migration of a single *Strongyloides* larva which progresses through the skin at approximately 10 cm/h. There are two zones: the zone of progression which is red, raised, and itchy, and the zone of resolution which is broader (12 mm rather than the narrower 2 mm progression zone), red, but not raised. The lesions may last for 12–48 hours, resolving with no sequelae. During intestinal infection, patients may complain of symptoms resembling peptic ulceration associated with malaise, abdominal pain, and diarrhoea.

The hyperinfection syndrome occurs when the host immune defence fails to such an extent that the auto-infection cycle continues in an uncontrolled manner. This syndrome arises usually when patients are treated with immunosuppressing agents such as corticosteroids or cytotoxic drugs, but may arise due to immunosuppressing conditions such as malignant disease, protein-calorie malnutrition, and severe burns. Hyperinfection syndrome has also been described in association with defects of humoral immunity and HTLV-1 infection, although there is no excess of cases in patients with AIDS despite the defect in cell-mediated immunity in that condition. This syndrome is characterized by pneumonitis, intestinal malabsorption, paralytic ileus, and meningitis. Invasion of the body with many larvae carrying with them gut bacteria results in Gram-negative septicaemia. Patients are febrile and may exhibit dyspnoea, haemoptysis, cough, cyanosis, diarrhoea, progressive lethargy, and coma.

2.3 Diagnostic tests

An eosinophilia, often greater than 50% may be present during the early phases of infection but can be absent in cases of hyperinfection. Examination of a direct saline wet preparation of stool for *Strongyloides* larvae will diagnose approximately 25% of cases. *Strongyloides* larvae are concentrated by the formol ether technique, but their motility ceases, making detection difficult. The yield can be improved culturing the stool to recover rhabditoid larvae (*Protocol 5*) (17).

Protocol 5. Detection of *Strongyloides stercoralis* by faecal culture

Equipment and reagents

- Sterile 30 mm Petri dishes
- Sterile 90 mm Petri dishes
- Activated charcoal
- Microscope

Method

1. Mix approximately 20 g of faeces with an equal volume of activated charcoal. Add sufficient water to form a heavy paste.
2. Place the faecal charcoal suspension in the smaller Petri dish lid and place this in the larger Petri dish.
3. Add water to the outer dish to a depth of 5 mm. Replace the lid of the outer dish and seal with 'DANGER OF INFECTION' tape.
4. Place in a labelled outer container (tin box) and incubate for up to seven days at room temperature.
5. Examine the water in the outer Petri dish for the presence of motile rhabditiform and filariform larvae.

CAUTION: filariform larvae are highly infectious and able to infect through intact skin.

The traditional filter-paper culture method is less efficient than the formol ether concentration technique (17). A modification of the technique described in this chapter (*Protocol 5*) has been reported (17). Faeces are placed in a double-walled agar plate (the agar containing 0.5% beef extract, 1% peptone, 0.5% NaCl, and 1.5% agar), and 25% glycerine poured into the space between the walls. After culture at room temperature for 48 hours, the agar is inspected using a plate microscope for furrows left by migrating larvae, which can be collected with a Pasteur pipette for identification.

Sampling of the duodenal juice can performed by using the string test. Although the sensitivity of this technique has been disputed for the diagnosis of strongyloidiasis it has the added advantage of detecting giardia trophozoites which may be important in the differential diagnosis (see *Protocol 6*). Patients often find the procedure of the string test uncomfortable.

Protocol 6. Detection of *Strongyloides* larvae by 'string test'

Equipment and reagents

- Tongue depressors
- Duodenal string 'Enterotest®
- Plastic universal containers with conical bottom
- Benchtop centrifuge
- Microscope

Method

1. Fast the patient for at least 6 h. Seat the patient and allow them to gargle and swallow a little water.
2. Pull the line out from the Enterotest capsule to ensure that it will unwind freely. While holding a loop of the nylon thread the patient swallows the capsule washing it down with water.

Protocol 6. *Continued*

3. Attach the end of the string to the face using non-allergenic adhesive tape. Leave in place for 3–4 h.
4. Remove the line by applying a gentle pull with the patient's mouth open. During this process the capsule separates from the string and is passed per rectum.
5. The string is placed in 10 ml physiological saline and should be examined immediately. The specimen is mixed using a vortex mixer to loosen any adherent mucus, tipping the suspension into a Universal container.
6. Centrifuge at 4000 *g* for 10 min.
7. Pour off the supernatant and examine the whole deposit using the × 10 objective. This deposit should also be examined using the × 40 objective to note the presence of motile trophozoites of *Giardia lamblia*. (Chapter 5, *Figure 3*).

Immunodiagnosis of *Strongyloides* infections has a small but useful part to play, being used in the screening of patients with potential infection, most notably the Far East prisoners of war who have been shown to have suffered continuing symptoms from their initial infection acquired while prisoners of war under the Japanese. A proportion of patients with strongyloidiasis will react positively in the antibody capture ELISA using *Brugia pahangi* antigen. A specific *Strongyloides* antibody capture ELISA has been shown to have a sensitivity of 97% and specificity of 99% in comparison with standard parasitological techniques (see *Protocol 8*).

Antibody capture ELISA (18) has been shown to be superior to older techniques such as the indirect haemagglutination assay (19). Cross-reactions in patients infected with other parasitic infections is thought to be uncommon (18, 19), but may occur with ascariasis and loiasis.

Protocol 7. Preparation of antigen for *Strongyloides* ELISA

Equipment and reagents

- *Strongyloides* larvae[a] (*Protocol 5*)
- Sonicator
- Benchtop centrifuge
- High speed centrifuge
- Phosphate-buffered saline pH 7.2

Method

1. Wash *Strongyloides* larvae by centrifugation five times in PBS.
2. Sonicate in an ice-bath.
3. Extract antigen by incubating overnight in PBS at 4 °C.

4. Centrifuge at 17 000 *g* for 20 min at 4 °C.
5. Aspirate supernatant, estimate protein concentration (Lowry or similar method) and store at −70 °C until required.

[a] Several sources of antigen have been used successfully including stored rhabditiform larvae from human cases, see *Protocol 5*, *S. cebus* filariform larvae (L_3) from monkeys, *S. stercoralis* L_3 from experimentally infected dogs, or *S. ratti* L_3.

Protocol 8. *Strongyloides* antibody capture ELISA

1. Coat microtitre ELISA plates with *Strongyloides* antigen at the optimal concentration defined by chequerboard titration by overnight incubation in bicarbonate buffer 0.06 M, pH 9.6 at 4 °C.
2. Wash three times with PBS–0.05% (v/v) Tween-20.
3. Dilute serum samples 1:100[a] in PBS–1% BSA and incubate for 1 h.
4. Wash three times with PBS–Tween-20.
5. Add 100 μl peroxidase labelled anti-human IgG at 1:1000 dilution.
6. Wash three times with PBS–Tween-20.
7. Add peroxidase substrate (ATBS) following manufacturer's instructions, and incubate at 30 °C until control reference serum gives a standard reading at 405 nm[b,c].

[a] This dilution will vary in different assay systems and should be standardized by chequerboard titration.
[b] Reference positive and negative control sera should be included in each ELISA run.
[c] The cut-off value is calculated as three standard deviations above the mean of control negative sera.

3. *Trichinella*

3.1 Introduction

Infection with *Trichinella spirillis* is a zoonosis. The natural infection cycle is found in small rodents and in larger animals which prey on them or are fed these animals, e.g. bears, wild boar, or pigs. Human infection results when undercooked meat from infected animals is eaten. The usual food implicated is pork from pigs which have been fed waste in their diet.

The infective stage is the third stage larvae present in the muscles of infected animals. Infection results when these tissues are ingested and the larvae liberated by the acid/pepsin environment of the stomach. The larvae enter the small intestine and develop into adult male and female worms. The adults copulate in the crypts of the duodenum and jejunum and larvae are produced from the uterus of the female. These larvae invade the intestinal wall and migrate to striated muscle where they develop into infective L_3 stages within a host-derived structure known as the nurse cell. The adults are expelled from the intestine within three weeks of infection, but each adult female may produce up to 1000 larvae.

3.2 Clinical features

The presence of adult worms in the intestine may not produce any symptoms except in heavy infections when abdominal discomfort, crampy pains, and diarrhoea may be found. Most clinical symptoms are related to the acute phase of muscle invasion. Patients complain of weakness, malaise, headache, and myalgia. Most are febrile and periorbital oedema is a common sign, conjunctivitis and urticarial skin rashes may also be found. Rarely the central nervous system is involved when seizures or meningitis may develop.

3.3 Diagnosis

The diagnosis of trichinosis is often made clinically and requires a careful food history to elucidate evidence of exposure. An eosinophilia is usually present in the acute phase, and is accompanied by an elevation in muscle enzyme concentration in the blood: lactate dehydrogenase, and creatinine phosphokinase. The electromyogram may be abnormal and a muscle biopsy will demonstrate the presence of the L_3 in the tissues (Chapter 14, section 5.6.2). Serological tests can provide supportive evidence but are unable to distinguish acute and past infection.

Several different techniques have been described including skin testing, indirect immunofluorescence, and antibody capture ELISA. Many of these tests have been developed to screen pigs.

Enzyme-linked immunosorbent assays are now the method of choice for serological diagnosis (20). Several antigens are employed to capture antibody. These include crude worm extract (CWE) which is derived from a pepsin digest of infected muscle (20). Assays using this antigen are usually more sensitive than other techniques (21). One such antibody capture ELISA was evaluated in an outbreak of 117 cases of trichinosis in Thailand where the infecting episode had been identified clearly. The IgG assay detected 68% of patients by day 23 and 100% by 50 days after infection. An IgM assay was positive in 93% by day 57 (22).

Like many other helminths the larval stage of *Trichinella* excretes excretory–secretory (ES) antigens. Assays using ES antigens lack the sensitivity of crude worm extract assays but are more specific (23).

More specific antigens for diagnosis have been identified by Western blotting (21). This study identified antigens which cross-reacted with other parasites and this activity was due to the presence of phosphorylcholine in the parasite antigens. Most of the antigens which were recognized by infected animals and humans shared a single antigenic determinant which could be purified from phosphorylcholine antigens by affinity chromatography. This antigen had an apparent molecular weight of 45 kd. An antibody capture ELISA using this antigen has been shown to be more specific than an assay using crude worm extract, but with similar sensitivity.

An immunoradiometric assay (IRMA) has been described which detects circulating *Trichinella* ES antigen (24). This assay correctly identified 47% of patients with clinical acute trichinosis. In comparison an antigen capture ELISA using *Trichinella* ES antigen and confirmed by inhibition with monoclonal antibodies correctly identified all of the patients.

References

1. Sprent, J. F. A. (1958). *Parasitology*, **48**, 184.
2. Maizels, R. M. and Robertson, B. D. (1990). In *Parasitic nematodes* (ed. M. W. Kennedy), pp. Taylor and Francis: London.
3. Gillespie, S. H. (1988). *Parasitol. Today*, **4**, 180.
4. Molk, R. (1983). *Ann. Ophthalmol.*, **15**, 216.
5. Woodruff, A. W. (1970). *Br. Med. J.*, **3**, 663.
6. Sadum, E. H., Norman, L., and Allain, D. (1957). *Am. J. Trop. Med. Hyg.*, **6**, 562.
7. Glickman, L. T., Schantz, P. M., Dombroske, R., and Cypress, R. H. (1978). *Am. J. Trop. Med. Hyg.*, **27**, 492.
8. de Savigny, D. H., Voller, A., and Woodruff, A. W. (1979). *J. Clin. Pathol.*, **32**, 284.
9. Josephs, D. S., Bhinder, P., and Thompson, A. R. (1981). *Public Health (London)*, **95**, 273.
10. Glickman, L. T., Grieve, R. B., Laura, S. S., and Jones, D. L. (1985). *J. Clin. Path.*, **38**, 103.
11. Matsumuru, K., Kazuta, Y., Endo, R., and Tanaka, K. (1984). *Immunology*, **51**, 609.
12. Robertson, B. D., *et al.* (1988). *Clin. Exp. Immunol.*, **74**, 236.
13. Gillespie, S. H., *et al.* (1993). *J. Clin. Pathol.*, **46**, 551.
14. Gillespie, S. H., Pereira, M., and Ramsay, A. S. (1991). *Public Health* (*London*), **105**, 335.
15. Beaver, P. C., Jung, R. C., and Capp, E. W. (1984). In *Clinical parasitology*. Lea & Febiger: Philadelphia.
16. Gill, G. V. and Bell, D. R. (1972). *Br. Med. J.*, **2**, 572.
17. Arakaki, T. (1990). *J. Parasitol.*, **76**, 425.
18. Bailey, J. W. (1989). *Ann. Trop. Med. Parasitol.*, **83**, 241.
19. Gam, A. A., Neva, F. A., and Krotoski, W. A. (1987). *Am. J. Trop. Med. Hyg.*, **37**, 157.
20. van Knapen, F., Franchimont, J. H., Ruitenberg, E. J., Baldelli, B., Gibson, T. E., Gottal, C., *et al.* (1980). *Vet. Parasitol.*, **7**, 109.
21. Homan, W. L., Derksen, A. C., and van Knapen, F. (1992). *Parasitol. Res.*, **78**, 112.

22. Morakote, N., Khamboongrang, C., Siriprasert, V., Suphawitayanukul, S., Marcanantachoti, S., and Thamasonthi W. (1991). *Trop. Med. Parasitol.*, **42**, 172.
23. Gamble, H. R., Rapic, D., Marinculic, A., and Murrell, K. D. (1988). *Vet. Parasitol.*, **30**, 131.
24. Ivanoska, D., Cuperlovic, K., Gamble, H. R., and Murrell, K. D. (1989). *J. Parasitol.*, **75**, 38.

10

Schistosomiasis

IAN MARSHALL

1. Introduction

Schistosomes are digenetic trematodes belonging to the phylum Platyhelminthes (flatworms) and infect more than 200 million people in 76 countries in the tropics and subtropics. Although 18 species of the genus *Schistosoma* are currently recognized, the majority are parasites of animals other than humans. Most infections in humans can be accounted for by *Schistosoma haematobium*, *S. japonicum*, and *S. mansoni*, together with a minor contribution from *S. intercalatum* and *S. mekongi*. The distribution of the clinically significant species of *Schistosoma* is shown in *Figure 1*.

Unusually for flatworms, schistosomes are dioecious, in which the cylindrical female resides in a ventral groove of the male, the gynaecophoral canal. Paired worms, 1–2 cm in length, live in, and feed on, blood, typically in venules around the intestine or bladder depending on the species (see *Table 1*).

Laboratory diagnosis relies heavily on the detection of parasite eggs in urine or faeces. Each egg is released in the terminal venules around the intestine or bladder. A combination of enzymes secreted across the shell by an enclosed ciliated larva, the miracidium, and the constant muscular movements of the host, ensure that a proportion of eggs reach the lumen of the appropriate organ.

2. Life cycle

In endemic areas, providing eggs reach fresh water soon after being passed, the enclosed miracidia hatch and need to penetrate the tissues of certain species of aquatic or amphibious snail to continue development. Inside the snail, asexual reproduction takes place and after a few weeks, large numbers of forked tailed cercariae, each up to 0.5 mm long, break out of the host tissues into the surrounding water. When humans make contact with water infested with cercariae, infection may occur, through penetration of intact skin. The parasites locate and passively migrate in the blood system, and a

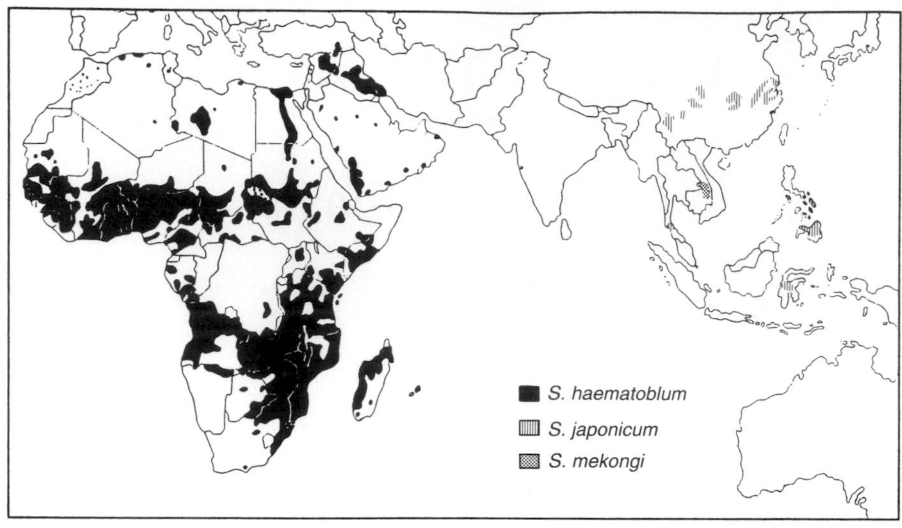

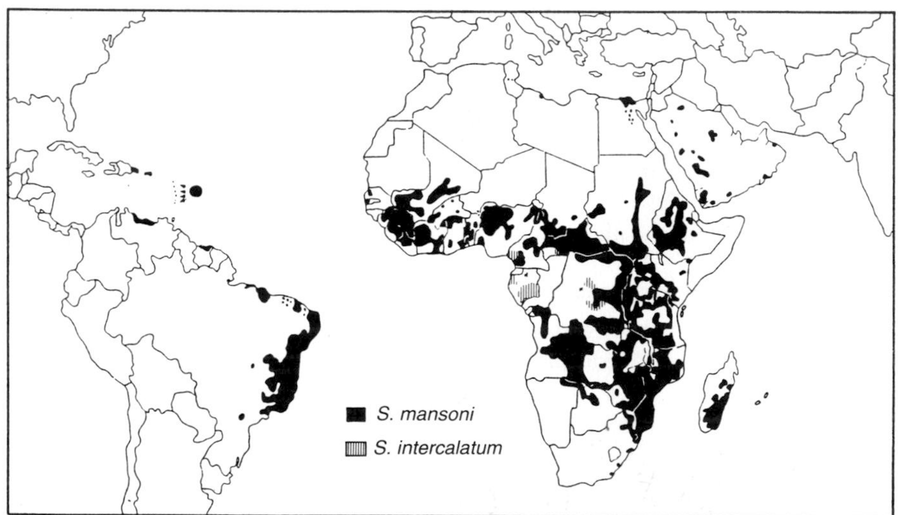

Figure 1. World distribution of clinically important *Schistosoma* spp. Reproduced by permission from *The control of schistosomiasis*; report of a WHO Expert Committee, Geneva, World Health Organization (WHO Technical Report Series, No. 728), 1985.

proportion will eventually reach the portal system of the liver, where pairing takes place. This process is essential for maturation of the female. Males then migrate against the blood flow, each carrying a female in the gynaecophoral canal, to their preferred site around the bladder or intestine. Eggs may be found in faeces or urine from approximately four weeks after infection.

Table 1. Schistosomes: some important features

Species	Geographical distribution	Location in humans	Approx. size of eggs	Egg location	Spine
S. haematobium	Africa, Arabia	Vesical veins	140 μm	Urine	Terminal
S. intercalatum	Limited foci, W. and C. Africa	Mesenteric veins	175 μm	Faeces	Terminal
S. japonicum	Mainly China, Philippines, Indonesia	Mesenteric veins	85 μm	Faeces	Vestigial
S. mansoni	Africa, Arabia, S. America, Caribbean	Mesenteric veins	135 μm	Faeces	Lateral

3. Clinical aspects

The majority of people infected with schistosomes, whether they are from or visitors to endemic areas are asymptomatic. Where symptoms develop they are related to the life cycle in the human host and/or to the intensity of infection.

The penetration of cercariae through the skin may result in an itchy, papular rash, known as swimmers itch. This condition may be due to the human schistosomes and those which develop in birds, or mammals other than humans. The cercariae of these species can penetrate human skin, but die shortly afterwards. A few weeks after infection a generalized immune complex disease may develop, particularly in visitors to endemic areas who may have been exposed to large numbers of cercariae over a limited period. This condition is sometimes referred to as 'Katayama fever', after a prefecture in Japan where it was first observed. It is thought to be due to an initial antigen excess as the worms develop and begin to produce eggs. It is usually self-limiting but severe disease may develop. The passage of eggs through the wall of the intestine or bladder leads to blood loss. This is characterized by bloody diarrhoea or haematuria. The latter is significant for the diagnosis of *S. haematobium*, at least in endemic areas.

The most important pathology induced by schistosomes is that related to worm eggs which fail to reach the outside world. Eggs released in venules around the bladder (*S. haematobium*) or gut (other species) may be swept to the lungs or liver in the respective venous drainage, where they become trapped; eggs can also stick in the gut or bladder wall. In contrast to adult schistosomes which are able to evade the host immune mechanisms eggs containing developing miracidia become the foci of inflammation. This leads to the development of circumoval granulomas. These lesions heal by resolution or fibrosis but, if egg production remains unchecked, obstructive pathology will increase. Eggs retained in the bladder or adjacent organs can lead to obstructive uropathy; in heavy, long-standing infection with *S. mansoni* and *S. japonicum*, fibrosis of liver and spleen leads to portal hypertension. This is complicated by ascites, hepatic failure, and oesophageal varices. Eggs may be found in virtually any organ of the body and occasionally, worms may be located in unusual sites, for example the spinal canal and central nervous system, where they can cause transverse myelitis or epilepsy.

4. Treatment

The objective is to eliminate all worms, and praziquantel has superseded other drugs for the treatment of schistosome infections. A single oral dose of 40 mg/kg is usually adequate, and the drug is effective against all species of schistosome infecting humans. Other drugs which may be considered are species-specific and not as effective as praziquantel in a single oral dose.

Treatment is justified if eggs containing a miracidium are observed, or, if active infection is strongly suspected on clinical grounds, in the absence of eggs, further details are given elsewhere (1, 2).

5. Diagnosis

The location of adult worms precludes a role in direct diagnosis of schistosomiasis. However eggs released by females can be detected in urine (*S. haematobium*) and faeces (other species), or rectal biopsy (all species). There is evidence that the number of eggs excreted is directly proportional to the worm burden, and may thus reflect the intensity of infection.

Indirect evidence for the presence of schistosomes can be obtained through immunodiagnosis on blood or urine or, for *S. haematobium* only, by the detection of haematuria and/or proteinuria. The most important approach to diagnosis is the detection of schistosome eggs in urine, faeces, or biopsy specimens.

A limited number of methods which the author considers appropriate for laboratories in developed countries, outside endemic areas, are given in detail. Readers must be aware that the reasons for, and the approach to, laboratory diagnosis, may be very different in endemic and non-endemic areas, or between developing and developed countries. In the UK for example, concern is solely with the detection and treatment of the infected individual; in endemic areas, although individuals are important, the diagnosis and control of schistosomiasis in the community is emphasised.

5.1 Diagnosis of infections due to *S. haematobium*

The clearest demonstration of an active infection is through the detection of living eggs in urine, although occasionally, eggs may be found in faeces.

5.1.1 General considerations

It has been repeatedly shown that a maximum concentration of eggs occurs in urine which is passed between approximately 10.00 and 14.00. It is preferable to obtain such a specimen, which ideally should be the total volume passed. Patients should **not** be asked for the terminal few drops of urine and **nor** should they be asked to exercise immediately before the passing of urine. There is no reliable relationship between egg concentration and these factors. Examination of a single urine specimen is not reliable for excluding a schistosome infection, and up to four specimens, passed on different days, may be necessary.

Dead eggs may be shed from the bladder wall over many months after the elimination of a schistosome infection and must not be confused with live eggs. The latter are translucent, very pale yellow to colourless, and contain a fully developed miracidium (*Figure 2*), movement within or of which, may

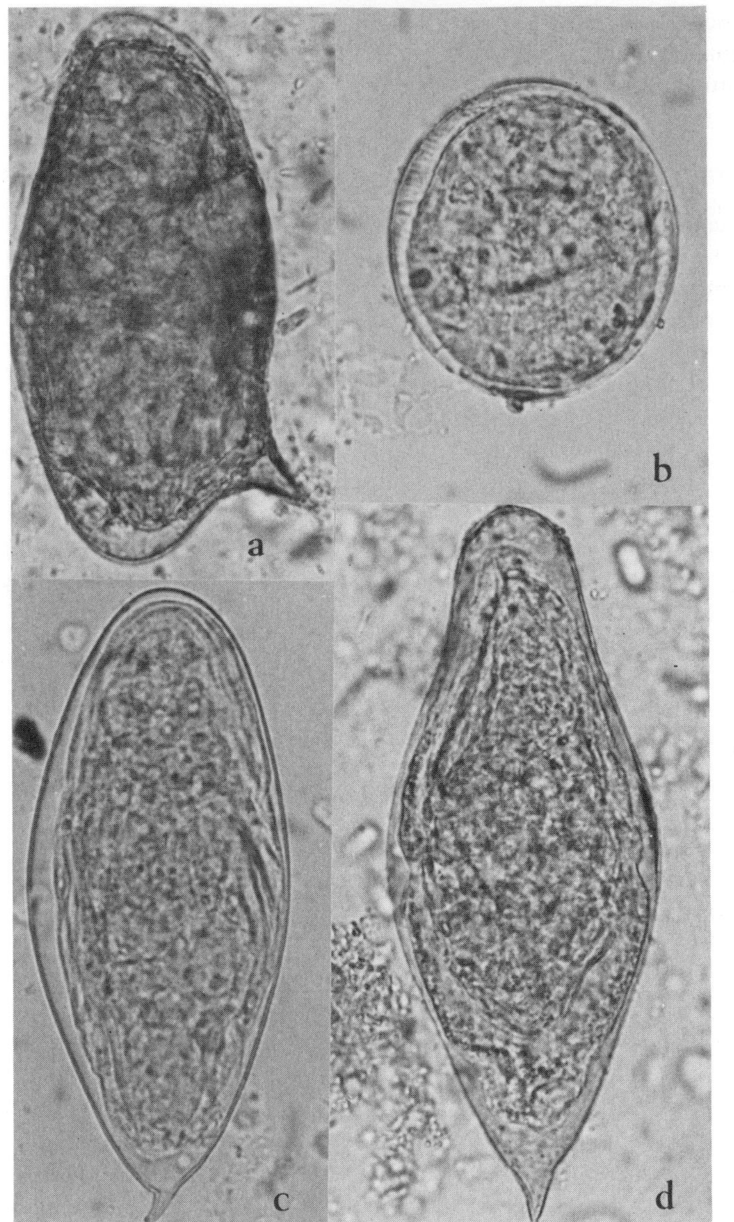

Figure 2. Eggs of schistosomes as seen with ×40 objective. (a) *S. mansoni*; (b) *S. japonicum*; (c) *S. haematobium*; (d) *S. intercalatum*. For typical sizes, see *Table 1*.

be observed in a fresh specimen. In contrast, dead eggs are generally opaque, have no miracidium, and often appear black in colour. There are no grounds for treatment if the only indication of infection is the presence of dead eggs. Rarely, eggs of *S. mansoni* have been found in urine.

5.1.2 Recommended methods for the detection of eggs in urine

- sedimentation by gravity or centrifugation
- filtration
- a combination of sedimentation and filtration

A number of factors can influence the choice of method. Sedimentation is cheaper in terms of materials, but may be more expensive in technician time if the volume of urine is large, eggs are absent or few in number, or the precipitate extensive. Although filters are expensive, the technique of filtration provides a rapid result, which is also semi-quantitative.

i. Sedimentation

A simple method giving a qualitative result. There is some evidence that the centrifugation of preserved urine gives a better recovery of absolute numbers of eggs, compared with filtration (*Protocol 1*) (3).

Protocol 1. Sedimentation of urine

Equipment

- Urine glass or similar container with conical base
- Bench centrifuge
- Pasteur pipette
- Microscope

Method

1. Place urine sample in appropriate container, according to volume.
2. Allow to sediment by gravity for 15–60 min, depending on container.[a]
3. Aspirate supernatant taking care not to disturb precipitate.
4. Examine precipitate under microscope, ×10 objective, and confirm eggs with miracidia under ×40 if necessary when specimen can be reported as positive.

[a] Alternatively, centrifuge at 600 *g* for 10–15 min.

ii. Filtration

After the first description of urine filtration for the diagnosis of *S. haematobium* (4), a number of simplified methods followed. The first of these involved the use of paper filters which required fixation and various stains to visualize the eggs (5–8). Specimens on polycarbonate filters (Nucleopore

TM), which provide an alternative to paper, do not require fixing or staining and the filters are easier to handle (9). Reusable polyamide filters (Nytrel TM) have been described (10, 11), although their reuse has been questioned recently (12, 13). Filtration offers the possibility of a semi-quantitative estimate of egg excretion and the following method is based on that routinely used in the diagnostic clinic at the Liverpool School (*Figure 3*) (*Protocol 2*).

Protocol 2. Filtration of urine

Equipment

- 25 mm diameter Swinnex filter holder (Millipore)
- 25 mm diameter Nucleopore membrane, 12 μm pore size (Bibby Sterilin; Nucleopore Corp.)
- Microscope
- Syringe, 10 ml or greater

Method

1. Take up a **random** aliquot (10 ml) or alternatively, the total urine specimen, into an appropriate syringe.[a]
2. Inject the urine through the filter holder.
3. Remove the syringe, fill with air, and inject through the filter holder, to expel excess urine and fix eggs to filter. Repeat once.
4. Open the filter holder and carefully remove the filter with fine forceps and place face upwards on to a clean slide.
5. Pipette a drop of saline on to the filter to prevent drying and examine immediately for eggs, using the ×10 objective, confirming under ×40 if necessary.

[a] A short, plastic extension tube can be fitted to the syringe to avoid contamination of the latter with urine, and removed prior to injection of urine through filter. However, eggs may stick to the inside wall.

Providing the whole of the filter is scanned and the volume of urine injected through the filter is known, a semi-quantitative estimate of egg excretion can be determined. It is conventional to express this as eggs per 10 ml urine. After examination, the filter can be preserved if required. The filter should be placed **face down** on to a clean glass slide and one or two drops of glycerine added. The preparation can be maintained in this condition for several months if kept in an air tight box and may be used for internal quality control.

iii. Filtration and sedimentation

This can be used if a large volume of urine is available and greater sensitivity is required. The sample should be sedimented as in *Protocol 1* and aspirated, leaving approximately 10–100 ml, depending on the amount of precipitate, which is then injected through the filter as in *Protocol 2*.

5.1.3 Indirect methods of diagnosis for *S. haematobium*

It is well established that haematuria and proteinuria are common features of infection with *S. haematobium*. The concentration of blood may be so great as to be clearly visible in the urine specimen, a condition referred to as macrohaematuria. In contrast, much lower levels of blood (microhaematuria) require specific detection; reagent dipsticks provide a simple and rapid method. In recent years, studies in several countries in which *S. haematobium* is endemic, have revealed a close relationship between the level of egg excretion and that of protein or blood, particularly the latter as detected by reagent sticks (Boehringer-Mannheim). Day to day and circadian variations in haematuria have been observed (14, 15). However, the precise relationship varies from country to country and, although in some studies a single dipstick has proved more sensitive than a single filtration, this is not always the case. It is not possible, therefore, to recommend this form of diagnosis as an alternative to direct methods, but reagent sticks to detect blood should be used in egg-free urine as a supplementary test. It is not necessary to routinely test for proteinuria.

These recommendations may not be appropriate in areas endemic for schistosomiasis in developing countries. Haematuria, which can be used in the evaluation of the control of *S. haematobium*, is becoming an increasingly important and reliable diagnostic tool. Dipsticks are cheap, quick, and easy to use, and are suitable for community surveys in rural areas where laboratory facilities are frequently absent.

5.2 Diagnosis of infection due to other species

The eggs of *S. japonicum*, *S. mansoni*, and *S. intercalatum* can be detected in faeces, although those of *S. mansoni* have been found rarely in urine. As with *S. haematobium*, the most convincing demonstration of an active infection is the presence of living eggs (*Figure 2*).

5.2.1 General considerations

It is **unsafe** to assume a random distribution of eggs in faeces, aliquots must be obtained from different parts of the specimen. Egg production varies from day to day although there is no recognized pattern of release, in contrast to that of *S. haematobium* eggs in urine. Absence of eggs in a single faecal specimen does not necessarily imply absence of active infection; three to five tests, on faeces passed on different days, may be needed.

A variety of methods for the detection of eggs in faeces has been developed, none of them entirely satisfactory for schistosomes. These range from the thin faecal smear in saline which uses approximately 2 mg of stool, to those involving dilution and/or sedimentation, filtration, or flotation with 1–2 g.

The thin smear technique is insensitive and is only reliable for the heaviest infections. However, thick smears which utilize up to 50 mg stool per preparation are much more appropriate. Flotation in saturated salt or zinc sulfate solutions is inappropriate due to the weight of schistosome eggs; sedimentation techniques are, however, useful.

Problems with early methods (particularly sensitivity) are discussed elsewhere (16, 17). The method based on the sedimentation of faeces in an acid–ether–xylol mixture (AEX) which is claimed to be sensitive to 10 eggs/g (16) is a considerable improvement on dilution methods (18). Bell (17) describes a filtration method based on sampling from large volumes of comminuted stool, filtering through paper, and staining with ninhydrin to visualize eggs of *S. mansoni*; sensitivity is superior to previous methods. However, both AEX and filtration are unacceptably cumbersome and are not recommended here.

5.2.2 Recommended methods for the detection of eggs in faeces

- formol ethyl acetate sedimentation
- Kato thick smear
- potassium hydroxide (KOH) digestion

Laboratories outside endemic areas can expect to examine specimens for the presence of schistosome eggs. For this reason, a simple, qualitative sedimentation technique (formol ethyl acetate), which has the advantage of detecting a wide-range of helminth eggs, larvae, and protozoan cysts, is strongly recommended. However, in the event that semi-quantitative data may be required, two further techniques are included although neither detect as wide a range of parasites.

i. Formol ethyl acetate sedimentation

Ethyl acetate is a less flammable alternative to methyl ether, recommended for a sedimentation technique modified for the recovery of schistosome eggs by Ritchie (19), but which had been developed some 40 years earlier. Ridley and Hawgood (20) simplified Ritchies' method whilst Allen and Ridley (21) reported further modifications which resulted in a sevenfold increase in the recovery of schistosome eggs. The later changes involved the substitution of formol saline with formol water and an increase in the centrifugation speed, both of which are included in this protocol. However, the precise way in which this technique is carried out varies between laboratories and no particular protocol can be regarded as superior. The method is described in Chapter 5, *Protocol 2*.

It is sometimes recommended that stool samples treated by this protocol should undergo one or more preliminary washes in physiological saline or water, according to whether the stool was fresh or preserved respectively, prior to the addition of 10% formalin. Each wash is achieved by emulsifying the sample in the appropriate solute, sieving, centrifuging at low speed for one minute, and discarding the supernatant. Washing but not sieving could be repeated if the supernatant is very turbid. Thereafter, following the addition of 10% formol water, proceed with the protocol. This adds to the workload of a busy laboratory, but can result in a cleaner final precipitate, aid diagnosis, and may improve recovery.

ii. Kato thick smear

In 1954, two Japanese workers, Kato and Miura, described a thick smear technique for the detection of helminth eggs which uses up to 50 mg of faeces, or 25 times that in the average thin smear. A series of modifications have resulted in the method being commonly used for the parasitological diagnosis of schistosome infections in endemic areas. The procedure yields semi-quantitative data and has contributed significantly to the understanding of aspects of epidemiology and control of schistosomiasis. The technique is currently recommended by the World Health Organization (WHO) for the diagnosis of *S. intercalatum*, *S. japonicum*, and *S. mansoni* (22).

The principle of the method is based on the clearing of a thick faecal smear with glycerine in the presence of a background stain, usually malachite green. The eggs appear unstained although miracidia are not visible. Katz *et al.* (23), described the use of a disposable cardboard template ($3 \times 4 \times 1.37$ mm thick) with a central hole 6 mm in diameter, which, when placed over a microscope slide and filled with faeces, contained an average of 43.7 mg. Reusable plastic or stainless steel templates are now commonly used in survey work and have greatly facilitated a quantitative approach to estimates of egg excretion and are easily manufactured locally. The method is often referred to as the modified Kato, or the Kato/Katz. However, outside endemic areas semi-quantitative data is not often required and a plug of faeces can always be weighed as an alternative method. Ovo-FEC kits for 100 or 500 examinations are available commercially (Boehringer-Mannheim Bioquimica) which contain reusable templates but according to WHO the stain solution may be defective.

Protocol 3. The Kato thick smear technique

Equipment and reagents

- Malachite green/glycerine: 1 vol. 3% aqueous stain, 100 vol. distilled water, 100 vol. glycerine
- Water wettable cellophane strips cut into 22 × 30 mm rectangles, stored in the stain[a]
- 105 mesh, stainless steel or nylon sieve
- Template, optional, and microscope slides
- Filter-papers or paper towelling
- Spatulas
- Microscope

Method

1. Mesh a portion of faeces, either by pressing the sieve down on faeces placed on filter-paper or paper towelling, or by pushing the sample through the sieve with a spatula, to remove fibre and other coarse debris.[b] Take care not to disperse faecal droplets.

Protocol 3. *Continued*

2. Place template, if used, in the middle of a clean microscope slide and fill with meshed faeces; or place faeces directly on to slide. Make two preparations.
3. Carefully remove template and place a glycerine/malachite green soaked cellophane strip over each plug of stool.
4. Invert each slide and press on an absorbent surface on a bench top to spread the faeces under the coverslip.
5. Position slides **with smear uppermost** to facilitate clearing of specimen and leave for 1–24 h.
6. Examine for eggs under × 10 objective.

[a] Important, these coverslips should be stored in the malachite green/glycerine solution for a minimum of 24 h prior to use. They can be stored in the stain for months without deterioration, preferably in a screw-capped jar or similar, away from stong light. If difficulty is experienced in obtaining cellophane, further information is available from: Chief, Schistosomiasis and other Trematode Infections, WHO, 1211 Geneva 27, Switzerland.

[b] The second option is preferable. Firmly attach the sieve to a support; see *Figure 3*, in which stainless steel mesh is welded to a home-made metal loop.

If quantitative data are required, both slides should be read fully. Assuming 50 mg of stool has been used for each, total eggs observed multiplied by ten convert the count to eggs per gram. Always prepare two slides, if possible, to increase sensitivity as it is important to detect low levels of infection in non-endemic areas. This does not always apply to community-based studies. If a qualitative result is required, searching can stop as soon as the first egg is observed. Most other helminth eggs can be detected in Kato slides, although hookworm eggs tend to collapse within one hour.

Teesdale *et al.* (24) have shown that drier stools from the same person produce up to seven times more eggs than wet specimens. These authors used a 'glass sandwich' technique based on Kato, in which 40 mg of meshed faeces was spread between two glass slides without stain or glycerine, and read immediately, before drying. This alternative is worth considering if wettable cellophane is unavailable.

Conventional Kato slides can be stored for weeks, or even many months, provided that they are prevented from drying out. The author has read preparations over two-years-old, in which some eggs remain clearly visible being useful for 'in-house' training or quality control.

Optimum clearing times have rarely been evaluated and are likely to vary with the amount and nature of stool, and a possible delay of several hours before diagnosis is a potential disadvantage. Also, very hard stools or diarrhoeic specimens can be difficult to process with the Kato method. Kato slides are more difficult to read than a sediment from the formol ethyl acetate technique.

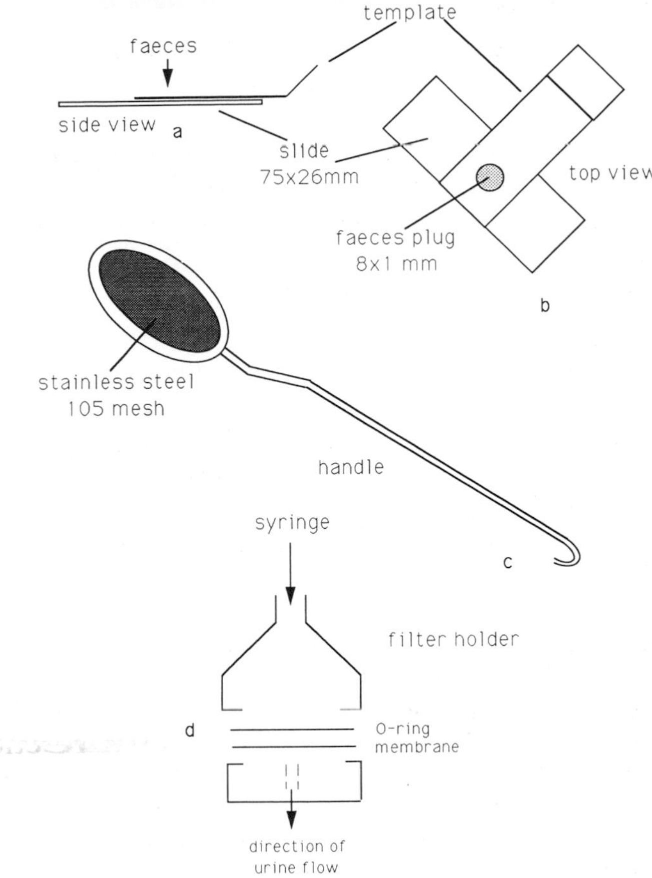

Figure 3. Diagrams showing typical materials for the diagnosis of: (a)–(c) schistosome eggs in stool using a modified Kato; (d) *S. haematobium* in urine by filtration.

iii. KOH digestion

Some of the problems associated with the Kato technique stimulated the development of an alternative method, based on KOH digestion of a larger amount of faeces, followed by random sampling of the filtered digest for egg counts (25). Approximately 300 mg faeces was digested and aliquots equivalent to 50 mg screened for eggs. A preliminary evaluation in Zambia, where the method was developed, showed KOH digestion to be more sensitive than locally used Kato/Katz, for *S. mansoni*; the KOH/Kato ratio for the geometric mean number of eggs per gram, in stools positive by both methods, was 3.5 (25). The digestion method was developed specifically for the detection of schistosome eggs, although those of other species, with the exception of *Taenia saginata*, survive just as well (*Protocol 4*).

Protocol 4. KOH digestion technique

Equipment and reagents

- 4% potassium hydroxide (KOH)
- 1 ml and 20 ml syringes, or automatic equivalents
- Aspirator
- Filter and filter holder (a stainless steel filter, 50 mesh, secured by heat to the barrel of a disposable 10 ml syringe sectioned at the 7 ml graduation, is ideal)
- Two plastic Universals with fitted spoon and conical base
- Spatula Sedgwick–Rafter counting cell (Fisons; Ernest F. Fullam)

Method

Before commencing the digestion, remove spoon from one of the Universals and calibrate to 6 ml with water.

1. Dispense approximately 20 ml 4% KOH into the Universal with fitted spoon.

2. Leaving the spoon in the lid, prepare a level spoon of faeces with the spatula. This will weigh about 300 mg, regardless of the nature of the specimen.

3. Replace the lid and spoon into the KOH, secure, and leave overnight at room temperature.

4. Shake digest vigorously to disperse the faecal material.

5. Place the filter/filter holder into the calibrated Universal and pour the digest through. Wash digest Universal with 1–2 ml 4% KOH and pour through filter.

6. Agitate the filter holder vertically in the filtrate to free any eggs which may be trapped in the coarse debris.

7. Remove filter and replace cap on Universal. Leave to sediment for 15 min.

8. Aspirate the filtrate to the 6 ml calibration.

9. Agitate the remaining filtrate and remove a random 1 ml aliquot (equivalent to 50 mg faeces).

10. Dispense into counting chamber and search for eggs with ×4 objective, confirming under ×10 if necessary.

11. Repeat steps **9** and **10** for semi-quantitative estimate of egg positive specimen.

If quantitative data are required, the number of eggs per gram faeces should be calculated as in the Kato technique (*Protocol 3*). Eggs do not adhere to the equipment and are rarely found in the aspirated filtrate. Miracidia can be seen in mature eggs, in contrast to Kato, although the eggs themselves begin to be digested within a few days at room temperature. KOH at this concentration is caustic and should be handled with care, but a range of faecal bacteria are destroyed within minutes of its addition. The aliquot size for screening can be varied easily, according to the number of eggs and/or degree of turbidity, and digestion time could be substantially reduced by increasing temperature.

Unless semi-quantitative data are required, formol ethyl acetate sedimentation is recommended. The choice between the two quantitative techniques described is less clear. There is considerably more information available for the modified Kato.

5.3 Indirect methods

Indirect methods for the diagnosis of intestinal schistosomiases involve immunodiagnosis, briefly covered in section 5.5.

5.4 Direct methods for all species

Two methods involving the detection of eggs are theoretically available for all species of schistosomes infecting humans:

- rectal biopsy
- miracidial hatching test

5.4.1 Rectal biopsy

Not to be recommended as a routine diagnostic test; it is invasive, involving the taking of one or more snips from the rectum. Also, an egg positive biopsy does not necessarily indicate an active infection, as it can be difficult to detect living eggs. In a study on expatriates returning to Britain, Harries *et al.* (27) reported that of 15 patients in whom eggs of *S. haematobium* were restricted to rectal snips, only four were positive for blood and/or protein by reagent stick. It is likely that a number of these patients were not actively infected. The same authors reported that 61% of patients were rectal snip positive for *S. mansoni* but in only 39% could eggs be detected in stool. However, the significance of these results regarding active infection is unclear as most patients were asymptomatic, and symptoms which were present were usually non-specific.

Harries and Speare (28) recommended up to four snips per egg negative patient but, as in the expatriate study, details of faecal screening methods used for comparison were not provided. Rectal snips can have a supporting role in the laboratory diagnosis of schistosomiasis, but only when other direct investigations are negative and where infection is suspected on case history or clinical grounds.

5.4.2 Miracidial hatching test

If a fresh specimen of urine containing viable schistosome eggs is sedimented as in *Protocol 1*, aspirated without disturbing the sediment, and topped up with fresh water, miracidia will hatch if the suspension is placed under strong light. Similarly, fresh faeces can be comminuted as in Chapter 5, *Protocol 2* and sedimented two or three times in physiological saline (a urine glass is ideal for this) before the addition of water and light to stimulate hatching. The active, ciliated larvae swim towards the light and can be concentrated easily, a feature which greatly increases sensitivity.

However, miracidial hatching is not recommended as a routine diagnostic here, for the following reasons:

(a) The need for a fresh specimen.
(b) Laborious, particularly with faeces; some larvae may take several hours to hatch.
(c) It is of potential advantage only when there are very few eggs, which may not be detected by other methods but, very small numbers of miracidia may be difficult for inexperienced workers to identify; ciliate contaminants may cause confusion.
(d) In the authors experience, miracidia become lethargic in distilled water and some tap-waters and some eggs may not hatch at all.

In endemic areas, miracidial hatching tests may have a role in the evaluation of community-based chemotherapy, particularly when very few viable eggs are being excreted.

5.5 Indirect methods for all species: immunodiagnosis

The ideal immunodiagnostic test should be capable of detecting current infections quickly and easily, and be specific, highly sensitive, cheap, robust, and reproducible. To date, the immunodiagnosis of schistosome infections (and that of many other parasites) falls short of these goals, although new technologies are likely to improve the position within the present decade. Many serological tests carried out in laboratories throughout the world involve the use of crude antigen extracts for the detection of antibodies. Problems with specificity and sensitivity led to the identification and purification of particular schistosome antigens for use with ELISA, radioimmunoassay, IFA, and other tests. Although some of these developments produced improvements, the general problem with antibody detection remains; results often reflect the history of a patient rather than current status of infection, and titres can remain high months after successful treatment.

Thus, increasing efforts are being directed toward the identification of specific schistosome antigens, and the advent of monoclonal antibodies is proving useful in their detection. For example, a number of proteoglycan antigens, including circulating anodic antigen (CAA), have been identified in sera from schistosome positive patients. Monoclonal antibodies have been produced against these and recently, De Jonge *et al.* (29) reported for the first time, the presence of CAA in the urine of patients infected with *S.*

mansoni and/or *S. haematobium*. A positive correlation with eggs of the former in stool, but not of the latter in urine, was noted.

Non-invasive immunodiagnostic tests would be a valuable development and, for schistosomes, it is likely that investigations of antigens in faeces will also occur. Although it is not possible to recommend any method in the present context, new technologies involving dipsticks, dot blots, and other approaches, have great potential. Hommel (30) considers that characteristics of new methods are likely to facilitate the production of tests for the patients own use, a development for which there would be a big demand in industrialized countries.

References

1. Rollinson, D. and Simpson, A. J. G. (ed.) (1987). *The biology of Schistosomes, from genes to latrines*. Academic Press, London and New York.
2. Jordan, P. and Webbe, G. (ed.) (1982). *Schistosomiasis: epidemiology, treatment and control*. Heinemann, London.
3. Richards, F. O. Jr., Hassan, F., Cline, B. L., and El Alamy, M. A. (1984). *Am. J. Trop. Med. Hyg.*, **33**, 857.
4. Bradley, D. J. (1965). *Bull. Wld. Hlth. Org.*, **33**, 503.
5. Dazo, B. C. and Biles, J. E. (1974). *Bull. Wld. Hlth. Org.*, **51**, 399.
6. Plouvier, S., Leroy, J. C., and Colette, J. (1975). *Med. Trop.*, **35**, 229.
7. Wilkins, H. A. (1977). *Ann. Trop. Med. Parasitol.*, **71**, 53.
8. Scott, J. A., Senker, K., and England, E. C. (1982). *Bull. Wld. Hlth. Org.*, **60**, 89.
9. Peters, P. A., Warren, K. S., and Mahmoud, A. F. F. (1976). *J. Parasitol.*, **62**, 154.
10. Mott, K. E., Baltes, R., Bambagha, J., and Baldassini, B. (1982). *Trop. Med. Parasitol.*, **33**, 227.
11. Mott, K. E. (1983). *Bull. Soc. Pathol. Exot.*, **76**, 101.
12. Braun-Munzinger, R. A. (1986). *Parasitol. Today*, **2**, 82.
13. Mshinda, H., Lengeler, C., Hatz, C., and de Savigny, D. (1989). *J. Parasitol.*, **75**, 476.
14. Wilkins, H. A., Goll, P., Marshall, T. F. De C., and Moore, P. (1979). *Trans. R. Soc. Trop. Med. Hyg.*, **73**, 74.
15. Feldmeier, H., Doehring, E., and Daffalla, A. A. (1982). *Trans. R. Soc. Trop. Med. Hyg.*, **76**, 416.
16. Loughlin, E. H. and Stoll, N. R. (1946). *Am. J. Trop. Med.*, **26**, 517.
17. Bell, D. R. (1963). *Bull. Wld. Hlth. Org.*, **29**, 525.
18. Stoll, N. R. (1923). *Am. J. Hyg.*, **3**, 59.
19. Ritchie, L. S. (1948). *Bull. US Army Med. Dep.*, **8**, 326.
20. Ridley, D. S. and Hawgood, B. C. (1956). *J. Clin. Pathol.*, **9**, 74.
21. Allen, A. V. H. and Ridley, D. S. (1970). *J. Clin. Pathol.*, **23**, 545.
22. WHO Technical Report Series, No. 728. (1985). The Control of Schistosomiasis. World Health Organization, Geneva.
23. Katz, N., Chaves, A., and Pellegrino, J. (1972). *Rev. Inst. Med. Trop. São Paulo*, **14**, 397.

24. Teesdale, C. H., Fahringer, K., and Chitsulo, L. (1985). *Trans. R. Soc. Trop. Med. Hyg.*, **79**, 369.
25. Marshall, I., Morrison, J. A., and Nyirenda, W. (1989). *Ann. Trop. Med. Parasitol.*, **83**, 31.
26. Cheever, A. W. (1968). *Bull. Wld. Hlth. Org.*, **39**, 328.
27. Harries, A. D., Fryatt, R., Walker, J., Chiodini, P. L., and Bryceson, A. D. M. (1986). *Lancet*, **330**, 86.
28. Harries, A. D. and Speare, R. (1988). *Trans. R. Soc. Trop. Med. Hyg.*, **82**, 720.
29. De Jonge, N., Fillié, Y. E., Hilberath, G. W., Krijger, F. W., Lengeler, C., De Savigny, D. H., *et al.* (1989). *Am. J. Trop. Med. Hyg.*, **41**, 563.
30. Hommel, M. (1991). *Trans. R. Soc. Trop. Med. Hyg.*, **85**, 151.

11

Hydatidosis and cysticercosis—larval cestodes

PHILIP S. CRAIG, MICHAEL T. ROGAN, and JAMES C. ALLAN

1. Introduction

Hydatidosis and cysticercosis are the names given to human or animal infection with the larval cystic stages of taeniid tapeworms belonging to the genera *Echinococcus* and *Taenia*. The most important species for public health are, in order, *E. granulosus* (the cause of cystic hydatid disease), *T. solium* (the cause of neurocysticercosis), and *E. multilocularis* (the cause of alveolar hydatid disease). These cestodes are transmitted in life cycles involving two mammalian hosts (*Table 1*) (1, 2). *T. solium* (with *T. saginata*) is unique among parasitic zoonoses in that man comprises the sole definitive host in nature. Apart from these species a few rare larval cestode zoonotic infections have been reported and these are the cause of polycystic hydatidosis, coenurosis, and sparganosis (see section 5).

1.1 Distribution

E. granulosus occurs on every continent and may be transmitted in arctic, temperate, and tropical regions, and is endemic in many developed as well as developing countries. Highly endemic areas include the countries of the

Table 1. Life cycles of major larval cestode species

Species	Definitive hosts	Infective stage	Intermediate hosts	Disease in man
E. granulosus	Dog, wild canids	Eggs in faeces	Horse, sheep, cow, etc. Wild herbivores (man)	Cystic hydatidosis/ echinococcosis
E. multilocularis	Fox, dog	Eggs in faeces	Wild rodents (man)	Alveolar hydatidosis/ echinococcosis
T. solium	Man	Eggs in faeces	Pig (man)	Cysticercosis neurocysticercosis

Mediterranean littoral (including north Africa), regions of countries in East Africa, Argentina, Chile, Uruguay, Russia, CIS, the Middle East, China, Mongolia, and parts of Australasia. Domestic transmission between dogs and sheep is the most important cycle in relation to human infection. Prevalence of human cystic hydatidosis between 1%–5% is very significant, as are annual incidences > 10/100 000, which frequently are above 50/100 000 for example in parts of Spain, Algeria, Argentina, or China, and may be > 200/100 000 in some foci such as northwest Kenya. *E. granulosus* is also endemic in parts of western Europe and western USA.

E. multilocularis is much less widespread than *E. granulosus* and is confined to the northern hemisphere, where transmission occurs primarily in wild-life cycles between foxes and arvicolid rodents (e.g. voles), domestic dogs may also be infected; important endemic areas include central western Europe, north and eastern Russia, northern China and Japan, Alaska, and parts of USA and Canada. In endemic foci, annual incidence rates of alveolar hydatidosis are generally much lower than for cystic hydatidosis (e.g. 0.18/100 000 in Switzerland), but may reach >60/100 000 in hyperendemic foci such as occur in parts of Alaska, northern Siberia, and central China. The greater severity of alveolar hydatid disease may result in higher morbidity and higher case fatality rates.

T. solium is particularly prevalent in Mexico, Central America, South America, South Africa, China, and non-Islamic South East Asia, and is cyclically transmitted between humans and pigs. In Mexico 7%–10% of admissions to neurological wards are due to neurocysticercosis. Prevalence of human cysticercosis may reach 2%–4% of routine autopsies in highly endemic countries like Mexico or Brazil. It is likely that the disease is grossly underreported in most endemic regions.

1.2 Pathology

These larval cestodes in man are usually characterized by slow growing, fluid-filled cysts (metacestode) containing one scolex (protoscolex) in the case of *T. solium* or many protoscoleces in the case of *E. granulosus*. Alveolar hydatids in humans, in contrast to rodent infection, are usually devoid of protoscoleces. Protoscoleces develop into the adult tapeworm when ingested by the definitive host, i.e. in the gut of man for *T. solium*, and canids for *E. granulosus*. *Echinococcus* protoscoleces also have the remarkable ability to develop independently in the cystic direction, this can result in secondary echinococcosis following cyst rupture or surgical spillage, a condition characterized by multiple cyst formation which is difficult to treat. In all three species, humans (adults or children) become infected by these larval cestodes through ingestion of eggs passed in faeces of infected definitive hosts. Main risk factors include contact with dogs or foxes in *Echinococcus* endemic areas, or contact with human tapeworm carriers in *T. solium* regions.

Human cystic and alveolar hydatidosis are chronic diseases usually affecting the liver (about 70% for *E. granulosus* and > 99% for *E. multilocularis*) or lungs (about 10%–25% for *E. granulosus*). Cystic hydatids are usually unilocular and may vary in size from only a few centimetres to > 30 cm containing many litres of fluid. In contrast, human alveolar hydatidosis is characterized by a solid tumour-like multivesiculated mass which progressively invades surrounding tissues by exogenous budding; in chronic infections formation of a central necrotic cavity is common and metastatic foci may occur in lungs and brain.

In human cysticercosis due to *T. solium*, the common cellulose-type cysts (0.5–1 cm in size) are most frequently found in striated muscle, subcutaneous tissues (where they are often palpable), the brain parenchyma, or the eye. A large ($\gg$ 1 cm) multilobulated cyst form of *T. solium* (racemose form) can occur particularly in brain ventricles, but the scolex in such cysts are usually degenerate or absent. Neurocysticercosis due to involvement of the CNS is common in humans.

Clinical symptoms and pathology of these chronic larval cestode infections is usually related to site, size, and condition of the cysts and especially pressure effects of the space-occupying lesion. For example, focal epilepsy is quite common in neurocysticercosis, while bile duct obstruction may occur in hepatic hydatidosis. Occasionally rupture of *E. granulosus* cysts may precipitate acute anaphylaxis. The period between infection and clinical manifestation is very variable and may be many years and consequently a proportion of cystic hydatidosis and cysticercosis cases are completely asymptomatic. Alveolar hydatidosis will invariably present with progressive liver destruction and is often considered the most lethal of parasitic helminth infections of man.

Clinical diagnosis of hydatidosis and cysticercosis may be difficult and relies on detection of space-occupying masses primarily with X-ray, ultrasound, NMR or CT scan (see section 3), although images may also be difficult to interpret. Larval cestodes are among the few parasitic infections where the basis for laboratory diagnosis is primarily serology. Surgery still remains the main form of treatment for hydatidosis and neurocysticercosis, however medical treatment with benzimidazole drugs (for echinococcosis and cysticercosis) and praziquantel (for cysticercosis) has a beneficial effect in about 70% of cystic hydatid and neurocysticercosis cases. Albendazole treatment for alveolar hydatidosis is beneficial in approximately 40% of cases.

2. Parasitological diagnosis

Direct parasitological diagnosis of human hydatid disease or cysticercosis is rarely possible due to the tissue location of cysts. However post-surgical or biopsy identification of parasitic stages and associated cyst membranes may be important.

2.1 Hydatidosis

Occasionally pulmonary cysts of *E. granulosus* can rupture and intact protoscoleces and hooks (sometimes cyst membrane) can be coughed up in sputum.

Microscopical examination of diluted, centrifuged sputum can therefore reveal these structures (*Figure 1*). Biopsy of suspected hydatid cysts is not recommended due to chances of disseminating secondary echinococcosis (through ability of protoscoleces and germinal membrane to independently vesiculate), or of causing anaphylaxis due to fluid spillage (for *E. granulosus*). Nevertheless hydatid cyst fluid is sometimes aspirated during exploratory laparotomy or after fine needle puncture under ultrasound guidance and may be sent to the laboratory for examination (see also section 4.2.1).

2.1.1 Microscopical examination of fluid samples from suspected hydatid cysts

If a suspected hydatid cyst, or its contents, is removed at surgery then any aspirated fluid can be examined for parasitological evidence as to the nature of the lesion. The fibrous host capsule of an *E. granulosus* hydatid cyst surrounds a flimsy white endocyst membrane of parasite origin which can often be removed intact with forceps once most of the fluid has been aspirated. Numerous brood capsules containing protoscoleces, may be attached to this membrane, pieces of which can be cut off and sectioned for histology. Clear fluid, which does not contain pus, should be centrifuged at 3000 *g* for 10 min and the resulting pellet examined unstained under a microscope with a × 10 objective lens. If protoscoleces or brood capsules (*Figure 1a*) are present then diagnosis of hydatidosis can be confirmed. Additionally the presence of rostellar hooks (*Figure 1b* and *Table 3*) is an indication that protoscoleces are, or were present. If protoscoleces are present then it is advisable to determine whether these are alive or not. Viability can be assessed by incubating the parasites in a 0.1% solution of eosin in PBS. Protoscoleces which take up the stain are judged to be dead whilst those which exclude it are alive. Additionally activity of the parasite excretory system, as determined by flickering movements in the flame cells, is an indication of parasite viability. There are 30 of these cells in each protoscolex and they are most easily visualized near the periphery of the organism.

If the contents of the cyst are putrid then these should be poured into a Petri dish and examined for the the presence of protoscoleces, hooks, or very small (1–20 mm) spherical cysts which are known as daughter cysts. The occurrence of any of these structures is indicative of a hydatid cyst due to *E. granulosus*. The absence of parasite material in fluid samples does not mean that the cyst is not a hydatid and in all cases a portion of the wall of the cyst should be taken for histological examination.

2.1.2 Histology of hydatid cyst tissue

Suspected cyst tissue should be fixed in 10% neutral buffered formalin and embedded in wax for sectioning. Sections should then be depariffinized and

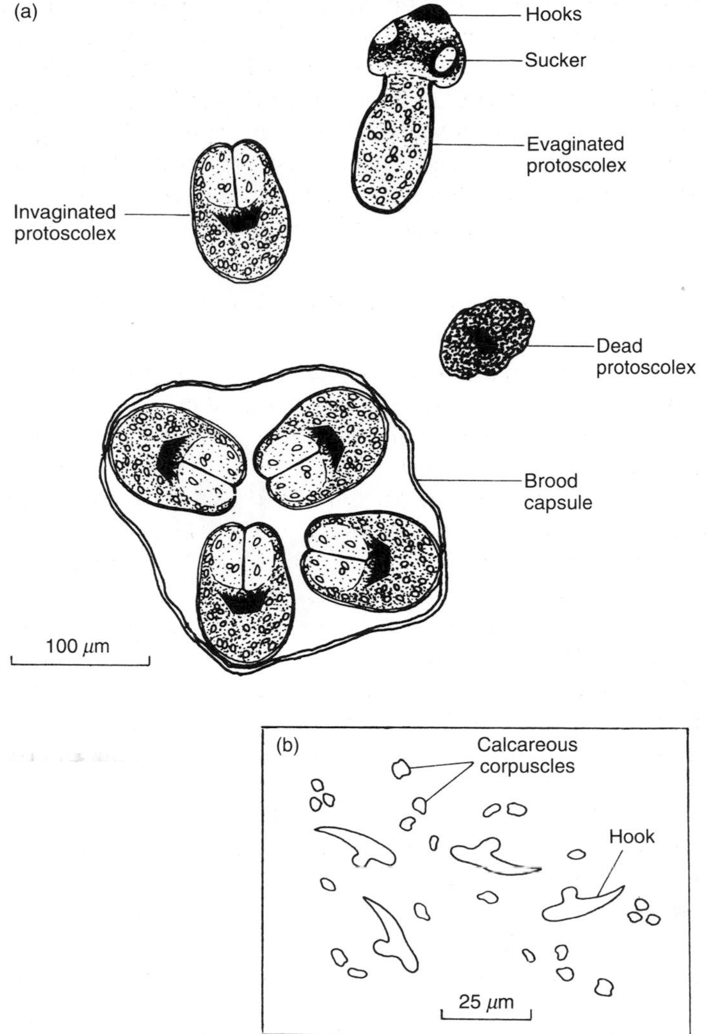

Figure 1. Microscopical appearance of hydatid cyst contents as may be apparent in biopsy samples or sputum. (a) Protoscoleces and brood capsule. (b) Degenerate contents of a hydatid cyst.

stained with haematoxylin/eosin or periodic acid–Schiff reagent (PAS). For PAS staining:

- hydrate tissues/sections
- incubate in 0.5% periodic acid for 5 min
- wash and incubate in Schiff reagent for 20–30 min
- wash and counterstain with methyl green for 30–60 sec

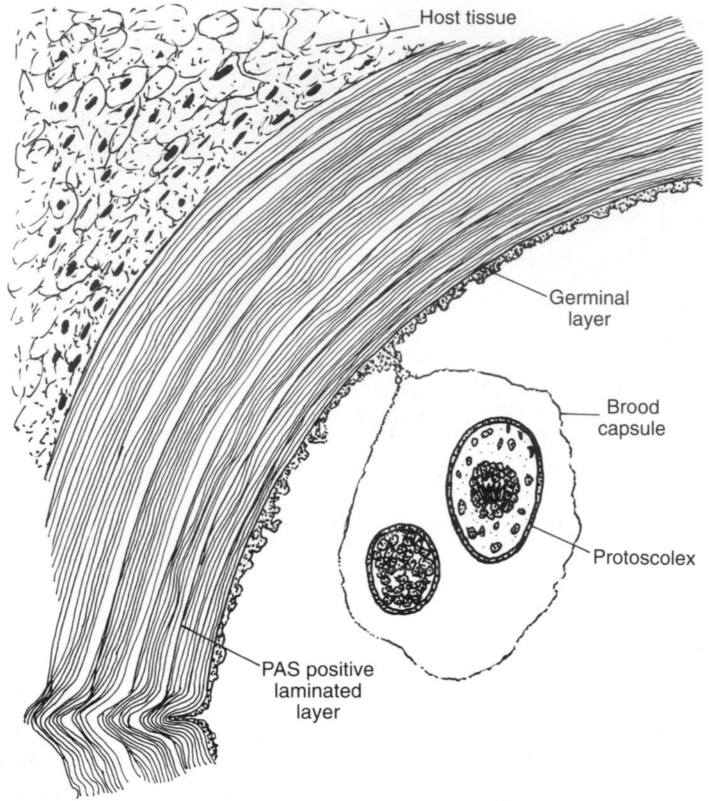

Figure 2. Histological appearance of sectioned *E. granulosus* hydatid cyst.

Hydatid cysts can be identified by the presence of a thick (0.2–2 mm) laminated layer (*Figure 2*) which appears striated and stains positively with the PAS reaction. This laminated layer is unique to the genus *Echinococcus* which makes it a diagnostic feature that other larval cestodes like *Taenia solium* do not possess. In healthy cysts, a thin (10–20 μm) germinal layer may be present on the inside edge of the laminated layer. This layer gives rise to the brood capsules and protoscoleces which may also be apparent in good sections. Small, translucent calcareous corpuscles (~ 5 μm in size) are usually visible in the protoscolex and often in the cystic mass of (~12 μm in size). Calcareous corpuscles are characteristic of tapeworms in general. Where cysts are showing signs of degeneration then the laminated layer may be the only recognizable structure. The fibrous host capsule present around cysts of *E. granulosus* is less prominent in cysts of *E. multilocularis*, also in the latter species the laminated layer is significantly thinner but will stain strongly in PAS, and protoscoleces are usually absent (*Figure 3*).

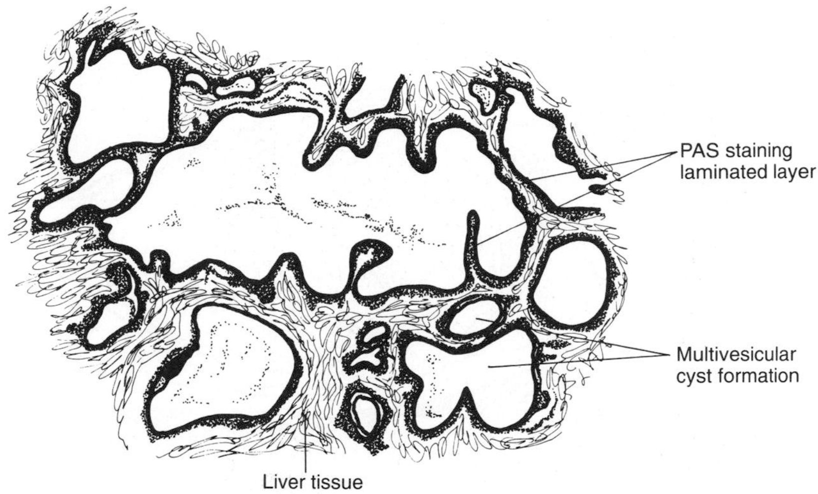

Figure 3. Histological appearance of sectioned *E. multilocularis* alveolar hydatid cyst in human liver.

2.2 Cysticercosis

Cysticercosis due to *T. solium* is usually quite distinct parasitologically from cystic or alveolar hydatidosis. However, the large racemose form of *T. solium* in the brain may be difficult to differentiate in patients from cerebral cystic hydatidosis, or more rarely from brain coenurosis due to *T. multiceps* (section 5) unless the laminated layer of the latter is visible through imaging techniques (section 4).

2.2.1 Biopsy

Biopsy is most useful in the diagnosis of subcutaneous cysts where whole or partial cyst recovery is possible. Grossly the presence of two rows of large and small hooks (hooks have the same general appearance as *Echinococcus* but are six times larger (*Table 3*), and four suckers on a single scolex within a fluid-filled thin-walled cyst is characteristic. With *T. solium* infections there is no danger of disseminating disease as for *Echinococcus*.

2.2.2 Histology of cysticercus

Tissue sections of cysticerci should be fixed and stained as in section 2.1. After histological processing typical presentation shows a space between host tissue and a folded host capsule, within which the cysticercus appears as a network of folds and spiral canals sometimes with part of the scolex (with associated hooks and suckers) visible (*Figure 4*). Calcareous corpuscles may also be present, and degenerating cysts show considerable cellular infiltration.

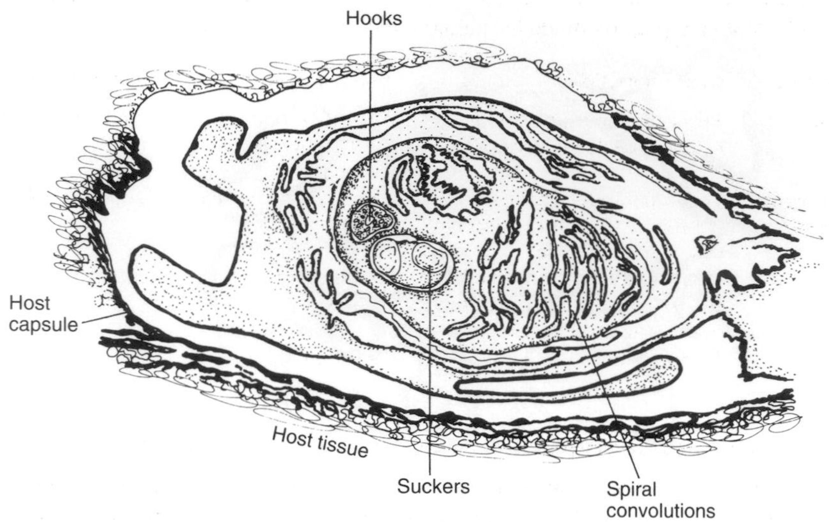

Figure 4. Histological appearance of sectioned *T. solium* cysticercus in muscle tissue.

3. Imaging

A variety of sensitive methods are available for identifying space-occupying masses in internal organs/tissues and most have been applied in the diagnosis of hydatidosis and cysticercosis. The four main imaging methods and their value is summarized in *Table 2*.

In most clinical cases of suspected larval cestode infection serological (and occasionally parasitological) diagnosis will be requested in support of a presumptive diagnosis based on imaging methods and patient history.

4. Immunodiagnosis

Due to the organ or tissue location of larval cestode cysts and the invariable lack of direct parasitological evidence of infection, immunodiagnostic methods are extremely useful in the diagnosis of both hydatidosis and cysticercosis. A variety of immunological techniques have been applied in the diagnosis of these parasitic helminth infections. These rely on the detection of anti-parasite antibodies or parasite antigen in host body fluids, or antigen (or DNA) directly in parasite material obtained post-surgically or from biopsy.

Unfortunately there has been duplication in the nomenclature of the immunodominant antigens in *Echinococcus* and *T. solium*. A lipoprotein antigen in hydatid fluid has been called antigen B, as has a para myosin-rich antigen purified from cyst membranes of *T. solium*. We shall refer to the *E. granulosus* antigen as EgB and the *T. solium* antigen as TsB.

Table 2. Main imaging methods for human larval cestode infections

Method	Cystic hydatid	Alveolar hydatid	Neurocysticercosis
X-ray	Primarily for lung cysts or calcified cysts elsewhere	Primarily for calcified liver and brain lesions	Calcified brain and muscle cysts
Ultrasound scanning	Liver and abdominal cysts, laminated layer and daughter cysts characteristic	Liver cystic masses	Occular cysts
CT scan	Liver, abdominal organs, bone, brain, laminated and daughter cysts characteristic	Liver and brain lesions	Brain cysts
NMR	As for CT scan	As for CT scan	As for CT scan

4.1 Antibody detection in cystic hydatid disease

Over the past 50 years a wide variety of immunological tests have been used to detect IgG, IgA, IgM, and IgE antibody responses in patients with cystic hydatid disease. These have principally included the complement fixation test, the indirect haemagglutination (IHA) or latex agglutination test, the Casoni intradermal test, the ELISA and various precipitation tests reviewed elsewhere (3). IgG responses are most suitable for detecting infection although levels may remain high for sometime after surgical removal of the cyst or following chemotherapy (*Protocol 1* and section 4.4).

Cyst fluid, protoscoleces, and cyst membrane antigens have all been employed in diagnosis and crude cyst fluid appears to be the most suitable in terms of immunogenicity and availability. The use of this complex mixture of proteins as an antigen source does, however, produce varying proportions of both false positive and false negative results, and it is now widely accepted that the sensitivity and specificity of diagnosis can be improved by the application of two or more diagnostic methods. Additionally the use of more purified fractions of cyst fluid antigens may improve specificity.

Hydatid cyst fluid contains two major lipoprotein antigens referred to as Antigen 5 and Antigen B (EgB) as well as several other components, some of which are of host origin. Antibodies to Antigen 5 in precipitation tests have previously been considered to be specific for *Echinococcus granulosus* although it is now known that a certain proportion of cross-reactions occur with sera from people infected with other species of *Echinococcus* and cysticercosis due to *Taenia solium*. The specificity of these tests, however, is high. In more sensitive diagnostic tests, Antigen 5 possesses a phosphorylcholine moiety which may be responsible for a proportion of the cross-reactions with other infections. Antigen B, however, is now thought to be highly genus-specific for *Echinococcus* some cross-reaction with cysticeriosis and a semi-purified preparation of this antigen may be preferable in some situations (*Protocol 2*).

The quality of cyst fluid antigens can vary between hydatid cysts particularly in terms of different host species and cyst condition. Clear fluid from fertile cysts (containing protoscoleces) of sheep, horse, camel, or human origin is antigenically most suitable. It is important, however, that if human cyst fluid is used then contaminating host immunoglobulins must first be removed. Cyst fluid batches should be aspirated from recently slaughtered animals, centrifuged at 1000 *g* for 15 minutes and checked for reactivity with known positive sera before their application in routine diagnostic procedures. Samples can be kept at −20 °C as a crude fluid or be dialysed against distilled water and lyophilized.

Diagnostic procedures should be designed so that suspected sera are screened with a sensitive method and confirmed with a more specific test. The current recommendation is that the ELISA test provides a sensitive initial screening technique which requires low quantities of antigen and sera. IgG is the dominant class of specific antibody in cystic hydatidosis. Positive samples with this assay should then be subjected to the 'Arc 5' or 'DD5' precipitation tests or assessment by immunoblotting. It must be noted that the location of cysts in a patient may affect the antibody response. Pulmonary cysts, for example, tend to be associated with a lower immunoreactivity than hepatic cysts.

Protocol 1. ELISA for antibody detection

1. Disposable polystyrene microtitre plates are sensitized overnight at 4 °C by coating each well with 50 or 100 μl of cyst fluid antigen at a total protein concentration of 5–10 μg/ml in 0.05 M bicarbonate–carbonate buffer pH 9.6.
2. Wash plates with PBS–Tween (0.1%) and block for 1 h either with PBS–0.3% Tween or 1% bovine serum albumin (BSA).
3. Sera to be tested are titrated in doubling dilutions (in PBS–0.1% Tween) from 1/20 onwards, in 50 μl–100 μl volumes, in duplicate. For large scale sero-epidemiological studies a single dilution (1/100) of each test sera in triplicate is recommended. Incubate sera for 1.5 h at room temperature (20 °C) or for 1 h at 37 °C.
4. Wash the wells and incubate for the same times as above, with the optimum concentration of enzyme-conjugated anti-human IgG (as determined by chequerboard titration).
5. Plates are subsequently washed and developed with substrate.
6. The optical density (O.D.) of the plates are then read after a suitable time interval (10–30 min) on a microplate spectrophotometer at the relevant wavelength. It is important that the appropriate control wells (i.e. no antigen, no sera etc.) are included in each plate.

4.1.1 Determination of positive samples in ELISA test

For sera which have been titrated the reciprocal of the final dilution which gives a positive reaction is the antibody titre. This can then be compared with titrations of known negative and known positive sera to establish a positive/negative cut-off titre.

In plates where only one serum dilution is used, a large number of samples, in several plates, can be directly compared, if O.D. readings are taken at exactly the same time. Since day to day fluctuations in the enzyme reaction may occur it is better to relate O.D. values of test sera to that of a reference serum included in each ELISA run. A positive/negative cut-off value must be calculated by assaying a number of known negative sera. A standard cut-off level is usually calculated as the mean O.D. plus three standard deviations of the negative controls. The sensitivity of the ELISA with crude cyst fluid antigen is approximately 80%–90% while specificity is approximately 75%–90%. Notable cross-reactions occur with a proportion of sera from people with alveolar hydatidosis, cysticercosis, filariasis, fascioliasis and schistosomiasis.

In areas where there is a possibility of infection with other parasitic helminths it may be preferable to carry out the above ELISA using a more specific *Echinococcus* semi-purified preparation of Antigen B as described by Oriol *et al.* (4).

Protocol 2. Preparation of an Antigen B (EgB) fraction of hydatid fluid

1. Hydatid fluid may be obtained from infected animals at slaughter. Centrifuge 100 ml of hydatid fluid at 1000 *g* for 15 min, and dialyse against 0.005 M acetate buffer pH 5.0 overnight at 4 °C.
2. Remove precipitate by centrifugation at 50 000 *g* for 30 min and re-suspend in 10 ml of 0.2 M phosphate buffer pH 8.0.
3. Mix solution with ammonium sulfate to 40% saturation, hold for 60 min, and centrifuge to remove the resulting precipitated globulin fraction.
4. Cover supernatant loosely with aluminium foil and boil at 100 °C for 15 min in a water-bath.
5. Centrifuge solution at 50 000 *g* for 60 min and remove the resulting supernatant containing Antigen B(EgB).
6. Estimate protein and dilute to 5 μg/ml for the sensitization of ELISA plates.

The EgB ELISA has recently been adapted as a rapid dot ELISA for field use. This assay can be done in approximately 30 minutes with whole blood samples. Good results have been obtained in field trials, although the test has not yet been fully evaluated (*Protocol 3*) (5).

Protocol 3. The EgB dot ELISA

1. 2 μl of the EgB fraction (1–2 μg protein) is dotted on to nitrocellulose strips and allowed to dry for 1 h.
2. Block reactive sites on strips with 5% skimmed milk in PBS for 30 min, and wash in PBS–0.1% Tween. Strips can be stored dry for several weeks at 4 °C.
3. Add 20 μl of sera or 50 μl of whole blood to 2 ml of PBS–0.1% Tween and incubate strips for 10 min, with regular agitation, in ten trough rack trays.
4. Wash strips in PBS–Tween and incubate for 10 min in a 1/1000 dilution of horse-radish peroxidase-conjugated, anti-human IgG.
5. Wash strips and incubate with 4-chloro-1-naphthol substrate solution and read visually after 10 min.
6. Positive results occur as blue coloured spots on the nitrocellulose strips. Sera which give positive results in a microtitre or dot blot ELISA should then be tested by additional diagnostic methods such as precipitation tests or immunoblotting.

4.1.2 Precipitation tests

The original identification of antibodies to Antigen 5 was performed by immunoelectrophoresis where sera from hydatid patients gave a distinct precipitation arc (arc 5) with hydatid fluid. This test has now been developed into a double diffusion test (DD5) (6) which is simpler. The test relies on a precipitation arc against cyst fluid which shows identity with an arc produced by a control reference serum against Antigen 5. The control sera is raised in sheep by immunization with sheep hydatid cyst fluid. The resulting antibodies are diluted until only arc 5 is revealed against hydatid fluid antigen. Reference sera can also be raised in rabbits (see *Protocol 7A*) but the resulting antibody must be absorbed against sheep serum proteins.

Protocol 4. The DD5 test

The precipitation reactions are carried out in 1.2% agarose gels in PBS.

1. Pour gels on glass slides or plates and cut wells for antigen, test sera, and reference sera as shown in *Figure 5*.
2. Add 150 μl of test sera, 50 μl of arc 5 reference sera, and 3 μl of hydatid fluid antigen (50 mg lyophilized antigen/ml PBS) to the corresponding wells, and place slides in a humidified chamber for 48 h at room temperature.

3. Wash slides in several changes of PBS over 36 h and dry at 37 °C.
4. Stain gels with Amido black or Coomassie blue to reveal precipitation arcs.

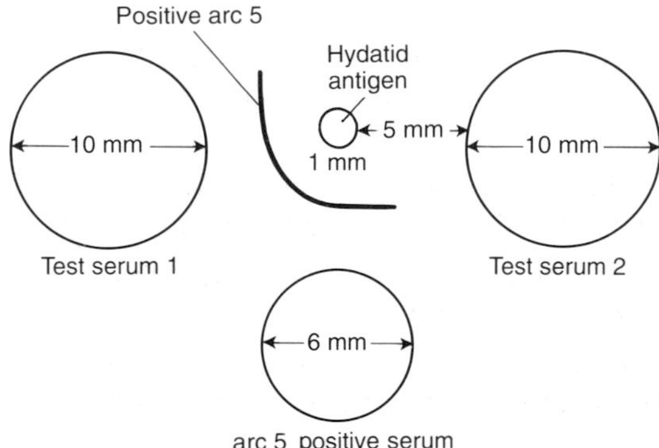

Figure 5. Diagram of agar gel for testing two sera by the double (DD5) test. Test serum 1 gives a positive precipitation arc which has identity with the arc 5 reference serum.

Positive sera are those which show a precipitin line of identity with the arc 5 control serum (*Figure 5*). The sensitivity of the DD5 test is approximately 66–75%, but it is highly specific with cross-reactions only with *E. multilocularis*, *E. vogeli*, and occasionally cysticercosis.

4.1.3 Immunoblotting

When hydatid fluid is separated by SDS-polyacrylamide gel electrophoresis, specific protein bands corresponding to subunits of the major parasite antigens can be recognized. Transfer of the separated proteins to nitrocellulose allows immunoblotting (Western blotting) with suspected sera to be carried out. *Protocol 5* shows the procedure for immunoblotting patients.

Protocol 5. Immunoblotting

1. Dialyse hydatid cyst fluid against distilled water and concentrate by lyophilization. Reconstitute antigen to approximately one tenth the original volume in PBS.
2. Run antigen preparation under either non-reducing or reducing conditions, preferably on 5%–20% gradient polyacrylamide gels (alternatively 12.5% gels can be used although the separation is not so good). 10–20 μg protein per lane or 200–300 μg per solid comb, is recommended for each gel.

Protocol 5. *Continued*

3. After gel electrophoresis, transfer proteins electrophoretically on to nitrocellulose paper.
4. Cut paper into strips and block with 5% skimmed milk for 1 h.
5. Incubate strips with the test sera at a dilution of 1/25–1/100 in PBS–Tween for 2 h at room temperature, or 1 h at 37 °C, or overnight at 4 °C, with constant agitation.
6. Incubate nitrocellulose strips with a peroxidase-conjugated anti-human IgG at an appropriate dilution (usually 1/1000) for 2 h at room temperature or 1 h at 37 °C.
7. The reaction is visualized using either 4-chloro-1-naphthol or diaminobenzidine (DAB) as a substrate.

4.1.4 Determination of positive results for immunoblotting

Under non-reducing conditions, the most frequently recognized protein bands for hydatid sera, lie in the 52–62 kd region and are thought to represent subunits of Antigen 5. Under reducing conditions this becomes a major subunit of 38 kd (*Figure 6*). Although recognized by the majority of hydatid sera, these bands are also recognized by sera from patients with other infections. The lower molecular weight bands in the 8–24 kd region show little change by reduction and appear to be more specific for *Echinococcus* and represent subunits of Antigen B. The lowest of these bands (approximately 8 kd) is thought to be most specific and is recognized by 78% of hydatid patients (7). This band is not species-specific but does appear to be highly genus-specific. It does not appear to be recognized by most sera from cysticercosis patients and is therefore a useful technique in helping to distinguish between the two diseases.

In conclusion, recognition of Antigen 5 in precipitation reactions can still be considered to be a specific indication of hydatid infection although occasional cross-reactions with cysticercosis cases do exist. In other diagnostic tests, e.g. ELISA, recognition of Antigen B is considered to be more useful. It should be noted that a proportion of patients with hydatid disease show a low antibody response and may be considered to be false negatives. It is therefore important that methods to detect both circulating antibody and circulating antigen be combined with imaging techniques such as ultrasound to reduce the proportion of false negative results.

4.1.5 Antibody detection in alveolar hydatidosis

Most people (> 98%) with active alveolar hydatidosis exhibit a good IgG antibody response and therefore immunodiagnostic sensitivity is not as prob-

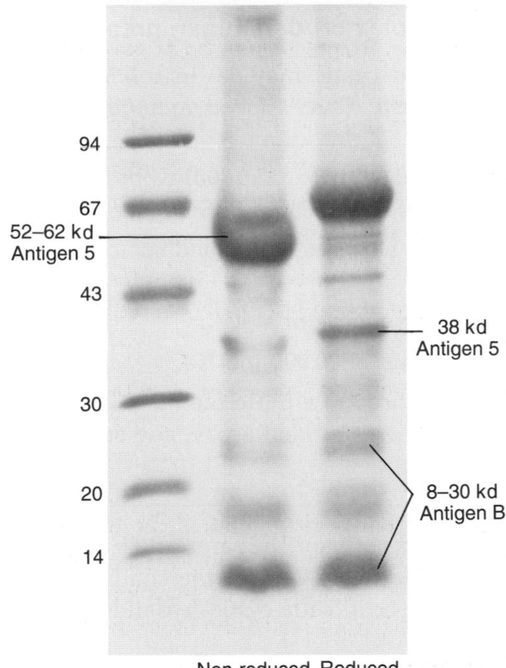

Figure 6. SDS–PAGE analysis of cystic hydatid fluid antigens under reducing and non-reducing conditions. Antigen 5 is represented by a 52–62 kd band in non-reduced conditions which becomes reduced to a major subunit of 38 kd. Antigen B consists of bands in the 8–24 kd region under both conditions.

lematical as for cystic hydatidosis. Until recently serum antibodies in suspected alveolar hydatid patients were invariably detected using crude cyst fluid preparations of *E. granulosus* (generally in an indirect haemagglutination test or arc 5 IEP) which contain cross-reactive antigens, and are easier to obtain.

E. multilocularis cysts and protoscoleces can be made available in the laboratory by intraperitoneal passage of cyst homogenate or protoscoleces (approx. 1000–2000) to form secondary echinococcosis in cotton rats (*Sigmodon hispidus*) or gerbils (*Meriones unguiculatus*). Protoscoleces usually develop by four to six months post-infection.

Crude somatic extracts of *E. multilocularis* protoscoleces or cyst masses are useful and very sensitive in tests like ELISA, although specificity is about 85%. Secretory–excretory (ES) antigens collected from *in vitro* maintenance of viable protoscoleces have also been reported as highly sensitive and specific for *E. multilocularis* antibody detection (8).

Protocol 6. Protoscolex crude antigen preparation (EmP)

1. Dice rodent-derived cystic material in 0.1 M PBS pH 7.2 and pass through a 100 mesh sieve. Sieved material is made up largely of protoscoleces.
2. Wash protoscoleces (approx. 150 000) twice in PBS by centrifugation at 1000 *g* and resuspend in 5 ml PBS containing 0.1 mg/ml Aprotinin.
3. Freeze–thaw pellet twice at −70 °C and sonicate on ice, 10 sec cycles, six times.
4. Stir sonicate gently overnight at 4 °C.
5. Centrifuge for 30 min at 20 000 *g* (4 °C).
6. Filter supernatant through a 5 μm membrane, determine total protein by the Biorad or Lowry protein assay, and store in aliquots at −20 °C or −70 °C.

The crude protoscolex antigen preparation (EmP) or a cyst mass homogenate can be used in the ELISA under the conditions described in *Protocol 1*. Cross-reactions can occur with cystic hydatidosis and to a lesser extent cysticercosis.

A species-specific polypeptide antigen designated Em2 (54 kd) has been purified from a crude *E. multilocularis* cyst extract (rodent-derived) by immunoaffinity absorption against rabbit anti-*E. granulosus* hydatid fluid IgG coupled to CNBr–Sepharose 4B (9). Em2 ELISA has been shown to have an overall sensitivity of 93% and a specificity of 100%, and also to be useful in post-operative follow-up (see section 4.4).

Protocol 7. Preparation of immunoaffinity purified antigen

A. *Rabbit antisera*

1. Immunize rabbit subcutaneously/intramuscularly with 0.5–1.0 mg protein of crude E granulosis hydatid fluid in 0.5 ml PBS emulsified in 0.5 ml Freund's Complete Adjuvant.
2. Administer three boosts of the same quantities in Freund's Incomplete Adjuvant at ten day intervals.
3. Bleed 10 days after final boost and separate off serum.
4. Prepare an IgG fraction from serum by low pH elution (0.2 M glycine–HCl pH 3.0) from an equal volume of Protein A–Sepharose CL4B (Pharmacia).
5. Concentrate IgG by ultrafiltration (30 000 Dalton membrane) or vacuum dialysis.

B. *Preparation of immunoaffinity column (Protein A IgG column)*

Either couple hyperimmune rabbit IgG to CNBr-activated Sepharose 4B (Pharmacia) according to manufacturer's recommendations, or couple IgG to Protein A–Sephrose 4B. The advantage of the latter method is that IgG is coupled to Sepharose via its Fc portion and therefore antibody is optimally presented (10).

1. Mix 10 mg/ml IgG in PBS pH 7.2 with swollen Protein A–Sepharose CL4B gel for 20 min at room temperature.
2. Centrifuge at 800 *g* for 60 sec and remove supernatant (determine unbound IgG by absorption at $O.D._{280}$).
3. Wash gel three times in 0.2 M triethanolamine pH 8.3 (with HCl).
4. Resuspend in 30 mM dimethylpimelimidate in 0.2 M triethanolamine pH 8.3 and mix for 45 min at room temperature.
5. Spin as above, remove supernatant, and terminate reaction by adding an equal volume of 0.2 M ethanolamine pH 8.0 to the Sepharose and mixing for 10 min.
6. Wash the gel four times in 0.15 m PBS pH 7.2, and remove unfixed IgG with one wash of 0.2 M glycine–HCl pH 3.0.

C. *Immunoaffinity absorption of EmP*

1. Mix EmP or crude cyst homogenate (in 0.15 M PBS pH 7.2) with anti-hydatid fluid Sepharose equivalent to approx. 30% of total IgG coupled, for 3–4 h at 4 °C.
2. Centrifuge at 800 *g* for 3 min.
3. Supernatant represents antigen EmP absorbed once.
4. Regenerate Sepharose by washing in elution buffer (0.2 M glycine–HCl pH 3.0) followed by 0.15 M PBS pH 7.2.
5. Repeat steps **1–3** to produce a doubly absorbed Em antigen preparation.
6. Concentrate supernatant by vacuum dialysis if necessary, and store at −20 °C or −70 °C.
7. Use in ELISA or dot ELISA as outlined in *Protocols 1* and *3* respectively. It is also possible to use IgG–Sepharose linked to IgG purified from sera of human cystic hydatid disease patients and use as an additional absorption step for the Em preparation.

4.1.6 Antibody detection in *T. solium* cysticercosis

The detection of anti-parasite antibodies, in sera or cerebrospinal fluid (CSF), has been carried out by a variety of techniques. Many laboratories have reported using the IHA as an initial screening technique but other techniques are becoming more commonly used. As the basis of initial screening the ELISA test is one of the most rapid and robust. Dependent upon the antigen used, the test has been shown to be highly sensitive detecting over 80% of infected individuals. In general there is a greater sensitivity for antibodies in CSF compared to serum. As for human hydatidosis there appears to be no correlation between antibody response and the clinical status of the disease.

Standardization of reagents for use in immunoassays is important if results are to be compared between different laboratories. Use of crude saline extracts by homogenization of whole cysticerci (derived from infected pigs) as a source of antigen have, however, been shown to cross-react with sera from patients with other diseases creating a problem with specificity. A refinement of this technique has involved the use of a partially purified antigen known as antigen B (TsB). The methods for the production of crude *T. solium* extract and antigen B (TsB) are listed below. Serial titration of sera and CSF's against reference positive and negative samples is recommended in ELISA, with the latter starting at a 1:2 dilution. Immunoblot analysis normally uses sera diluted to 1:100 and CSF to 1:20. The normal antigen concentration for coating the ELISA plate is in the region of 5 μg to 10 μg total protein/ml.

Since *T. solium* is non-endemic or has extremely low prevalence in most of the developed world the amount of effort involved in the preparation of antigens for serodiagnosis of a few imported cases is probably excessive. For this reason it is common for sera to be sent to national or regional screening centres.

Protocol 8. Preparation of crude cyst extract of *T. solium*

1. Excise whole cysticerci from pig muscle and remove from host capsule. Wash overnight at 4 °C in 0.15 M PBS pH 7.2.
2. Homogenize on ice in PBS containing 0.1 mg/ml Aprotinin. Leave mixture stirring gently overnight at 4 °C.
3. Centrifuge at 25 000 *g* at 4 °C, collect supernatant, determine protein concentration, and store at −20 °C or −70 °C.

Protocol 9. Preparation of antigen B (TsB) from cysts

1. Homogenize solid parts of cysticerci on ice in 0.2 M 2-mercaptoethanol (Sigma) in 0.45 M NaCl containing 0.1 mg/ml Aprotinin.
2. Centrifuge homogenate at 25 000 *g* for 60 min at 4 °C, dialyse overnight in 0.5 M acetic acid pH 2.3, and re-centrifuge.
3. Adjust protein concentration to 0.5 mg/ml and precipitate TsB with NaCl to a final concentration of 0.86 M and resuspended in 0.5 M acetic acid.

Antigen B of *T. solium* has the advantage of being more specific than the crude extract but this antigen cross-reacts with sera from patients with other infections, particularly hydatidosis. It is therefore important that serology based on this antigen is interpreted in combination with the clinical features and image scanning to confirm the diagnosis. As an alternative to ELISA the immunoelectrophoresis (IEP) technique can be used. This technique is reported to be highly specific, sera from patients detecting eight antigens in the crude antigen extract (11). The sensitivity of IEP is lower than ELISA at around 50%.

If further analysis of serum antibodies is necessary immunoblotting (Western blot) can be employed. This has the advantage of of characterizing the response to a much greater degree than is possible with ELISA. Antigen TsB is recognized by over 80% of patient serum and is present as a doublet between 95 kd and 105 kd. But once again sera from patients with other conditions, particularly hydatidosis, may cross-react with this antigen.

Recently there have been refinements to the immunoblot technique which give good sensitivity and specificity. The most promising has been developed by the Centres for Disease Control, Atlanta, USA, and involves recognition of a group of *T. solium* glycoproteins by patient serum or CSF. This test has been reported to have a sensitivity of 98% and a specificity of 100% (12). A series of seven antigens are considered to be diagnostic for cysticercosis, no one serum will recognize all the antigens but recognition of any one is indicative of a positive diagnosis. These antigens are termed GP 50, GP 42, GP 24, GP 21, GP 18, GP 14, and GP 13, the number represents the kd value. The antigen itself is, however, relatively complicated to prepare and the method is described below.

Protocol 10. Preparation of glycoprotein antigen extract from cysticerci

A. *Isolation of glycoprotein*

1. Porcine cysts (stored frozen, preferably in 1 g–20 g batches in liquid nitrogen) are thawed in 5 vol. (1/5 w/v) of sucrose/Hepes/PMSF buffer (0.05 M Hepes-NaOH, 0.25 M sucrose, 2.0 mM EDTA, 5 mM PMSF, pH 7.2) at 37 °C. PMSF or benzyl sulfonyl fluoride is incorporated into buffers at 5 mM.
2. Homogenize cyst suspensions on ice.
3. Centrifuge at 500 *g* for 20 min at 4 °C. Remove cloudy supernatant and re-homogenize the pellet in 5 vol. of sucrose/Hepes/PMSF buffer. After re-centrifugation the first and second supernatants are combined (this is termed the 0.5 KG supernatant and the combined pellet the 0.5 KG ppt).

Protocol 10. *Continued*

4. Centrifuge the 0.5 KG supernatant at 250 000 *g* for 2 h to yield a dense pellet and a clear supernatant. Aspirate the lipid scum on top of the supernatant and remove any adherent residues with a cotton wool swab.
5. Resuspend the pellet left after the 250 000 *g* centrifugation in 10–20 ml urea/PMSF buffer (8 M urea, 0.05 M Tris–HCl, 5 mM PMSF, pH 8.0) by gentle repeated passage through a 13 gauge cannula and syringe. Sonicate this suspension on ice at 100% power, 20% pulse duty cycle for 5 min, and stir for 30 min at 4 °C.
6. Centrifuge the urea extract at 48 000 *g* for 20 min. Discard pellet and desalt supernatant through a Sephadex G25 (Pharmacia) column equilibrated with 0.2 M NaCl, 0.05 M Tris–HCl pH 8.0 (NaCl/Tris). The desalted fraction is known as 250 KG PS.
7. Concentrate the 250 000 *g* supernatant by ultrafiltration through a YM 10 membrane (Amicon), desalt through G25 into NaCl/Tris. This fraction is referred to as the 250 KG SUP.
8. Combine the 250 KG PS and 250 KG SUP to give a single fraction known as LL-P.
9. Equilibrate a lentil-lectin Sepharose 4B column (Pharmacia) with NaCl/Tris. Prepare 1 ml of lectin gel/3 mg of protein in the solution. Purge lectin columns with two alternating cycles of NaCl/Tris (baseline buffer) and the highest concentration of elution buffer (0.2 M α-methylmannoside, 0.2 M NaCl, 0.05 M Tris–HCl pH 8.0).
10. Load samples (equilibrated in NaCl/Tris baseline buffer) on to columns (ascending). Purge unbound materials with six to eight bed volumes of NaCl/Tris buffer.
11. Elute bound glycoproteins stepwise. Firstly with five bed volumes of 0.005 M and then 0.2 M solutions of α-methyl-mannoside in 0.2 M NaCl, 0.05 M Tris–HCl pH 8.0. The fraction eluted with 0.2 M α-methylmannoside contains the glycoproteins for immunoblotting and is termed LL-GP. If concentration is necessary this can be accomplished by ultrafiltration through a YM 10 membrane (Amicon). Storage should be carried out by adding 0.77 vol. of glycerol and mixing thoroughly, aliquoting, and storage in liquid nitrogen. Aliquots can then be kept at −20 °C (at which temperature it is not frozen and is stable for months).

B. *Immunoblot parameters*

1. Heat LL-GP (about 0.5–0.1 μg/μl protein) at 65 °C in the presence of 1% SDS, 0.1% bromophenol blue (w/v), 0.01 M Tris–HCl pH 8.0 for 15–20 min non-reducing conditions.

2. Dilute treated antigens in 6% glycerol in H_2O until the final protein concentration ≈ 0.1 μg/μl and the SDS concentration is $\leqslant 0.1\%$.
3. Run samples by SDS–PAGE in 0.1% SDS, 0.025% (w/v) bromophenol blue, 1% glycerol, 0.0025 M Tris–HCl pH 8.0 and blot on to nitrocellulose. The optimum antigen dilution is recommended to be in the range of 20–80 ng/μl per millimetre of gel.
4. Probe with sera diluted 1:50 or CSF diluted 1:10.

Recently a number of immunodiagnostic tests based on the detection of cysticercus antibodies in undiluted saliva have been developed. These have demonstrated good sensitivity in both immunoblot and ELISA (13, 14).

4.2 Antigen detection

Detection of circulating antigen or circulating specific immune complexes can also be a useful immunodiagnostic approach for larval cestodes infections particularly when specific antibodies can not be detected or are at low/borderline levels in suspected patient serum. Apart from individual variation in host antibody responses, the site and condition of cystic metacestodes may account for low antibody titres, e.g. pulmonary cystic hydatidosis and calcifying cysts. In neurocysticercosis use of CSF is generally more sensitive than serum for both antigen and antibody detection.

While not yet fully assessed serum antigen detection is potentially more useful than antibody detection in assessment of post-surgical/chemotherapy follow-up (section 4.4). In general, however, it appears that circulating antigen assays for larval cestodiases are less sensitive and less reliable than those for antibody detection. Circulating antigen tests have been used in the diagnosis of cystic hydatidosis using serum samples and with CSF for neurocysticercosis. A number of immunoassays have been applied to detect circulating antigens but the ELISA has proved most useful because it is so adaptable and very sensitive. Of course parasite-specific antigen can also be detected directly in *E. granulosus* hydatid fluid which is sometimes collected during surgery or after biopsy (section 4.2.2).

4.2.1 Antigen detection in cystic hydatidosis

Circulating antigens (CAg) have been detected by ELISA in 33%–85% of patients with cystic hydatid disease (15, 16). However, a significant proportion of serum antigen is complexed with antibody (both IgG or IgM) to form soluble immune complexes. Up to 57% of antibody negative (or with borderline titres) of cystic hydatid patients were positive for specific antigen in 3% polyethylene glycol (PEG 6000) precipitated immune complexes. Detection of CAg by capture antibody ELISA or in 3% PEG precipitates has proved useful to us and others (17) in establishing diagnosis of cystic hydatidosis in several antibody seronegative patients. A capture ELISA using rabbit anti-

E. granulosus cyst fluid IgG was more sensitive than antibody detection in assessment of surgical treatment. Serum antigen has been detected at concentrations of up to 270 ng/ml serum (15).

Protocol 11. Capture ELISA for serum antigen in cystic hydatidosis

1. Raise rabbit antisera against sheep, horse, or bovine hydatid cyst fluid and prepare IgG fraction (as in *Protocol 7*).
2. Remove cross-reactive anti-'host' (sheep, horse, or bovine antibodies) by absorption against respective host species serum coupled to CNBr–Sepharose (as described in *Protocol 7B* and *C*).
3. Conjugate 8 mg IgG to 4 mg of horse-radish peroxidase (HRPO) after Wilson and Nakane (18) as follows:
   (a) Dissolve HRPO in 1 ml distilled water, add 200 μl of freshly prepared 0.1 M sodium periodate (Sigma) and mix for 20 min at room temperature.
   (b) Dialyse HRPO solution against excess 1 mM sodium acetate buffer pH 4.4 overnight 4 °C.
   (c) Add 20 μl of 0.2 M sodium carbonate/bicarbonate buffer pH 9.6 (BCB) to raise pH to 9–9.5.
   (d) Immediately add 8 mg IgG in 1 ml of 0.1 M BCB pH 9.6 and mix, end over end, for 2 h room temperature.
   (e) Add 0.1 ml freshly prepared sodium borohydride (4 mg/ml distilled water) to reduce any free enzyme, and leave for 2 h at 4 °C.
   (f) Dialyse IgG–HRPO solution overnight against excess 0.15 M PBS pH 7.2 at 4 °C.
   (g) Aliquot conjugate and store at −20 °C or −70 °C until used (avoid freezing and thawing more than once).
4. Coat wells of ELISA microtitre tray, e.g. Immulon no.1 (Dynatech Ltd.) with optimal concentration determined by chequerboard titration (usually 10–20 μg IgG/ml) of unlabelled IgG antisera in 0.05 M BCB pH 9.6 overnight 4 °C.
5. Wash and block as *Protocol 1*.
6. Add duplicate sera (samples and controls) neat or diluted no less than 1:5 in PBS–0.1% Tween-20 and incubate for 2 h at room temperature.
7. Wash wells.
8. Add HRPO-conjugated anti-hydatid fluid IgG at optimum concentration (determined by chequerboard titration) for 1 h at room temperature.
9. Wash.

10. Develop using substrates recommended in *Protocol 1*.
11. Read optical density of wells between 30–60 min (at relevant wavelength). Determine optimal end-point by use of control positive of serially diluted hydatid cyst fluid in normal human sera. A standard curve can be constructed with known protein concentrations of hydatid fluid, therefore relative serum concentration values for CAg can be determined.

4.2.2 Specific antigen detection in cystic hydatid fluid samples

Samples of fluid from suspected hydatid cysts are often taken during exploratory surgery or before cyst removal particularly when hydatid serology is negative. Where protoscoleces have not been aspirated or the cyst is sterile (no protoscoleces), and where histology can not be carried out, it is possible to check the cyst fluid sample for presence of *Echinococcus* antigens. Previous reports have used the DD5 test (section 4.1) (19) and a simple ELISA without a capture antibody (20) (*Protocol 12*).

Protocol 12. ELISA for antigen detection in hydatid fluid samples

1. Coat ELISA plate with centrifuged (1000 $g \times 10$ min) cyst fluid sample(s) diluted (from 1:10) in BCB pH 9.6, incubate overnight 4°C.
2. Wash and block as before.
3. Add optimal dilution of HRPO-conjugated rabbit anti-hydatid cyst fluid and incubate 1 h room temperature.
4. Wash.
5. Develop with substrate as described in *Protocol 1*. Include a known hydatid fluid sample from human or animal infection as a positive control.

4.2.3 Antigen detection in neurocysticercosis

The demonstration of parasite-specific antigens in CSF has been undertaken as a means of diagnosing 'current' infection with neurocysticercosis, the argument being that secreted parasite antigens will only be present if the parasites were viable as opposed to antibodies which may persist for considerable periods after the death of the parasites. These tests have, however, generally been shown to be less sensitive than those involving antibody detection. Tests based on detection of circulating parasite antigens have used polyclonal antibodies raised in rabbits against the metacestode (crude cyst extract or TsB) (21), and monoclonal antibodies against *T. solium* cyst fluid or surface glycoprotein of *T. saginata* (22). A capture ELISA similar to that described in *Protocol 11* with appropriate antisera can be used with CSF samples neat or diluted 1:2. The sensitivity of CAg-ELISA, based on a polyclonal anti-metacestode, for CSF from neurocysticercosis patients is approximately 77% (21).

4.3 Critical diagnostic pathways for laboratory diagnosis of hydatidosis and cysticercosis

4.3.1 Cystic hydatidosis (*E. granulosus*)

i. Serodiagnosis

(a) Carry out ELISA for IgG serum antibody detection using crude hydatid fluid antigen preparation or purified EgB antigen. Use latter in dot ELISA if access to only basic laboratory facilities (*Protocols 1, 2,* and *3*).

(b) Carry out DD5 test as a second serum antibody test (*Protocol 4*).

(c) Carry out immunoblotting of serum sample against crude hydatid fluid for confirmation of antibody recognition of the 8–24 kd antigen subunits (*Protocol 5*).

(d) If all antibody tests negative or inconclusive carry out CAg-ELISA on serum sample (*Protocol 11*).

(e) If all serological tests negative, test cyst fluid sample (if available) for presence of *Echinococcus* antigen (*Protocol 12*).

ii. Surgical or biopsy sample

(a) Check cyst aspirate for presence of protoscoleces, hooks, and brood capsules; carry out histology of cyst membranes (sections 2.1.1, 2.1.2, and *Figures 1–3*).

(b) In the absence of parasitological evidence carry out ELISA for *Echinococcus* antigen detection with cyst fluid sample (*Protocol 12*).

4.3.2 Alveolar hydatidosis (*E. multilocularis*)

i. Serodiagnosis

(a) Carry out ELISA for IgG antibody detection using crude, EmP, cyst homogenate or the more specific Em2 antigen (hydatid fluid antigen can be used if *E. multilocularis* antigens unavailable) (*Protocols 1, 6,* and *7*).

(b) Use dot ELISA with EmP or Em2 antigen if only access to basic laboratory facilities (*Protocols 1, 3, 6,* and *7*).

ii. Surgical or biopsy sample

(a) Check gross specimen and histology of tissue sections for characteristic morphology—thin laminated layer, germinal membrane, and lack of host capsule (section 2.1.2).

(b) Subject fine needle biopsy material to PCR reaction for DNA amplification and probe with pAL1 DNA probe (23), if facilities available.

4.3.3 Cysticercosis (*T. solium*)

i. Serodiagnosis

(a) If cysticercus glycoprotein purified extract available carry out immunoblotting with sera or CSF to identify specific Gp 42–Gp13 antigens (*Protocols 5*, and *10*).

(b) Carry out ELISA for IgG antibody detection in serum or CSF (more sensitive) using crude cyst extract or TsB antigen if (a) not possible (*Protocols 1*, *8*, and *9*).

(c) If serum and CSF seronegative, test CSF for circulating antigen by capture ELISA.

ii. Surgical or biopsy sample

(a) Examine fresh or fixed specimen under a dissecting microscope for characteristic cysticercus gross morphology.

(b) Check histology of tissue sections for characteristic appearance (*Figure 4*).

4.4 Post-treatment follow-up by serology

Surgery and increasingly chemotherapy are the main forms of treatment of human hydatidosis and cysticercosis. Evaluation of surgical treatment and particularly benzimidazole chemotherapy of hydatidosis is often difficult, and in many patients uncertainty exists about cure. Secondary echinococcosis associated with surgical spillage or recurrence after chemotherapy may not become apparent until several years later.

Difficulties for anti-hydatid chemotherapy include failure to obtain proof of parasite viability before and after chemotherapy, and lack of knowledge about the natural history of untreated hydatid disease. Numbers, size, site, and condition of cyst masses may vary considerably, and imaging methods do not always indicate clear changes in cyst contents, structure, or size in patients during or after chemotherapy.

Post-surgical follow-up by serology for antibody detection has by and large not been very useful, mainly because of the residual nature of antibodies even after complete surgical removal of cysts in some cases. The complement fixation test (CFT) appears most useful for post-surgical follow-up of cystic hydatidosis, as CFT antibody titres often decrease significantly by three months after successful surgery (24). For alveolar hydatidosis the Em2 ELISA is probably currently most appropriate for correlation with successful resection of hepatic cyst lesions, as negative seroconversion occurs in some patients within one year after successful resection (25).

Circulating antigen (CAg) (*Protocol 11*) and circulating immune complex (CIC) assays based on ELISA have been partially assessed in relation to surgical and chemotherapeutic treatment of cystic hydatidosis (15, 16). Levels of serum antigen were observed to become negative in two patients by ten days and ten months following surgical removal of liver cysts. Levels of IgM-specific CICs also decrease more rapidly than antibodies (IgG or IgM) following successful cystic hydatid surgery. IgM–CICs are detected by the capture ELISA of *Protocol 11* but where the anti-cyst fluid IgG enzyme conjugate is replaced with anti-human IgG or IgM enzyme conjugates.

Assessment of benzimidazole drug therapy for human hydatidosis with the aid of serology is more difficult and still requires further research. Difficulties arise because degenerate or dead cyst material may still stimulate antibody responses. The serial variation in antibody levels (especially CFT titres) during and after chemotherapy is more useful than absolute values, and this also applies to CAg and IgM–CIC values. We have observed significant variability between different patients undergoing albendazole chemotherapy. In some cystic hydatid patients where chemotherapy had a major effect on hepatic cysts, levels of CAg, IgM–CICs, and IgG antibodies increased soon after the onset of chemotherapy, and only the first two parameters decreased to near background levels by 12–18 months after treatment.

Serologic follow-up of praziquantel treated neurocysticercosis patients using an IgG ELISA showed an initial rise in antibody levels followed by a steady decline in most cases and negative seroconversion in a few patients. Corticosteroid cover in a number of patients appeared to suppress the elevation of antibody levels (26).

5. Rare larval cestode infections in man

More than 95% of all human larval cestode infections are due to *E. granulosus*, *T. solium*, or *E. multilocularis*. Rare larval cestode infections can be realistically divided into three other diseases namely, polycystic hydatidosis, coenurosis, and sparganosis.

5.1 Polycystic hydatidosis—*E. vogeli*

Less than 30 cases of *E. vogeli* hydatidosis have been reported and all originate in northern South America. The parasite is primarily transmitted in a sylvatic cycle between the bush dog (*Speothos venaticus*) and the large rodent (*Cuniculus paca*). Human infections have occurred in Columbia, Venezuela, Ecuador, Panama, Argentina, and probably Brazil; they are most likely as a result of semi-domestic transmission via dogs in association with forested regions. In man cysts are usually found in or connected to the liver. Morphologically the cysts appear between the cystic and alveolar forms of *Echinococcus*, i.e. they consist of small fluid-filled chambers surrounded by a fibrous host capsule, usually containing some brood capsules and protoscoleces, and with laminated layers of variable thickness, but as in alveolar hydatidosis, a semi-fluid matrix with exogenous budding may occur and often with some central necrosis. Hook size in protoscoleces of *E. vogeli* is significantly larger than for *E. granulosus* or *E. multilocularis* (see *Table 3*).

Table 3. Larval scolex hook sizes

Species	Mean length μm (range)	
	Large hooks	**Small hooks**
E. granulosus	30 (19–44)	25 (17–31)
E. multilocularis	27.5 (25–30)	24 (21–27)
E. vogeli	40.5 (38–46)	33 (30–37)
T. solium	184 (163–198)	123 (104–134)
T. multiceps	167 (157–177)	125 (109–136)
T. serialis	156 (145–170)	111 (45–125)
T. brauni	145 (139–150)	108 (102–114)

Antibody responses have been detected using haemagglutination and arc 5 IEP tests and will cross-react with *E. granulosus* antigens.

5.2 Coenurosis—*T. multiceps, T. serialis, T. brauni*

Human coenurosis usually occurs as a result of infection with the larval stage of one of three main *Taenia* species in which adult tapeworms are parasitic in domestic or wild canids. A hundred or so human infections have been described, with *T. multiceps* being the most frequently diagnosed (27). *T. multiceps* and *T. serialis* have a cosmopolitan distribution including Europe and USA, while *T. brauni* appears to be restricted to Africa. Infection is through ingestion of *Taenia* eggs passed in definitive host faeces. Coenuri in man are found in the brain, spinal cord, eye, subcutaneous and muscular tissues, they generally vary in size from 1–5 cm and are usually fluid-filled containing numerous protoscoleces (brood capsules and laminated layer are absent). Protoscoleces are much more like those of *T. solium* than *Echinococcus*, and are usually arranged in scattered groups on the germinal membrane of *T. multiceps* or in a radiating serial pattern for *T. serialis*. Multiple scoleces are often visible in histological sections. In the natural intermediate hosts (lagomorphs and rodents) *T. serialis* and *T. brauni* primarily locate intramuscularly or subcutaneously, while those of *T. multiceps* (sheep and goats) are almost always in the CNS. Comparative hook sizes are shown in *Table 3*. Sera from coenuriasis patients usually contain antibodies which are cross-reactive with *T. solium* antigens.

5.3 Sparganosis—*Spirometra* spp., *Diphyllobothrium* spp.

Sparganosis is a general term for human infection with the plerocercoid stages of pseudophyllidean cestodes usually belonging to the genera of *Spirometra* or less commonly *Diphyllobothrium*. In many cases the species is not known. Sparganosis has a wide geographical distribution but with most human infections occurring in the Far East especially Korea, China, and Thailand, but also in parts of Africa and S. America. The mode of infection is not always apparent and could be through drinking water containing infected copepods (first intermediate host), or more likely from eating secondary intermediate hosts which may be fish, amphibians, reptiles, or mammals infected with plerocercoids. Natural final hosts are usually carnivores including dogs and cats. Spargana usually locate in subcutaneous tissues as inflammatory nodules, and appear as white ribbon-like worms several centimetres in length. They possess a poorly developed scolex which lacks hooks or suckers. Histologically the body wall of spargana in tissue sections superficially resembles that of a cysticercus but without the spiral convoluted appearance. Sera from sparganum infected individuals may cross-react in antibody tests for cysticercosis.

Note added in proof

The recent development and application of specific recombinant antigens of *E. multilocularis* and *E. granulosus* for serum antibody detection has great potential for standardized immunodiagnosis of alveolar hydratosis. (28, 29).

References

1. Thompson, R. C. A. (ed.) (1986). *The biology of Echinococcus and hydatid disease*. George Allen and Unwin, London.
2. Gemmell, M., Matyas, Z., Pawlowski, Z., and Soulsby, E. J. L. (ed.) (1983). *Guidelines for surveillance, prevention and control of taeniasis/cysticercosis*. World Health Organization, Geneva.
3. Schantz, P. M. and Gottstein, B. (1986). In *Immunodiagnosis of parasitic diseases* (ed. C. F. Walls, and P. M. Schwartz, Vol. 1, pp. 69–107. Academic Press, New York.
4. Oriol, R., Williams, J. F., Perez-Esandi, M. V., and Oriol, C. (1971). *Am. J. Trop. Med. Hyg.*, **20**, 569.
5. Rogan, M. T., Craig, P. S., Zeghle, E., Romig, T., Lubano, G. M., and Liu, D. (1991). *Trans. R. Soc. Trop. Med. Hyg.*, **85**, 773.
6. Coltorti, E. A. and Varela-Diaz, V. M. (1978). *Trans. R. Soc. Trop. Med. Hyg.*, **72**, 226.
7. Maddison, S. E., Slemenda, S. B., Schantz, P. M., Fried, J. A., Wilson, M., and Tsang, V. C. W. (1989) *Am. J. Trop. Med. Hyg.*, **40**, 377.
8. Auer, H., Hermentin, K., and Aspock, H. (1988). *Zentbl. Bakt. Mikb. Hyg. A.*, **268**, 416.
9. Gottstein, B., Eckert, J., and Fey, H. (1983). *Zeit. Parasitkd.*, **69**, 347.
10. Parkhouse, R. M. E. (1984). *Br. Med. Bull.*, **40**, 297.
11. Flisser, A., Woodhouse, E., and Larralde, C. (1980). *Clin. exp. Immunol.*, **39**, 27.
12. Tsang, V. C. W., Brand, J. A., and Boyer, A. E. (1989). *J. Infect. Dis.*, **159**, 50.
13. Feldman,M., Plancarte, A., Sandoval, M., Wilson, M., and Flisser, A. (1990). *Trans. R. Soc. Trop. Med. Hyg.*, **84**, 559.

14. Acosta, E. (1990). *J. Clin. Lab. Anal.*, **4**, 90.
15. Gottstein, B. (1984). *Am. J. Trop. Med. Hyg.*, **33**, 1185.
16. Craig, P. S. (1986). *Parasite Immunol.*, **8**, 171.
17. Schantz, P. M. (1988). *N. Eng. J. Med.*, **318**, 1469.
18. Wilson, B. M. and Nakane, P. K. (1978). In *Immunofluorescence and related staining techniques* (ed. W. Knapp, K. Holubar, and G. Wicks), pp. 215–24. Elsevier/North Holland Biomedical Press, Amsterdam.
19. Guarnera, E. A. and Varela-Diaz, V. M. (1985). *Trans. R. Soc. Trop. Med. Hyg.*, **79**, 149.
20. Craig, P. S., Bailey, W., and Nelson, G. S. (1986). *Trans. R. Soc. Trop. Med. Hyg.*, **80**, 256.
21. Tellez-Giron, E., Ramos, M. C., Dufour, L., Alvarez, P., and Montante, M. (1987). *Am. J. Trop. Med. Hyg.*, **37**, 169.
22. Correa, D., *et al.* (1989). *Trans. R. Soc. Trop. Med. Hyg.*, **83**, 814.
23. Gottstein, B. and Mowatt, M. R. (1991). *Mol. Biochem. Parasitol.*, **66**, 183.
24. Wilcox, M. H., Bailey, J. W., and Morris, D. L. (1988). *J. R. Soc. Med.*, **81**, 714.
25. Gottstein, B., Tschudi, K., Eckert, J., and Ammann, R. (1989). *Trans. R. Soc. Trop. Med. Hyg.*, **83**, 389.
26. Cho, S. Y., Kim, S. I., and Kang, S. Y. (1986). *Korean J. Parasitol.*, **24**, 159.
27. Abuladze, K. I. (1970). In *Essentials of cestodology* (ed. K. I. Skrjabin), Vol. 4, pp. 383–90. Israel Program for Scientific Translations, Keter Press, Jerusalem.
28. Gottstein, B., Jacquier, P., Bresson-Hadim, S., and Eckert, J. (1993). *J. Clin. Microbiol.* **31**, 373.
29. Helbig, M., Frosch, P., Kern, P., and Frosch, M. (1993). *J. Clin. Microbiol.*, **31**, 3211.

12

Microfilariae

D. A. DENHAM

1. Introduction

The conventional method of detecting and counting microfilariae has been to prepare 'thick' smears of either measured or unmeasured quantities of blood. When I first started work on filariasis in the laboratory I found this technique laborious and slow and began using the chamber system which was subsequently described and evaluated by Denham *et al.* (1). Southgate (2) used the chamber under field conditions and compared its efficiency with that of thick blood smears made on unwashed new slides. As in our laboratory study they found the chamber detected consistently more microfilariae. Partono and Idris (3) have shown since that microfilariae are lost from thick smears if anticoagulated blood is uscd and this cxplains much of the differences between the counting chamber and thick smear methods found by Denham *et al.* (1). Partono and Idris (3) also showed that microfilariae were easily lost from corroded or unclean slides. Probably the major contribution that the paper on the chamber method made was to draw attention to the great care needed when examining blood for microfilariae. It was especially important in pointing out that thick blood smears should not be too small.

The most important advance in the diagnosis of onchocerciasis has been the development of the technique for the quantitative determination of skin microfilariae of *Onchocerca volvulus* described in section 5 and developed by Braun-Munzinger *et al.* (4). The following sections should enable the reader to learn to count and identify all the human microfilariae.

2. Methods of counting microfilariae

Several methods of counting microfilariae in blood have been reported in the literature. These methods depend on either preparing a stained slide or using live smear techniques. In the case of human filariasis, identification of microfilariae is easy if the correct stain is used (*Protocols 8* and *9*).

Protocol 1. Preparing conventional thick smears

1. Clean 75 × 25 mm glass slides very carefully. Slides should be washed with a detergent scouring powder, rinsed thoroughly in water, and rinsed in alcohol before being polished with a clean cloth. Any grease or detergent left on the slide will cause areas of the film to float off during subsequent treatment.
2. With an automatic pipette or a graduated pipette take a measured quantity of blood from a finger or ear lobe prick and prepare a rectangular smear on the clean glass slide using the end of the pipette. In the case of a 40 μl or 60 μl sample the smear should be 20 × 25 mm. If the smear is too small and, therefore too thick, microfilariae will tend to float off during the subsequent dehaemoglobinizing and staining procedures. It is better to make smears too big than too small even though it takes longer to examine large smears.
3. Allow the slide to dry in a dust-free and insect-free environment. A gauze covered box in an incubator or cupboard is perfect for this. In areas of very high humidity an electric light bulb in a cupboard is a useful drying cabinet. The hot bonnet of a vehicle can be used in the field. Remember that dust can be very confusing when stained and that ants, cockroaches, and other insects will eat thick blood smears. The slides should be dried for about 2 h or overnight. Do not leave them for more than 24 h as they become impossible to dehaemoglobinize after this and are then useless.
4. The smear is dehaemoglobinized by immersing the slide in a vertical position in clean tap-water in a staining jar. Watch carefully during this procedure. The blood cells lyse and pigment can be seen to fall away into the water. The whole process should take no more than a minute or two. The longer the slide remains in the water the more likelihood that microfilariae will float off. **Do not run water over the slide.**
5. Remove the slide from the water, allow to dry, and, only when thoroughly dry, immerse it in methanol for 2 sec. This fixes the smear and acts as a mordant and, therefore, permits good staining. Allow the slide to dry in air. The smear may be stored in this condition.
6. The smear can now be stained with either May–Grunwald Giemsa (*Protocol 8*) or Mayer's haemalum (*Protocol 9*).

2.1 Modified thick smear technique

This method (*Protocol 2*) was developed by Webber (5) and evaluated in the laboratory by Abaru and Denham (6).

The method was found to be as accurate as the counting chamber method and as permanent preparations are made the examination can be performed later. As glass slides cost quite a lot of money I have adopted a modification of this method for use in the field. A measured volume of blood is taken and mixed with clean water. The slide is then examined straight away (as described in *Protocol 3*) when the live microfilariae are easily seen and counted. The slide is then dried, rinsed in water, and fixed in methanol. It can then be taken back to the laboratory and stained. Slides on which no microfilariae are found can be washed and used again.

Protocol 2. Preparing thick smears

1. Clean slides as in *Protocol 1.*
2. Place two drops of distilled water on a slide.
3. Mix 40 or 60 μl of blood with the water. Allow it to dry in a dust-free environment.
4. Dip in water for a few seconds to remove haemoglobin.
5. Fix in methanol.
6. Stain with Giemsa or Mayer's haemalum (*Protocols 8* and *9*).

2.2 The counting chamber method

This method was developed in our laboratory to enable speedy, accurate, and immediate counts of microfilariae to be made when the identity of the microfilaria is known (1).

Protocol 3. Counting chamber method for enumeration of microfilariae

1. The counting chamber is prepared by marking a glass 76 × 25 mm slide with lines about 2 mm apart. These can be scratched on with a diamond pencil or etched with hydrofluric acid. Strips of glass (cut from another slide) are then placed on the slide in such a way that a well, approximately 20 × 30 mm, is formed. These strips are fixed to the slide using DPX, Canada Balsam or any slide mountant, or an epoxy resin. We use DPX as it can be easily cleaned from the slide. Once the cement has dried the slides are cleaned and are ready for use.
2. A measured volume of blood from a finger prick or ear lobe prick is taken. We routinely use between 20 μl and 100 μl measured with an automatic pipette. If 100 μl is used the red coloration due to haemoglobin is too dense in the size of cell chamber recommended above, so we use a larger chamber about 20 × 45 mm.
3. The measured volume of blood is discharged into a small volume of

Protocol 3. *Continued*

water in the counting chamber. Further water is added until the chamber is almost full. It is important that sufficient water is added to prevent a large concave meniscus forming as this obscures microfilariae on the edge of the slide. Equally the chamber should not be overfilled so that a convex meniscus is formed. **Do not** add a coverslip.

4. The microfilariae can now be easily seen at a magnification of × 30–40. When you start using this method use a slightly higher magnification then work down until you find your personal optimum. Good quality transillumination makes counting much easier and more accurate. But adjust the lighting so that the microfilariae can be seen easily.
5. Count the microfilariae using the slide markings as guide-lines. We use a hand-tally but it is not too difficult to count without one.

We have used this method to count microfilaria of several species and find it very reliable even in the hands of completely inexperienced people. We expect to take a blood sample and produce an accurate count within two minutes.

Some species of microfilaria die quickly in water, others live for a long time. For example *Brugia*, *Loa*, and *Wuchereria* all remain alive. *Dirofilaria immitis* always dies whereas *D. repens* remains alive.

If you are unable to examine the slide immediately take the blood sample and discharge it into 0.5–1.0 ml 3% acetic acid. The lysed blood is conveniently stored in a 1 ml vial. Samples taken in this way can be stored and examined months later.

3. Concentration techniques

Although the methods described above are useful for counting microfilariae when there are reasonable quantities, many patients with filarial infections have fewer than one microfilaria in 20 μl of blood. This can, to some extent, be overcome by taking 100 μl. To surmount this problem several concentration techniques have been employed.

Protocol 4. Knott's concentration technique for microfilariae in blood (7)

1. Take 1 ml of blood and mix it by inverting the test-tube several times with 10 ml of 2% formalin[a] in a 15 ml conical centrifuge tube. By this process the blood will be haemolysed and the microfilariae will be relaxed.
2. Leave the tube upright for 12–24 h. A small compact sediment of

leucocytes and microfilariae collects in the tip of the centrifuge tube. Alternatively, centrifuge at 1000 r.p.m. for 5 min.

3. Discard the supernatant.
4. Take up the deposit into a Pasteur pipette, place it on a microscope slide, and count the microfilariae.
5. If stained preparations are required, thin smears of the deposit in water can be spread over an area of 20 × 30 μm on an ordinary glass microscope slide and allowed to dry.
6. Stain with any of the stains indicated in *Protocols 8* and *9*.

[a] The substitution of 1% Teepol for the formalin solution produces very much cleaner preparations but microfilariae will tend to wash off the slides when being stained.

Whilst Knott's technique is efficient it is rather time-consuming and more recently two filtration concentration techniques have been described (*Protocols 4, 5, and 6*).

Protocol 5. Concentration by the Nuclepore filtration technique as developed by Dennis and Kean (8)

1. Take blood into a syringe by venepuncture using sodium citrate anticoagulant.
2. Place a Nuclepore 5 μm filter (Nuclepore Inc.), 25 mm in diameter, in a Swinnex filter holder (Millipore). For the smaller microfilariae use a 3 μm filter. The correct alignment of the membrane is helped if the surface of the filter holder is wet. Ensure that the rubber sealing ring is in the correct position.
3. Push the blood from the syringe directly through the filter.
4. Fill the syringe with 0.85% sodium chloride solution or water. Reattach it to the filter and push this fluid through.
5. Repeat this operation once or twice until no more red colouring from the blood is seen in the washings. The microfilariae are nearly all retained on the filter.
6. Fill the syringe with air and blow this through the filter. Do not retract the syringe plunger whilst it is attached to the filter as this will wreck the membrane. I find it very convenient to examine the membrane while it is fresh but it can be stained.
7. Pump methanol through the filter followed by air and remove the filter.
8. Dismantle the filter holder and remove the filter membrane and place it, sample side upwards, on a glass slide.

Protocol 5. *Continued*

9. Stain the membrane in hot, but not boiling, haematoxylin (*Protocol 9*) or Giemsa stain (*Protocol 8*).
10. Before mounting allow the stained filter to dry and clear it in xylol. Mount it in Euparal, DPX, or any conventional mountant. Kits for the membrane filtration are available from WHO.

Protocol 6. Millipore membrane filter technique, based on the work of Bell (9) developed by Desowitz and Southgate (10)

1. Take 1 ml of blood into a 10 ml syringe containing 2 ml of sodium citrate anticoagulant.
2. Take 7 ml of 1% Teepol in normal saline into the same syringe and rotate, or shake, the syringe until the blood is completely haemolysed. If you cannot examine the blood immediately store it with a few drops of saturated aqueous phenol solution added.
3. Remove the needle and replace it by a Swinnex filter holder containing a 25 mm diameter Millipore membrane of 5 μm porosity. Take great care to ensure that the membrane and rubber seal are correctly positioned.
4. Pass the haemolysed blood through the filter by steady pressure on the syringe plunger.
5. Wash the membrane by passing 5 ml of normal saline through the holder syringe.
6. Pass 10 ml of formol saline through the filter to fix any microfilariae collected on the membrane.
7. Wash the membrane again with two lots of 10 ml of distilled water.
8. Take the Swinnex filter holder apart and remove the Millipore membrane and place it in a small tube or on a slide for staining.
9. Stain the membrane in Giemsa stain or haemalum (*Protocols 8* and *9*). Rinse rapidly and allow to dry.
10. Place the filter on a microscope slide, add a few drops of immersion oil and coverslip, or, alternatively, make a permanent preparation with DPX or Green Euparal.
11. Scan the filter under a low power objective. We find that a total magnification of × 40–50 (i.e. a × 4 or 5 objective and a × 10 eyepiece) gives very satisfactory results.

4. Methods for obtaining microfilariae from the skin

Microfilariae of *Onchocerca volvulus* and *Mansonella streptocerca* in man have a tropism for the skin. Before subjecting man or animals to skin snip procedures it is important to have some idea of the distribution of the microfilariae in the skin. For example in West Africa the pelvic girdle is the most heavily parasitized area whereas in Guatemala microfilariae are most numerous around the trunk and head. The microfilariae of *O. volvulus* and *M. streptocerca* escape readily from skin snips (*Protocol 7*).

Protocol 7. The extraction of microfilariae from skin snips

1. Clean the appropriate area of skin with an antiseptic swab (e.g. 70% isopropranol) and allow it to dry.
2. Insert a sterile needle[a] almost horizontally into the superficial layer of the skin. Lift the point of the needle to raise a cone of skin about 2–3 mm in diameter. Slice off the cone of skin below the needle-point using a sterile razor-blade or scalpel. The snip should be bloodless but a small amount of blood and serum will ooze into the wound. (No local anaesthetic is necessary.)
3. Weigh the snip by placing it epidermis side down on a torsion balance, designed to weigh up to 10 mg. It is essential that the 'snip' is weighed as soon as possible as it will lose weight by evaporation.
4. Place the skin snip in 100 μl of physiological saline in a well of a microtitration plate. Keep a careful record of which well each sample has been placed in.
5. Cover the microtitration tray with a plastic tape to prevent evaporation.
6. Remove the skin snip and examine the fluid at least 6 h, preferably 24 h, later. This can be done in a microtitration tray using an inverted microscope but many people find it more convenient to pipette the fluid on to a slide. Examine under a magnification of × 40. The microfilariae can be counted and the result expressed as the number of microfilariae per milligram of skin. If the specimens can not be examined immediately a drop of formalin is added to each well and the tray re-sealed. Specimens preserved in this way can be kept for several months if the wells are prevented from drying out.
7. If microfilariae are found add a drop of serum and allow the preparation to dry. Fix with methanol and stain with either the Giemsa or haematoxylin methods outlined in *Protocols 8* and *9*. (This stage is

Protocol 7. *Continued*

essential where there is doubt about the identification of the microfilariae especially in areas where *O. volvulus* and *M. streptocerca* occur together.)

[a] A corneoscleral punch is very good for taking skin snips. It is much more expensive than the needle and razor-blade method but less frightening for the patient.

Protocol 8. Staining with Giemsa's stain

1. Prepare and dehaemoglobinize thick smears as indicated in *Protocol 1*.
2. Fix the thick smears in a few drops of methanol.
3. Pour off the methanol.
4. Using a 20 ml hypodermic syringe take up 15 ml of distilled water and 3 ml of concentrated Giemsa stain. Thoroughly mix by inverting the syringe several times.
5. Place the slide face downwards in a plastic Petri dish and inject the stain underneath. This allows minimal contact between the stain and the air and, thus, reduces the amount of deposit that is formed.
6. Leave the film in contact with the stain for 30 min.
7. Remove the slide from the plastic Petri dish and wash for 1 sec (**no longer**) by dipping in tap-water. Stand the slide in an upright position to drain and dry.
8. Place one drop of immersion oil on to the thick smear and spread this with your finger, or add a drop of xylol and use a coverslip.
9. Examine the slide under a good microscope using a magnification of between × 40 and × 75. If small microfilariae are expected use × 75.

Protocol 9. Staining microfilariae with haematoxylin

1. To prepare Mayer's acid haemalum, mix the following:
   - haematoxylin 1 g
   - sodium iodate 0.2 g
   - potassium alum 50 g
   - distilled water 1000 ml
2. Shake frequently over a period of several hours until the solution turns blue-violet in colour and then add:
   - chloral hydrate 50 g
   - citric acid 1 g

3. Thoroughly shake and then store in a borosilicate glass bottle. This stain lasts for at least three months. Whilst I recommend the use of Mayer's stain most of the alum haematoxylin stains, such as those of Erlich or Harris, give good results.
4. Prepare and dehaemoglobinize thick smears as in *Protocol 1*.
5. Pour some Mayer's haemalum on to the slide and heat until steam rises but do not allow the solution to boil.
6. Stain for 10–15 min.
7. Rinse the slide by dipping it in tap-water and examine under the low power of the microscope. If understained stain for a longer period. If overstained wash quickly in 1% HCl in ethanol. It is better to overstain and differentiate as this removes the blue background from the film.
8. Clear in toluene.
9. Mount in Canada Balsam or DPX.

5. The identification of microfilariae

The identification of microfilariae in human blood is really quite simple. One must remember that in most parts of the world the number of species likely to be present is very limited. Microfilariae in different geographical regions of the world are as follows:

(a) Africa: *Wuchereria bancrofti*, *Loa loa*, *Mansonella perstans*, *Mansonella streptocerca*, and *Onchocerca volvulus*.

(b) South and Central America: *Wuchereria bancrofti*, *Mansonella ozzardi*, *Mansonella perstans*, and *Onchocerca volvulus*.

(c) Indian sub-continent: *Wuchereria bancrofti* and *Brugia malayi*.

(d) South-East Asia and the Philippines: *Wuchereria bancrofti*, *Brugia malayi*, and *Brugia timori*.

(e) Central and Eastern Pacific area: *Wuchereria bancrofti* and *Brugia malayi*.

(f) China: *Wuchereria bancrofti* and *Brugia malayi*.

Many of the filariae exhibit diurnal/nocturnal periodicity. Thus in most places *W. bancrofti* and *B. malayi* is not found in the peripheral blood during the day. Blood samples should be taken as near midnight as possible. It is possible to bring microfilariae of these species into peripheral circulation during the day by giving 50 mg of diethylcarbamazine to the patient but there are never as many as at midnight. *Loa loa*, on the other hand, exhibits diurnal periodicity so that its microfilariae are maximal during the middle of the day and absent during the night.

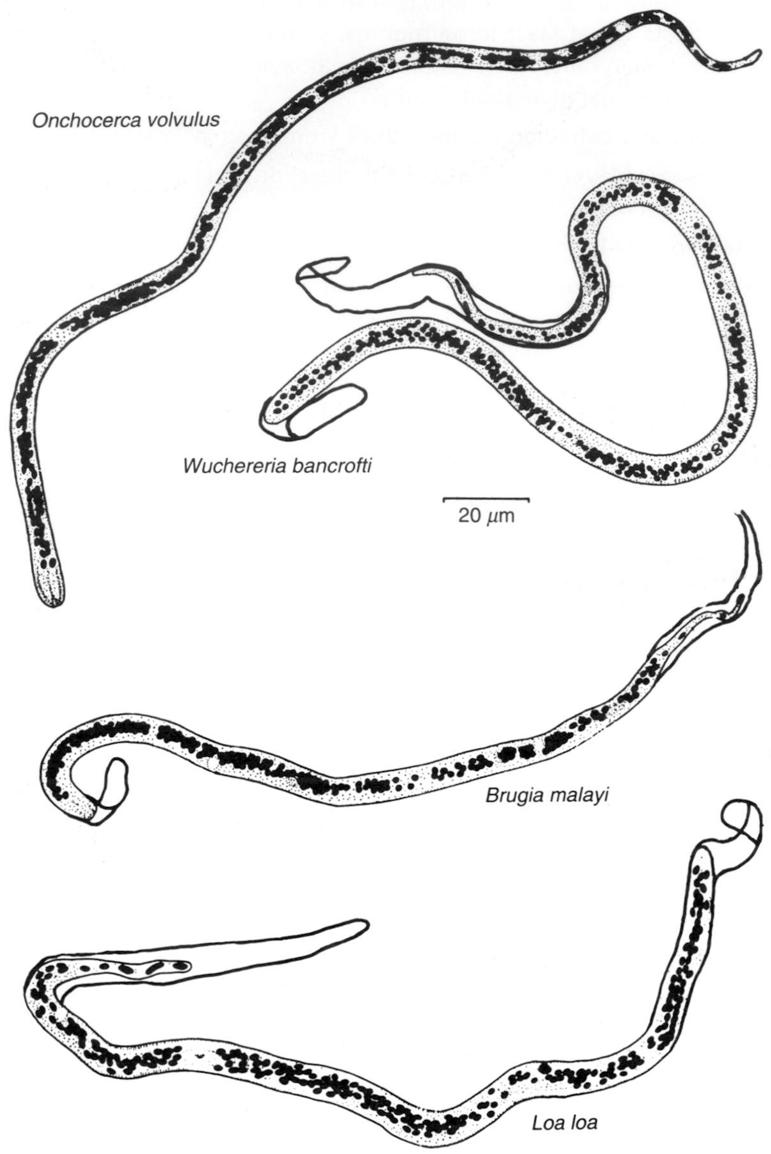

Figure 1. Drawings of the microfilariae found in the skin or blood of man. Note that the *Loa loa* must have been stained with haemalum as its sheath is visible.

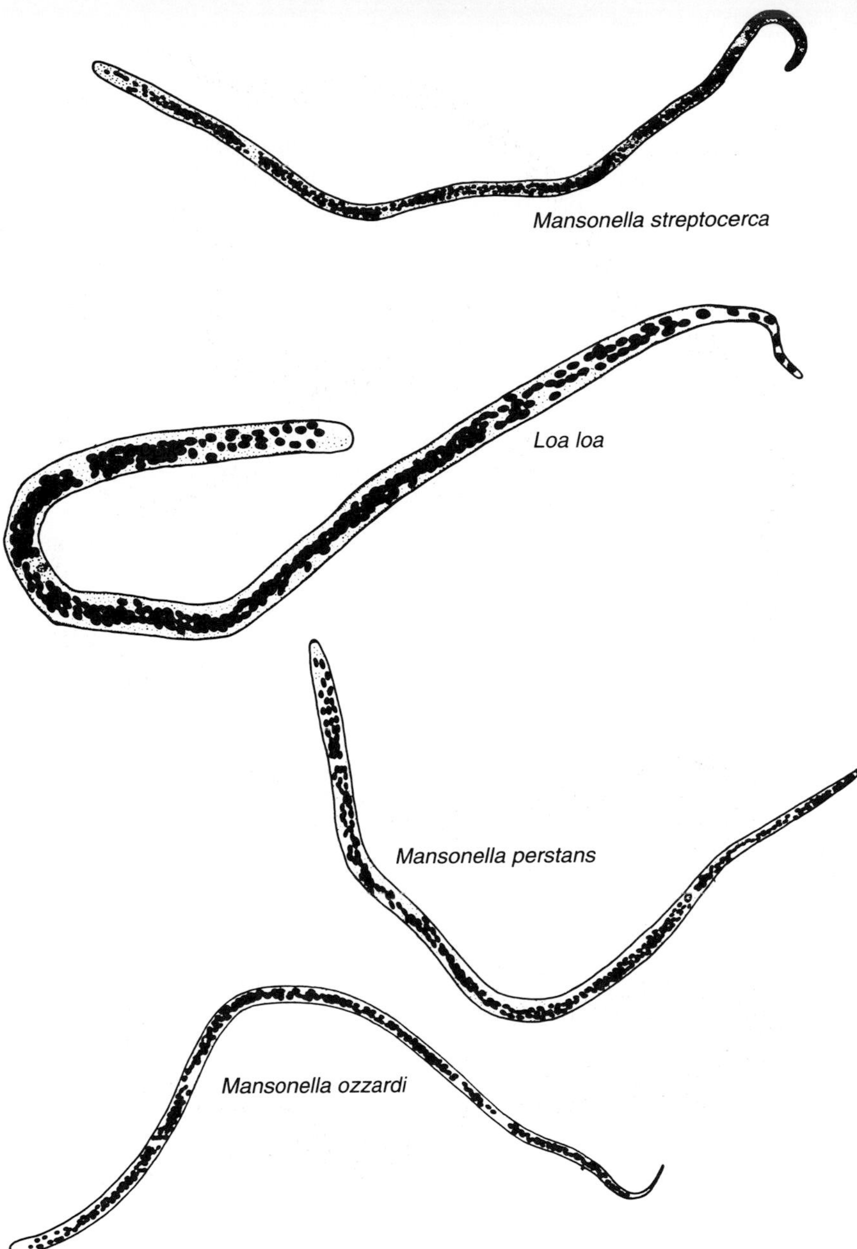

Figure 2. Drawings of the microfilariae found in the blood of man. Note that the *Loa loa* must have been stained with Giemsa as its sheath is invisible.

The morphological characteristics of the microfilariae found in man are shown in *Figures 1* and 2.

(a) *Wuchereria bancrofti*. The microfilaria is usually found in the blood and is 210–320 μm in length and nearly 10 μm in diameter. It has a loose sheath that, when stained with dilute Giemsa, is pale pinky-blue. The sheath does not always stain well. The nuclei are discrete. The tail end tapers evenly and there are no nuclei in the tip of the tail. When seen in a thick blood smear it usually lies in graceful curves. The microfilaria is illustrated in *Figure 1*.

(b) *Brugia malayi*. The microfilaria is found in the blood and is 170–260 μm in length and 5–6 μm in diameter. The sheath stains much more red than does that of *W. bancroft* in Giemsa stain. The nuclei are coarse and overlap. The tip of the tail contains a single nucleus and there is another nucleus just a little nearer the head (*Figure 1*). Quite often the sheath does not stain.

(c) *Loa loa*. Microfilariae are found in blood and cerebrospinal fluid and are 225–300 μm in length and 6–8 μm in diameter. The microfilaria is sheathed, **but the sheath does not stain with Giemsa.** It stains well with Mayer's stain. The nuclei are large and often overlap. The tail of the microfilaria is rather blunt and nuclei, that are large and flattened, extend right to its tip.

(d) *Mansonella perstans*. This small, often coiled, microfilaria is found in blood and is 190–240 μm long and 4 μm in diameter. The tail ends in a large rounded nucleus.

(e) *Mansonella streptocerca*. This small microfilaria is found in the skin. It is 180–240 μm long and 3 μm in diameter. The tail ends in a crook and terminates bluntly with nuclei to its tip.

(f) *Mansonella ozzardi*. This is usually found in the blood but accumulates in the skin. It is 175–240 μm in length and 5 μm in diameter. The tail is sharply pointed and there are nuclei in its tip. The tip of the tail is not easy to see in Giemsa stained preparations.

(g) *Onchocerca volvulus*. This microfilaria is normally found in the skin but may be found in the blood and urine. It is 280–330 μm long and 6–9 μm in diameter. The tail is sharply pointed and there are no nuclei in its tip. The cephalic space is one and a half to two times the width of the body.

Protocol 10. Key to the identification of microfilariae found in human blood stained with Giemsa

1. (a) Sheath present—**2.**

(b) Sheath absent—**3.**[a,b]

2. (a) Sheath stained red, nuclei in tip of tail—*Brugia* spp.
   (b) Sheath stained pale mauve, no nuclei in tip of tail—*Wuchereria bancrofti*.
3. (a) Nuclei not extending to tip of tail—**4.**
   (b) Nuclei extending to tip of tail—**6.**
4. (a) Microfilaria about 300 μm long—**5.**
   (b) Microfilaria 200–225 μm long—*Mansonella ozzardi*.
5. (a) Cephalic space more than one and a half times the diameter of the head—*Onchocerca volvulus*.[c]
   (b) Cephalic space less than, or equal to, the diameter of the head *Wuchereria bancrofti* (with no sheath).
6. (a) Microfilaria at least 260 μm long—**7.**
   (b) Microfilaria 200–225 μm long—**8.**
7. (a) Tail with a complete column of nuclei—*Loa loa*.
   (b) Tail with two isolated nuclei—*Brugia malayi*.
8. (a) Tail with prominent terminal nucleus—*Mansonella perstans*.
   (b) Tail with crook-shaped bend—*Mansonella streptocerca*.

[a] The sheath of *Loa loa* does not stain with Giemsa.
[b] Any sheathed microfilaria can lose its sheath.
[c] *Onchocerca volvulus* can be found in the blood.

Protocol 11. Key to the identification of microfilariae found in human blood stained with Mayer's haemalum

1. (a) Sheath present—**2.**
   (b) Sheath absent—**4.**
2. (a) Nuclei to tip of tail—**3.**
   (b) No nuclei in tip of tail—*Wuchereria bancrofti*.
3. (a) Sheath loosely applied, microfilaria over 250 μm long—*Loa loa*.
   (b) Two nuclei in tip of tail—*Brugia malayi*.
4. (a) Microfilaria more than 275 μm long—**5.**
   (b) Microfilaria less than 250 μm long—**6.**
5. (a) Cephalic space more than one and a half times the diameter of the head—*Onchocerca volvulus*.
   (b) Cephalic space less than, or equal to, the diameter of the head—*Wuchereria bancrofti* (with no sheath).

Protocol 11. *Continued*

6. (a) Nuclei to tip of tail—**7**.
   (b) No nuclei in tip of tail—*Mansonella ozzardi*.
7. (a) Tail straight with prominent terminal nucleus-—*Mansonella perstans*.
   (b) Tail bent into crook shape—*Mansonella streptocerca*.
8. (a) Microfilaria at least 260 μm long—**7**.
   (b) Microfilaria 200–225 μm long—**8**.
9. (a) Tail with a complete column of nuclei—*Loa loa*.
   (b) Tail with two isolated nuclei—*Brugia malayi*.
10. (a) Tail with prominent terminal nucleus—*Mansonella perstans*.
    (b) Tail with crook-shaped bend—*Mansonella streptocerca*.

References

1. Denham, D. A., Dennis, D. T., Ponnudurai, T., Nelson, G. S., and Guy, F. (1971). *Trans. R. Soc. Trop. Med. Hyg.*, **67**, 521.
2. Southgate, B. A. (1974). *Trans. R. Soc. Trop. Med. Hyg.*, **68**, 177.
3. Partono, F. and Idris, K. N. (1977). *SE Asian J. Trop. Med. Publ. Hlth.*, **8**, 158.
4. Braun-Munzinger, R. A., Scheiber, P., and Southgate, B. A. (1977). *Trans. R. Soc. Trop. Med. Hyg.*, **71**, 548.
5. Webber, R. H. (1976). *Trans. R. Soc. Trop. Med. Hyg.*, **70**, 537.
6. Abaru, D. A. and Denham, D. A. (1976). *Trans. R. Soc. Trop. Med. Hyg.*, **70**, 333.
7. Knott, J. (1939). *Trans. R. Soc. Trop. Med. Hyg.*, **33**, 191.
8. Dennis, D. T. and Kean, B. H. (1971). *J. Parasitol.*, **57**, 1146.
9. Bell, D. R. (1967). *Ann. Trop. Med. Parasitol.*, **61**, 220.
10. Desowitz, R. S. and Southgate, B. A. (1973). *SE Asian J. Trop. Med. Publ. Hlth.*, **4**, 179.

13

Diagnosis of intestinal helminth infections

D. A. DENHAM and R. R. SUSWILLO

1. Introduction

Intestinal helminths may cause minimal gastro-intestinal symptoms but many (e.g. *Ascaris*) have a major impact on human health compromising the nutritional status of children in developing countries (see Chapter 1)

Several species of nematodes, trematodes, and cestodes live in the human intestine and produce eggs which are passed in the faeces. Eggs of lung and liver flukes also are passed in the faeces. Parasitological diagnosis of most intestinal helminthic infections depends on finding and identifying these eggs. With the *Taenia* species, however, it is rare to find eggs in faeces as the proglottids are usually passed whole. Similarly, *Enterobius vermicularis* deposits its eggs on the perianal skin and eggs are seldom found in the faeces. *Strongyloides stercoralis* produces first stage larvae (L_1) instead of eggs.

The diagnosis of schistosomiasis is dealt with in Chapter 10.

2. Collection of faecal samples

Samples should always be collected into a clean, dry pot. Eggs are not uniformly distributed in the faecal mass so as large a sample as possible should be collected and mixed before the sample to be examined is removed.

2.1 Simple faecal smears

The simplest method of detecting worm eggs is to emulsify a small, unweighed portion of faeces on a slide with a small amount of saline and examine with a low power objective. Unfortunately, this method (which uses about 2 mg of faeces) is insensitive when dealing with parasites that produce relatively few eggs. It is probably adequate in an endemic area where worm burdens are likely to be high and costs must be kept to a minimum.

2.2 The 'Kato-Katz' thick faecal smear technique

Kato and Miura introduced a thick smear technique for the examination of faeces for the major schistosomiasis control programmes in Japan. By their method 50 mg samples can be examined. This is made possible by clearing the faecal smear under a cellophane coverslip impregnated with glycerine (*Protocol 1*) (1).

A number of modifications to this technique have been reported with the object of easily obtaining uniform amounts of faeces without the necessity of weighing each sample. Katz and his colleagues (2) used a template with a standard sized hole to give a known volume of faeces and this method is now widely adopted using commercially available plastic 'Kato-Katz' kits.

Protocol 1. Semi-quantitative technique for the enumeration of helminth ova

Equipment and reagents

- Template with central hole of such a size that it contains 50 mg of faeces
- Water wetable cellophane sheet cut into 22 × 30 mm rectangles
- Glycerine–malachite green solution: glycerine 100 ml, malachite green 3% aqueous solution 1 ml, distilled water 100 ml (the malachite green is not essential but provides a useful background and reduces the glare)
- Wooden applicator sticks
- Plastic tea strainer
- Microscope slides
- Absorbent paper

Method

1. Soak the cellophane squares in the glycerine–malachite green solution for at least 24 h. They may be stored in this solution.
2. Mix the faecal sample and push a portion through the tea strainer.
3. Place the template on a microscope slide and fill the hole of the template with strained faeces level with the surface.
4. Remove the template leaving 50 mg of faeces on the slide.
5. Cover the specimen with a glycerine soaked cellophane rectangle and invert the slide on to an absorbent paper surface.
6. Exert sufficient pressure on the slide to spread the sample almost to the edge of the coverslip.
7. Turn the slide so that the cellophane is uppermost and leave until the faecal smear has cleared.[a] Additional glycerine may be added to the edges of the cellophane to displace air bubbles and facilitate examination.
8. Examine the whole coverslip area at × 100 magnification (i.e. × 10 objective) and with the substage condenser closed enough to obtain

maximum definition. The whole coverslip area must be examined. Use higher magnification to check the identity of the eggs.

[a] The clearing process may be temporarily halted by inverting the slide on a smooth flat surface until required for examination. A number of slides can be prepared at one time and leaving them inverted, with two or three being left face upwards to clear. Hard stools present a problem because they may take up to 48 h to clear. One way of overcoming this is to mix the measured sample with glycerine before applying the cellophane.

An alternative method is the formol ether concentration method which is described in detail in Chapter 5, *Protocol 2*. This modification of the original method of Allen and Ridley (3) is now widely used as a standard diagnostic method. The increased yield of positive findings with all types of faecal parasites, the relatively clean deposit, and enhanced visibility of the structural details of the eggs obtained by formol ether concentration justify its use as a routine diagnostic procedure.

A heavy deposit, which renders the sample too opaque, may result from taking too large a specimen or, more likely from insufficiently vigorous shaking of the faeces in the formol ether mixture.

2.3 Zinc sulfate centrifugal flotation method

This method was developed by Faust to meet the needs of a clinical laboratory to obtain heavy concentrations of helminth eggs and protozoal cysts in a readily diagnosable condition.

Protocol 2. Zinc sulfate flotation method

Equipment and reagents

- 33% zinc sulfate in distilled water—if there is any difficulty in obtaining zinc sulfate a saturated solution of sodium chloride or magnesium sulfate can be used
- Tea strainer
- Centrifuge with 10 × 150 mm centrifuge tubes
- Pestle and mortar
- Wooden applicator sticks
- Small plastic bowls
- Large bacteriological loop (about 6 mm in diameter)

Method

1. Emulsify 5 g of faeces with water in the pestle and mortar.
2. Pour emulsion through the tea strainer into a plastic bowl.
3. Pour 10 ml of strained emulsion into a centrifuge tube.
4. Centrifuge for 5 min at 1000 *g*.
5. Discard supernatant.
6. Suspend deposit in a small volume of water and then fill tube with water.

Protocol 2. *Continued*

7. Centrifuge for 5 min at 1000 *g*.
8. Repeat this washing procedure until the supernatant is clear.
9. After the final centrifugation decant clear supernatant.
10. Suspend the deposit in a small volume of zinc sulfate solution and then fill with more zinc sulfate solution.
11. Centrifuge for 1 min at 1000 *g*.
12. Using the bacteriological loop remove surface material from the tube and place on a glass slide.[a]
13. Examine at × 100 magnification.

[a] If this method is used routinely for large numbers of specimens the following modification is very useful. Have the tops of the glass centrifuge tops ground flat. When filling the tube with zinc sulfate produce a slight positive meniscus and lay a coverslip on this. Centrifuge for 1 min at 1000 *g*. Remove coverslip and place on microscope slide and examine as before. **Thin-shelled eggs become rapidly deformed if left in concentrated solutions.**

3. The Harada–Mori technique for the development of infective larvae of hookworms and *Strongyloides stercoralis* larvae

To differentiate the human hookworms it is necessary to allow larvae to develop to the third stage (L_3). This method is a simple way of producing such larvae in a safe way (*Protocol 3*).

Protocol 3. Harada–Mori technique

Equipment and reagents

- Large test-tubes (180 × 18 mm)—wider bore tubes allow loading of more faeces thus increasing the sensitivity of the method
- Rack for tubes
- Pasteur pipettes long enough to reach the bottom of the tubes
- Filter-paper strips 150 × 15 mm folded longitudinally, or bigger if the tubes allow
- Cellophane for sealing tubes
- Incubator at 28 °C
- Wooden applicator sticks
- Beakers
- Forceps

Method

1. Place test-tubes in rack and add 5 ml of distilled water to each tube.
2. Smear the faeces along the filter-paper leaving 5 cm clear at one end. Use a generous amount of faeces but not such that it drains downwards when held vertically.

3. Insert the strip into a test-tube with the unsmeared portion reaching to the bottom of the tube.
4. Cover the top of the tube with cellophane and label.
5. Incubate at 28 °C for ten days. Four days is adequate for *S. stercoralis*.

CAUTION. From this time on wear gloves as L_3 larvae could be on any surface.

6. Remove and discard the cellophane and filter-paper strip with forceps.
7. Withdraw some fluid from the bottom of the tube and place in small Petri dish.
8. Examine at × 50 magnification for motile L_3.
9. Heat the L_3 in the tube at 50 °C for 15 min. This kills the larvae without distortion.
10. Transfer to centrifuge tube and centrifuge for 3 min at 1000 *g*.
11. Decant supernatant and transfer deposit to a glass slide.
12. Examine each L_3 with high power magnification to differentiate *Ancylostoma duodenale* and *Necator americanus* (4). Differentiation of hookworm and *S. stercoralis* larvae is made on the appearance of the buccal chamber (*Figure l* and section 4.4).

Note. Faeces should be cultured when they are as fresh as possible. Exposure to strong light or refrigeration will kill the developing larvae.

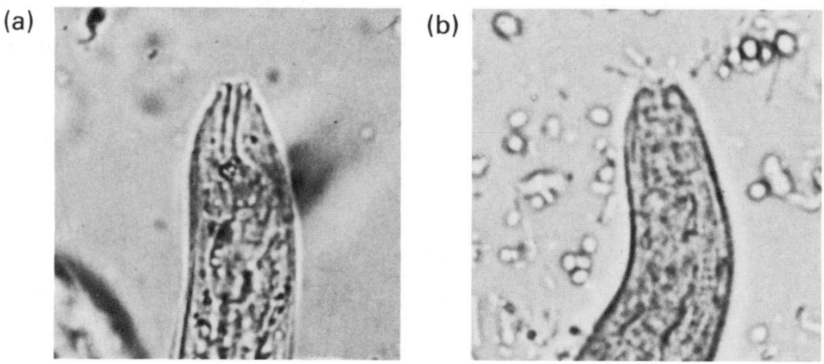

Figure 1. (a) Hookworm larva; (b) *Strongyloides* larva.

4. Identification of eggs

Helminth eggs are much easier to identify than protozoal cysts. They all have distinct shapes, colours, and most importantly, sizes. *Plate 1* shows the outline, colours, shapes, and sizes of many eggs that may be encountered in human faeces.

Some eggs, such as those of *Trichuris trichiura* (*Plate 4d*), are so distinctive that it is difficult to misidentify them. Others, such as *Ascaris lumbricoides* come in a variety of shapes and confuse the uninitiated (*Plate 4b* and *c*).

Size is a very important criterion for distinguishing eggs that at first sight appear identical. An eye-piece micrometer is vital. The *Paragonimus westermanni* (*Plate 5d*) and *Diphylobothrium latum* (*Figure 2*) eggs are operculated (i.e. have a small cap at one end from which the larval stage escapes), and are thin walled and pale. However, *Paragonimus* is 85 μm long and *Diphylobothrium* is 65 μm long. The smart brown operculate eggs of *Opisthorchis sinensis* (*Plate 5c*), *Heterophyes heterophyes*, and *Metagonimus yokogawi* (*Figure 3*) look very similar in colour, shape, and size, but *Opisthorchis* is slightly larger.

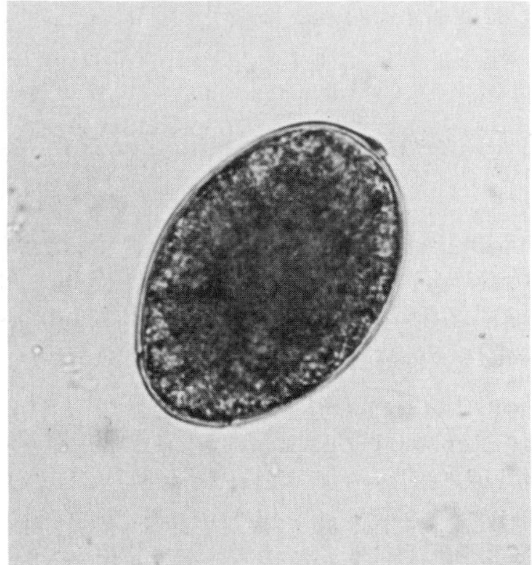

Figure 2. *Diphylobothrium latum* ovum (65 × 60 μm).

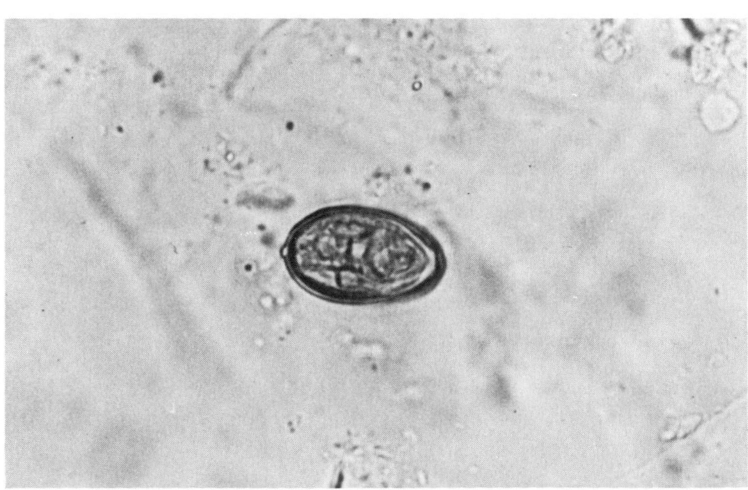

Figure 3. *Metagonimus yokogawi* ovum (27 × 12 μm).

It is not a good idea to use Lugol's iodine when searching for helminth eggs, although it helps in the identification of protozoan cysts (see Chapter 5).

Some nematode eggs embryonate rapidly and larvae may hatch out. If a sample has to be sent by post in warm weather it is a good idea to have half the sample fixed in formalin. Do not fix all of the sample as the remainder may be used for strongyloides and hookworm culture.

The following is a description of the eggs most commonly found in human faeces. These eggs are also illustrated in *Plates 4* and *5*.

4.1 Nematodes

(a) *Ascaris lumbricoides*. The eggs of the large roundworm come in two major variants. The fertile egg is 50–70 μm long and broadly ovoidal. It has a thick shell covered by a mammilated, yellow coat which may vary in thickness and contains a large unsegmented ovum (*Plate 4b*). The infertile egg is 85 μm long and rather narrower than the fertile egg. It has a thinner, irregular shell containing a mass of disorganized granules (*Plate 4c*). A third variant is the decorticated type which is colourless and has a smooth shell (*Figure 4*). Fertile eggs inadequately fixed in formalin can develop a fully formed larva after two to three weeks but this is unlikely to be confusing due to the long time needed for this development.

(b) *Trichuris trichiura*. This egg is barrel shaped with mucoid plugs at each end. The shell is smooth and rich brown and, when fresh, contains an unsegmented ovum (*Plate 4d*). In old faeces the ovum may divide into several cells.

(c) *Enterobius vermicularis*. This egg is colourless and asymmetrical with one

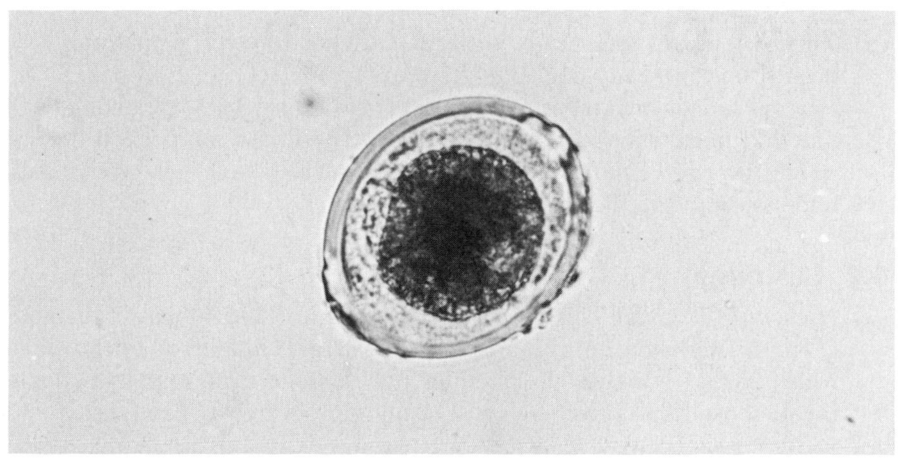

Figure 4. Decorticated ovum of *Ascoris lumbricoides* (55 × 45 μm).

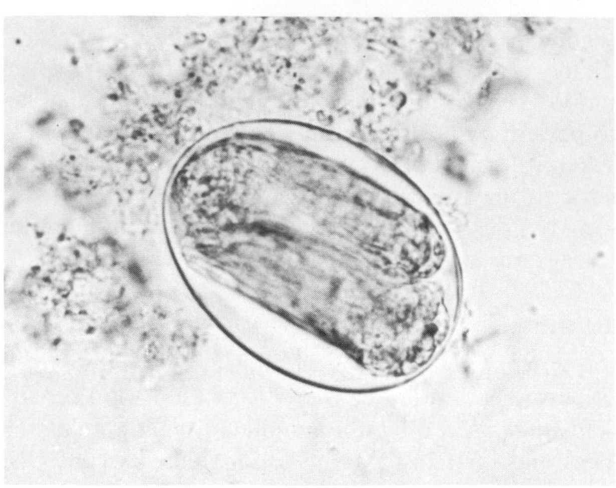

Figure 5. Developing hookworm ovum (60 × 40 μm).

side flattened (*Plate 4e*). The shell is thin walled and in this specimen, from a faecal concentrate, a folded larva can be seen. This rapidly develops to the infective stage.

(d) Hookworm eggs. The eggs of *Ancylostoma duodenale* and *Necator americanus* are indistinguishable (*Plate 4f*). Identification of the species involved depends upon culturing the infective larvae (see section 3). Remember both species may be present in the same patient. The eggs of the hookworms are 60 um in length, ovoidal, and colourless with a thin clear shell wall. Development is very rapid and if the sample has been kept warm for 24 hours the eggs may contain a larva (*Figure 5*) and L_1 will frequently hatch.

(e) *Trichostrongylus* species. A variety of trichostrongylid nematodes have been found infecting man but these are rarely seen in Europeans. The eggs are longer than those of hookworms (85 μm). They are ovoidal with one end more rounded than the other. There is a multicelled embryo inside the egg (*Figure 6*). The curvature of this large egg gives a false impression of the shell being double walled.

4.2 Cestodes

(a) *Hymenolepis nana*. This egg is almost spherical and 40 μm in diameter (*Plate 5a*). It has a thin colourless shell wall and contains an onchosphere which has six hooklets. Polar filaments emanate from opposite ends of the onchosphere. These are most easily seen in freshly fixed eggs.

(b) *Diphylobothrium latum* These eggs are 65 μm long and ovoidal with a thin double wall shell (*Figure 2*). There is a terminal operculum at one

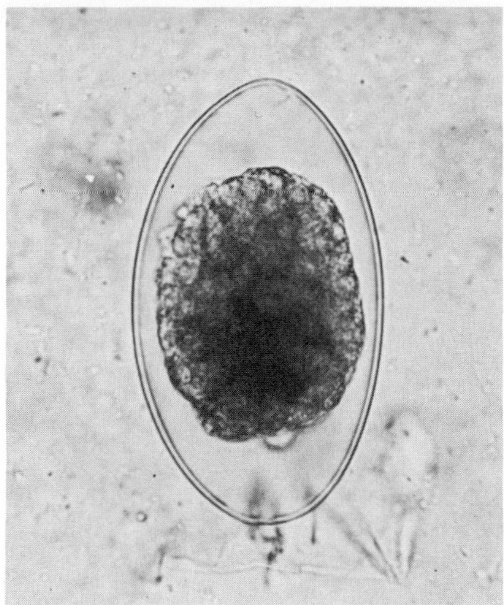

Figure 6. *Trichostrongylus colubriformis* ovum (85 × 40 μm).

end but is difficult to see. It often exhibits as an out of focus ridge on the shell near one end. A small knob may be seen at the other end of the shell. The egg contains an immature unsegmented embryo.

(c) *Taenia* species. The eggs of the two human species can not be differentiated (*Plate 5b*). They are spherical and 35 μm in diameter. The egg shell is thick and appears to have radial lines which are pores. The egg contains an onchosphere with six small hooks not all of which will be visible at any one time. The only way to differentiate *T. saginata* from *T. solium* is to recover proglottids and identify these (see section 4.6).

4.3 Trematodes

(a) *Opisthorchis sinensis*. This was previously called *Clonorchis*. The egg is 32 μm long and flask shaped (*Plate 5c*). It is yellow to brown in colour and has a prominent operculum at one end: at the opposite end a tiny terminal spine may be visible. Although the egg is passed fully embryonated the miracidium is only visible in freshly fixed eggs.

(b) *Heterophyes heterophyes* and *Metagonimus yokogawi*. These eggs are indistinguishable but the parasites occur in totally different parts of the world. They are 27 μm long (*Figure 3*) and slightly more ovoid than *O. sinensis*. A miracidium is present within the eggs but is quite difficult to see.

(c) *Fasciolopsis buski*. These eggs are very large being 140 μm in length. They are oval and yellow to brown in colour (*Figure 7*). The operculum is faintly visible. Agranular contents usually fill the egg.

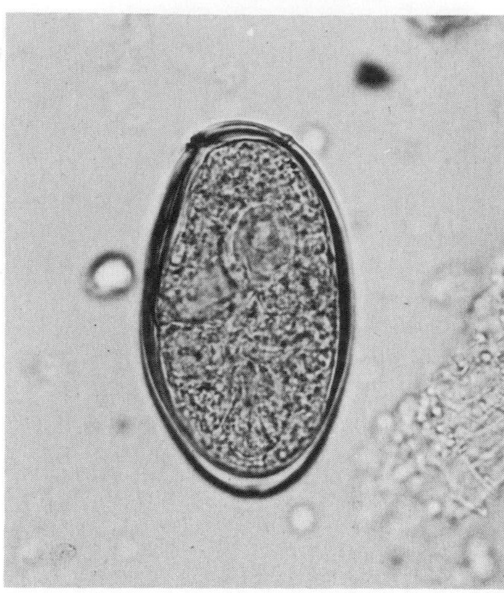

Figure 7. *Fasciolopsis buski* ovum (130–140 × 80–85 μm).

(d) *Fasciola hepatica*. The ova of this species are slightly larger (150 μm) than those of *F. buski*. Although infections with this liverfluke are quite common eggs are very rarely found in faeces in chronic fascioliasis. The acute clinical features of this disease may precede the appearance of eggs in the faeces by several weeks. For these reasons serology is frequently used to make a diagnosis and to monitor therapeutic response. A range of antibodies appear in patients two to four weeks from infection. An ELISA based on a crude *Fasciola* antigen preparation is available (5), in patients from areas of the world where *Schistosoma masoni* is endemic, a circumoval precipitin (COP) test should also be performed. A positive ELISA with a negative COP test strongly suggest fascioliasis. An immunoblot test for a 17 kd excretory–secretory antigen appears to be affected by concomitant schistosomiasis and may prove useful.

(e) *Paragonimus westermanni*. This egg is 85 μm long and yellow to brown with a very prominent operculum with ridges on the shell (*Plate 5d*). The shell is double walled and irregular being thickened at the end away from the operculum. These eggs will be more common in sputum than in faeces.

4.4 Differentiation of hookworm and *Strongyloides* L_1

If faeces arrive in the laboratory after a delayed journey it is possible that any hookworm eggs will have hatched into the L_1 or even developed to the L_2. As *Strongyloides stercoralis* larvae also develop rapidly in faeces there may be confusion between hookworms and *Strongyloides*.

Larvae (L_1) of *Strongyloides* are 250 μm long and those of hookworms almost 300 μm long but this has little practical significance as the larvae grow in culture. The only reliable way to differentiate the L_1 is to examine the buccal cavity. In hookworms this is deep and, because it is lined with refractile material is easy to see (*Figure 1*). In *Strongyloides* the buccal cavity is much shorter and difficult to see.

4.5 Differentiation of hookworm and *Strongyloides* L_3

It is possible to differentiate the two hookworms species at the L_3 stage.

It is important to note that the L_3 is surrounded by the cast cuticle of the L_2. This is called the sheath. The L_3 of *Strongyloides* has no sheath so there is no problem in differentiating the L_3 of this species from the hookworms.

The easiest way to differentiate the L_3 of the two hookworms is by examination of the tip of the tail of the larvae. The tail of *Ancylostoma* is blunt whilst that of *Necator* is sharply pointed. There is also a gap between the oesophagus and intestine in *Necator*. Confirmation of the differentiation can be obtained by measuring their length. The body (*not* the sheath) of the L_3 of *A. duodenale* is 660 μm long whilst that of *N. americanus* is only 590 μm long. This difference is also reflected in the length of the sheath which in *Ancylostoma* is 720 μm and in *Necator* 660 μm long.

Very rarely *Trichostrongylus* spp. L_3 will be found in faecal cultures. These are longer (750 μm) than hookworms and the tail has a knob at its extremity.

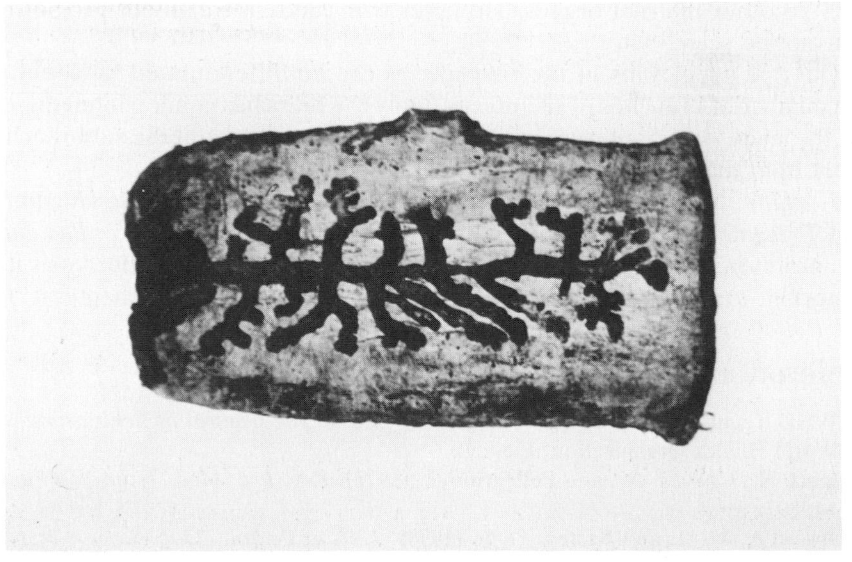

Figure 8. *Taenia solium* proglottid.

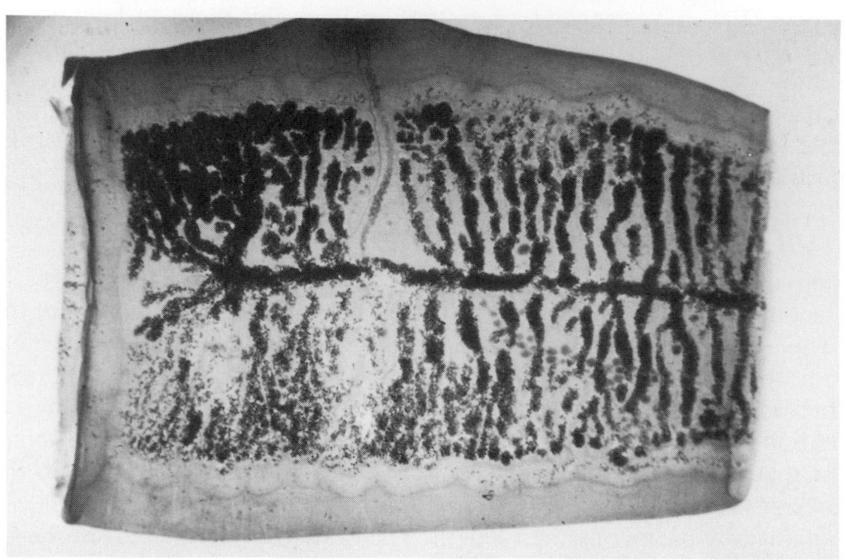

Figure 9. *Taenia saginata* proglottid.

4.6 Differentiation of the proglottids of *Taenia saginata* and *Taenia solium*

The proglottids of the two *Taenia* species are usually passed as fully developed 'ripe' proglottids with a multibranched uterus that is full of eggs and with no other internal organs. However with modern treatment proglottids may not be seen.

The ripe proglottids of the two species can be differentiated by counting the number of branches of the uterus. Only the branches coming immediately off the main, central uterus should be counted. Do not count the subbranches away from the central uterus.

T. solium has less than ten branches of the uterus **on each side** (*Figure 8*) and *T. saginata* has more than 16 branches **each side** (*Figure 9*). As *T. solium* is much more pathogenic because of the possibility of neurocysticercosis it is important to make the differentiation of the two species (see Chapter 11).

References

1. WHO Technical Report Series, No. 728. (1985). *The Control of Schistosomiasis*. World Health Organization, Geneva.
2. Katz, N., Chaves, A., and Pellegrino, J. (1972). *Rev. Inst. Med. Trop. São Paulo*, **14**, 397.
3. Allen, A. V. H. and Ridley, D. S. (1970). *J. Clin. Pathol.*, **23**, 545.
4. Ash, L. R. and Orihel, T. C. (1987). *Parasites: a guide to laboratory procedures and identification*. ASCP Press, Chicago.

5. Hillyer, G. V. (1986). In *Immunodiagnosis of parasitic diseases* (ed. K. W. Walls and P. M. Schantz), Vol. 1, pp. 39–68. Academic Press Inc., New York.

Further reading

1. Beaver, P. C., Jung, R. C., and Cupp, E. W. (1984). *Clinical parasitology*, 9th edn. Lea and Febiger, Philadelphia.

5. [illegible] (198[illegible]). [illegible] Academic Press, New York.

Further reading

1. [illegible]

14

Histopathology of parasitic diseases

N. FRANCIS

1. Introduction

Because of widespread international travel the diagnosis of imported diseases is a problem in hospitals outside their own geographical range. Added to this is the expanding population of HIV infected people in whom the diagnosis of opportunistic infections and unusual tissue responses to them is going to present an increasing problem across the UK and Europe. There are also a variety of parasitic infections indigenous to the UK which are discussed.

2. General considerations

The first step in histological diagnosis is obtaining an appropriate and adequate tissue sample. You should be in a position to give advice to clinicians on the best sort of tissue sample. In some infections the site and type of specimen may increase the chances of a positive diagnosis (see section 2.2.1 and under individual organisms).

2.1 Fixation and transport

Most specimens are fixed in an adequate amount of 10% formalin or neutral buffered formalin. The latter has the advantage of producing less formalin pigment and enables more reliable immunocytochemical studies to be carried out on paraffin sections. If electron microscopic studies are being performed a second specimen should be put in appropriate fixative and if handling specimens from other hospitals you should have a clearly established protocol and reliable method of transport (*Protocol 1*).

Protocol 1. Collection, fixation, and transport of specimens

1. For routine light microscopy put tissue samples (no larger than 1 cm diameter) in a container with six times the volume of fixative clearly labelled with the tissue sample type, site, and date. If samples are being stored fixative should be changed after four to seven days.

Protocol 1. *Continued*

2. For electron microscopy place fresh tissue in a drop of EM fixative and dissect into pieces (maximum smallest dimension 1 mm) handling gently with a pipette not forceps. Put in a labelled vial of EM fixative and leave at 4°C for 2–4 h. Change fixative to phosphate buffer and store in buffer at 4°C prior to transport. Fixative to be freshly made each week and buffers, stock solutions, fixatives, and tissue stored at 4°C. Do not allow tissue to freeze (as can occur in an aeroplane cargo hold).
   (a) 0.1 M phosphate buffer pH 7.2:
   - Stock solution a: $NaH_2PO_4H_20$—15.6 g in 500 ml distilled water
   - Stock solution b: $Na_2HPO_4H_20$—17.8 g in 500 ml distilled water
   - Mix 28 ml of solution a with 72 ml solution b and add 100 ml distilled water (solution b may need to be warmed and stirred first to dissolve all crystals).

   (b) EM fixative: (3% glutaraldehyde in phosphate buffer) 1.5 ml 50% glutaraldehyde + 23.5 ml 0.1 M phosphate buffer.
3. Transport tissue by courier to receiving laboratory which should give to the sender their: name, address, telephone and fax number and notify the name of the cargo agent to be used.

2.2 Examination and laboratory handling

2.2.1 Tissue sampling

Carefully examine and describe the specimen and, if appropriate, photograph. If an adult worm is seen in the specimen the blocks should be taken to ensure parts of the worm are not lost. Keep the intermediate spare sections in case the diagnostic area is absent from stained sections. Fresh imprints, smears, and aspiration specimens are quite frequently of value (see *Protocol 2*) but, if from high risk patients, handle in an appropriate safety cabinet. In the string test a nylon thread in gelatin capsule is swallowed by the patient, withdrawn, and uncoiled in the duodenum. Direct examination of the adherent mucus may reveal organisms not found in stools, particularly *Giardia* and *Strongyloides*.

Protocol 2. Imprints from fresh tissue and aspiration specimens

1. Smears and imprints: Lightly press or smear the surface of the specimen (freshly cut surface in the case of lymph nodes) on to a clean glass slide or one pre-coated with poly-L-lysine solution (Sigma Chemical Co. Ltd.) by dipping and drying overnight.
2. Aspirations: The clinician taking the specimen usually makes the

slides. Ensure that smears are thin and evenly spread. If fluids are received make cytological preparations and handle mucoid, bloody, or voluminous specimens appropriately (see Coleman and Chapman in further reading).

3. More than one slide should be prepared.
4. Rapidly fix for 10 min in methanol.
5. Make additional air dried smears.
6. Stain fixed slides (Giemsa and H&E) air dried (Romanowsky).
7. Retain spare slides of each type for other stains.
8. Put any remaining tissue in histological fixative.

2.2.2 Preservation of parasite specimens

You may want to preserve a parasite specimen (see *Protocol 3*) for a teaching collection, or for sending to one of the reference centres (see section 2.5) for confirmation of its identity.

Protocol 3. Preservation of parasite specimens

1. Make up a general fixative of equal parts of 10% formalin and 95% ethyl alcohol containing 5% acetic acid (5 parts glacial acetic acid and 95 parts formalin–alcohol).
2. Heat fixative to 63 °C.
3. Add specimen and swirl round, leave in fixative for 5–10 min until cool.
4. Store in a labelled specimen pot containing 5% glycerine in 70% alcohol for transport, storage, or display.

2.3 Microscopy

A good quality microscope with variable light source is essential. An oil immersion lens and ideally a high power dry (× 60) objective should be available. Calibrate the microscope for accurate sizing of any parasites found, using either the Vernier scale on the slide stage (usually accurate to within 0.1 mm), or for the smaller parasites an ocular micrometer disc calibrated against a stage micrometer slide for your own microscope.

2.4 Routine and special stains

A good haematoxylin and eosin stain is essential but when examining material for the presence of parasites other infectious agents may have to be excluded. You are therefore likely to perform bacterial and fungal stains in the differential diagnostic procedure together with stains that may aid the identification of parasites.

Stains commonly used in the diagnosis of parasitic infections are:

- Periodic acid Schiff with or without diastase
- Grocott (see Pneumocystis for rapid protocol)
- Ziehl–Neelsen
- Wade–Fite
- Giemsa
- Wright's
- Gram
- Romanowsky

The methods for all of the above are familiar to most laboratories and are well-described in standard texts (1).

To be reliable these stains need to be performed on a regular basis. If only performed at the time of a difficult diagnosis they may be at best unhelpful and at worst positively misleading. Methods for immunocytochemistry are widely available and should be consulted before starting this service. Where an antibody is of value it is indicated in the text (with the source).

2.5 Reference centres

Reference centres or expert opinions are useful for confirmation or assistance with unusual diagnostic problems and may be important where the outcome may alter patient management. As it is impractical to list all the available centres, it is suggested that you seek out a local or national expert and ask their advice, or get them to direct you to the most appropriate National or International reference centre.

3. Histopathology of infections caused by protozoa

3.1 Apicomplexa

3.1.1 Malaria (*Plasmodium* spp.)

During the process of development and shizogony in the deep vascular beds haemozoin pigment is produced. This has a granular blackish appearance, is birefringent, and can be found in infected red cells and in cells of the reticuloendothelial system. In long-standing infections the pigment may form large clumps. It is difficult or impossible to distinguish haemozoin from formalin or shistosomal pigment (all of which are acid haematin compounds). Differential bleaching of the pigment with picric acid (see *Protocol 4*) may help as well as allowing parasites to be seen more easily. Giemsa stain may help visualization of parasites, with or without prior picric acid treatment.

Protocol 4. Picric acid bleaching of haemozoin pigments

1. Take sections to absolute alcohol.
2. Transfer to a solution of equal parts picric acid (saturated in absolute alcohol) and absolute alcohol.
3. Leave for 15 min to overnight.
4. Rinse in 90% alcohol followed by 70% alcohol, and then wash well.
5. Stain with H&E or Giemsa.
   Formalin pigment is removed in 15 min to overnight (depending on amount), malarial pigment needs 12 h for removal.

The diagnosis of malaria is usually made on a blood film but may be an unexpected finding in a tissue sample. It is not usually possible to speciate the parasite in histological material. The main findings in sections are the presence of parasitized red cells and pigment. Capillaries or post-capillary venules contain parasitized red cells (PRBC), many of which are in close association with endothelial cells (*Plate 5e*).

In cerebral malaria (*P. falciparum*) the brain shows multiple petechial haemorrhages and focal haemorrhage, usually with a central small vessel containing PRBC. Ring haemorrhages are also seen in which there is a central zone of necrosis of the white matter. Durk's granulomas are thought to represent the healing of ring haemorrhages and consist of a central demyelinated focus with surrounding glial proliferation.

The spleen is always enlarged and often shows hyperplasia of lymphoid follicles with increased numbers of plasma cells around the penicillary arteries of the red pulp. The liver may show focal or widespread fatty change and in severe cases with high levels of parasitaemia may show pericentral liver cell necrosis, which may be due to shock rather than a direct effect of the parasites.

The kidney may show changes of acute tubular necrosis in patients with shock or heavy parasitaemia and a transient glomerulonephritis may occur in infection by *P. falciparum*. *P. malariae* is associated with quartan malarial nephropathy which is also caused by immune complexes. Malaria (and babesosis) in patients with HIV infections from endemic areas do not show different clinicopathological features from cases that are not infected.

3.1.2 Cryptosporidiosis (*Cryptosporidia* spp.)

This organism may cause self-limiting diarrhoea in immunocompetent patients or a persistent watery diarrhoea in the immunosuppressed. It has become the most widely recognized intestinal coccidial infection since the appearance of AIDS. The organism is located superficially on bowel epithelial cells and sometimes the biliary epithelium. Extraintestinal spread has been observed, notably to the bronchial tree. The tissue reaction may be minimal but there is usually some villus shortening and a chronic inflammatory infiltrate in the lamina propria. Focal acute inflammation and crypt abscesses may occur particularly in association with ruptured glands and there is often a periglandular accentuation of mononuclear cells and macrophages. Large bowel may show a reactive crypt hyperplasia. The cysts are about 4.5–6 μm in diameter and are usually seen easily with H&E staining (see *Plate 6c*), trophozoites are smaller. Both may be difficult to distinguish from mucin droplets or nuclear debris but use of Giemsa, Best's mucicarmine, or Alcian blue/neutral red may help distinguish them. A monoclonal antibody has been shown to work in paraffin sections but fails to stain trophozoites (2).

- Diagnosis. Stool examination using a modified Ziehl–Neelsen stain (which does not work in tissue sections) or biopsy.

3.1.3 Isospora (*Isopora belli*)

Relatively uncommon in the UK, but much more common in Africa as a cause of diarrhoea in patients with AIDS and in some groups of AIDS patients in the USA. It primarily infects the small bowel although it may be found in the large bowel and rarely spreads to extraintestinal sites. All stages of enterocyte intracytoplasmic development (zoites to gametocytes) can be seen as small bodies (3–20 μm diameter). Small bowel shows variable inflammation usually with eosinophils and a crypt hyperplastic atrophy but may show florid eosinophilic enteritis.

- Diagnosis. Stool microscopy (oocysts), duodenal aspirate, small bowel biopsy. Differential diagnosis: Sarcocystis see below, Microsporidia, and Toxoplasma are smaller.

3.1.4 Sarcocystis (*S. hominis, S. suihominis*)

May be difficult to differentiate from Isospora and will probably need referral. Sporozoites released from ingested sarcocyst enter the mucosa and parasitize cells of the lamina propria. Segmental eosinophilic or necrotizing enteritis may ensue. In sections the stages of development are found in the lamina propria cells, typically immediately below the enterocytes. Oocysts are similar to Isospora but more spheroidal and delicate.

3.1.5 Toxoplasmosis (*Toxoplasma gondii*)

Infection in developed countries is often asymptomatic. Congenital and acquired forms occur. After humans ingest infective oocysts or cysts, sporozoites are liberated in the intestinal tract, gain access to intestinal blood vessels, and thence to tissues. Intracellular multiplication takes place with the rapid proliferation of trophozoites (tachyzoites) which fill and eventually rupture the cell with infection of other cells. Some forms (bradyzoites) develop more slowly and become cysts in almost any tissue. In congenital infection, from transplacental spread, the placenta shows mild to severe inflammation with necrosis, vasculitis, and calcification and parasites are difficult to demonstrate. The changes in the infant are most marked in the brain which shows meningoencephalitis with dilation of the ventricles and usually hydrocephalus. Necrotic lesions, sometimes large, are randomly distributed and there is commonly calcification around the ventricles and cortex. The earliest reaction is aggregation of microglial cells in nodules with central neuronal degeneration. Bradyzoites and tachyzoites are relatively easily found and parasites are present in up to 20% of the nodules. Chorioretinitis, myocarditis, and other organ involvement are also common in congenital disease.

Acquired disease has become very much more common since the appearance of AIDS, in which central nervous system involvement is the most important manifestation. The brain is swollen and shows microscopic necrosis and inflammation in varying stages of organization. Vasculitis with thrombosis is common. Tachyzoites and bradyzoites are found. Myocarditis and ocular diseases also occur in acquired infection. Toxoplasmic lymphadenitis is common in immune competent children and adults producing enlarged nodes with follicular hyperplasia and a prominent epithelioid histiocytic infiltrate of the cortex and paracortex. Clusters of epithelioid cells encroach on, or are found within, the germinal centres. The subcapsular sinus is distended with mononuclear cells and occasionally epithelioid granulomas with Langhan's-type giant cells are present. Parasites are difficult to find in sections or imprint preparations. Toxoplasmic pneumonitis occurs but may have widespread areas of necrosis, parasites are usually abundant. Tachyzoites are crescentic $4–8 \times 2–3$ μm, with a blue stained cytoplasm, and dark red nucleus in H&E. Sizes, for imprint preparations, are larger than in sections. Cysts (40 μm with 1 μ membrane) (*Plate 6b*), containing bradyzoites/tachyzoites have a weakly positive PAS wall. Zoites in the cyst are strongly PAS positive. Monoclonal antibody (Bioquote) may be useful in staining zoites (3).

- Diagnosis. Tissue imprints (air dried) and stained with Wright's or alcohol fixed and Giemsa stained. Biopsy.

3.2 Microspora

3.2.1 Microsporidiosis (*Enterocytozoon bieneusi*)

Infection of the small intestine with this recently recognized organism has been suggested as possible cause of diarrhoea in patients with AIDS. They are found in 30% of patients in whom there is no other cause of diarrhoea (4). The spores are found in the apical part of the enterocytes as small haematoxyphilic bodies 0.5–1.5 μm on H&E stain (*Plate 6d*), and red with blue polarity with the Brown–Brenn Gram stain. Meronts may also be seen with difficulty. Small bowel Giemsa stained smears may be useful in identification. Organisms have been detected in the large bowel in two cases. The enterocytes usually show little damage but focal degeneration tufting and necrosis are seen (4). Stages other than spores are difficult to diagnose by light microscopy and electron microscopy is often required to confirm the diagnosis.

The related *E. cuniculi* and *E. hellem* may cause peritonitis, hepatitis, and conjunctival keratitis in patients with AIDS. Inflammation is scanty. Organisms (1–2 μm) are seen on Giemsa or Gram stain and electron microscopy will confirm diagnosis. *Septata intestinalis* has been found in HIV patients in association with diarrhoea. It differs from *E. bienensi* in that more enterocytes contain more spores, the prespore stages are less obvious and spores are found in lamina propria macrophages. Infection can become disseminated.

3.2.2 Pneumocystis (*Pneumocystis carinii*)

This organism's taxonomy is currently undecided showing some protozoal and some fungal characteristics. Asymptomatic infection is common and it is in the immunosuppressed host, particularly in patients infected with HIV, that clinical disease becomes apparent. The main site for infection is the lung although involvement of non-pulmonary sites does occur. The lung appears pale with pneumonic consolidation and less commonly cavitation, which may mimic tuberculosis. Trophozoites and spherical thick-walled cystic stages exist in the alveoli, the latter containing intracystic bodies that look like trophozoites. The characteristic microscopic appearance is an intra-alveolar foamy exudate, pink in H&E stains, in which the faintly basophilic intracystic bodies and trophozoites can be seen. The lung parenchymal changes range from very little to interstitial fibrosis. In the cavitating form there is often necrosis and a more marked inflammatory infiltrate. Cystic forms may infiltrate under the endothelium leading to occlusion of small vessels and are a potential route of dissemination to extrapulmonary sites.

Most cases are now diagnosed from induced sputum or broncho-alveolar lavage specimens but transbronchial biopsy specimens are still sometimes performed. Grocott and Giemsa stains are both reliable in showing the organism. The former stains the cyst walls and intracystic bodies, the latter will stain trophozoites. A rapid Grocott method can be used for urgent cases (see *Protocol 5*). Monoclonal antibodies (Dako) can also be used on smears, fluids, and sections which stains cysts and trophozoites (*Plate 6e*).

Protocol 5. Rapid Grocott staining method

1. Take test and control sections to distilled water.
2. Put slides in a 50 ml Coplin jar of 5% chromic acid solution (fresh).
3. Heat to 60 °C in a microwave oven for 2 min precisely.
4. Rinse in several changes of distilled water.
5. Transfer sections to a Coplin jar of hexamine silver (3% hexamine 50 ml; 5% borax × 2ml; 10% $AgNO_3$ 0.625 ml) at room temperature.
6. Heat to 60 °C in a microwave and check at 1 min intervals until control section is light brown (approx. 5–7 min).
7. Stop the reaction by washing well in distilled water.

8. Tone in 0.2% gold chloride solution if desired. Wash.
9. Fix silver in 5% sodium thiosulfate for 2 min. Wash.
10. Counterstain with 0.2% light green stain solution.
11. Wash, dehydrate, clear, and mount.

3.3 Flagellates

3.3.1 Giardiasis (*Giardia lamblia*)

Patients usually present with explosive and foul smelling diarrhoea due to infection of the small bowel. Parasites are found on the surface of the small bowel villi and in the crypts. Tissue invasion is not usually seen (reports of this remain to be verified). Changes in the mucosa range from normal to shortened villi with a variable inflammatory infiltrate of polymorphs and mononuclear cells. Nodular lymphoid hyperplasia may occur. The histological changes do not correlate with the number of organisms or the clinical severity. Although common in patients with HIV infection the severity and course do not differ from that in immunocompetent patients.

Trophozoites are identifiable in an H&E section as greyish-blue with a rounded anterior end with paired nuclei giving a 'monkey face' appearance and a tapering posterior end. They are often not seen as clearly as this description suggests and may appear elongated or sickle shaped (*Plate 6c*). Giemsa stain may help in the diagnosis. Cysts are not seen in tissue sections.

- Diagnosis. Stool microscopy, duodenal aspirate, touch imprint from small bowel biopsy, and routine histology.

3.3.2 Leishmaniasis (*Leishmania donavani* complex, *L. mexicana* complex, *L. brasiliensis* complex, *L. tropica*, *L. aethiopica*, *L. major* 'Old World complex')

Many of the cases seen in the UK are acquired in the Mediterranean region and Middle East. The different species are indistinguishable histologically and require isoenzyme or DNA probing to subclassify them. For a detailed clinicopathological review see Bryceson (5).

In cutaneous lesions the early nodules contain macrophages filled with *Leishmania* amastigotes, the Leishman–Donovan (L–D) bodies, and usually heal spontaneously. Ulceration is common and scarring may be marked. Necrotizing epithelioid granulomas or macrophage necrosis are common with numerous plasma cells, as the numbers of amastigotes decrease. Rarely a tuberculoid reaction may be seen with few plasma cells. Biopsies taken during the healing phase may have few organisms. The differential diagnosis then includes other causes of a granulomatous inflammation.

Visceral diseases occurs in two major forms. The first is widespread infiltration of macrophages in the reticulo-endothelial system with large numbers of organisms, usually with a plasmacytic infiltrate, expansion of lymphoid sinuses, infection of Kupffer cells, and occasionally hepatocytes. Alternatively limited involvement of liver, spleen, and lymph nodes with fewer parasites and more granulomas occurs. Epithelioid clusters and microgranulomas are found which may involve the germinal centres of lymph nodes as well as the paracortex. Caseation of these granulomas may develop. Over 100 cases of visceral Leishmaniasis have been reported in AIDS patients, occasionally in unusual settings, e.g. Kaposi's sarcoma. L–D bodies (1.5–3 μm) have an intracellular location in macrophages although other cell types may contain them, round nucleus with rod or oval-shaped kinetoplast attached to edge of the nucleus in colourless slightly refractile cytoplasm. The differential diagnosis is between *Toxoplasma gondii* zoites which are rarely intracellular, *Trypanosoma cruzi*, the same but does have a kinetoplast, *Histoplasma capsulatum*, when a fungal stain will distinguish them. Karyorrhectic cellular debris in areas of necrosis, when few organisms will be seen. Bacteria, a Gram stain will differentiate these from L–D bodies. Special stains may be helpful such as Giemsa staining of smears/biopsies. Monoclonal antibodies are helpful but not available for all species (6). Polyclonal are also helpful and show staining in and outside cells in late cases of cutaneous diseases when no L–D bodies are seen (7).

- Diagnosis. Dab smears from tissues with monoclonal antibodies, *in vitro* culture, Giemsa stained smears, biopsy.

3.3.3 Trichomonas (*Trichomonas vaginalis*)

T. vaginalis is the only species commonly causing symptoms of vaginitis with a discharge. It is not usually a diagnosis that is made by histopathological assessment but commonly on cytology.

3.3.4 Trypanosomiasis

i. Trypanosoma cruzi

This is rarely encountered in the UK but does enter the differential diagnosis of toxoplasmosis and leishmaniasis. Patients develop acute or chronic myocarditis, cerebral infiltration, destruction of parasympathetic nerve cells leading to megaoesophagus, and placental or congenital infection.

The aflagella trypomastigote stage enters the host cell cytoplasm where amastigote reproduction occurs resulting in liberation of flagellates and the destruction of the cell with chronic inflammation, cellular degeneration, and presence of amastigotes. Amastigotes (1–2 μm) are intracellular, extracellular forms are due to rupture of cells during processing. A pseudocept of *T. cruzi* in human heart muscle is shown in *Plate 3d*.

- Diagnosis. Blood films, blood culture, serology. Biopsies or tissue specimens should be received fresh, imprint slides made, and Giemsa stained. Amastigotes are larger (2–4 μm) in imprints.

ii. Trypanosoma brucei complex

Sleeping sickness may present with the inoculation site chancre which shows oedema, intense inflammation, tissue damage, and vasculitis. Trypomastigotes are found in the interstitium. They gain access via dermal lymphatics to lymph nodes where a sinus histiocytosis, plasmacytosis, and mononuclear cell expansion are seen. This transforms to a depleted stage later in the disease. Parasites are found in large numbers in lymph nodes. With spread to other organs a mononuclear cell myocarditis and meningoencephalitis develop. The latter shows perivascular and meningeal infiltrates of lymphocytes, macrophages, and plasma cells which may contain large Russell bodies known as Mott cells, highly suggestive of the infection. Neuronal destruction, demyelination, haemorrhage, and obliterated vessels may be seen.

- Diagnosis. Blood films, lymph node, or CSF smears for flagellates. Lymph node or bone marrow aspirates for trypomastigotes.

3.4 Amoeba

3.4.1 *Entamoeba histolytica*

Many people carry *E. histolytica* without symptoms. A relatively small number develop colitis where the trophozoites reside and develop into cysts which are passed in the stool. The pathogenicity of *E. histolytica* is of some debate but appears to be related to their isoenzyme patterns (zymodeme type) (8). The histological evidence of the prescence of a pathogenic strain is phagocytosis of red cells by the trophozoites and tissue invasion. The latter may lead to bloodstream spread and metastatic lesions in the liver, lung, brain, and other organs.

The colonic appearance ranges from normal to extensively ulcerated. The ulcers may be small or large with necrosis, are typically perpendicular to the long axis, flask shaped with undermining of the adjacent mucosa, and may perforate. In early inflammation the epithelial cells lyse with acute inflammation and necrosis which progresses to ulceration. Amoebae are found at the junction of necrotic and viable mucosa. In deep ulcers they are also found in muscle and serosal tissue as the trophozoites follow the line of least resistance.

Vascular thrombi and necrosis commonly accompany this process and infective emboli are disseminated in this way and by direct invasion of larger vessels. Amoebomas develop in a small percentage of patients, most commonly in the caecum, when they consist of central necrosis, granulation tissue, and surrounding fibrosis. Recent metastatic lesions usually consist of a single abscess containing central brownish necrotic debris often likened to 'anchovy paste'. They result from a microinfarct due to infected thromboemboli in the small portal vessels, are usually single and most often in the right lobe. Older lesions have a better developed irregular outer fibrous wall.

Trophozoites are hard to find and are located in the wall of the abscess. Lesions in the lung and pleura develop more rapidly and are therefore often less well defined than in the liver.

Cutaneous lesions due to a primary focus, an abscess draining to skin or surgical transfer, present as ulcers, pseudocondylomata, or as cervical and vaginal ulceration, which may mimic carcinoma. In H&E sections (best for morphology) trophozoites are 15–25 μm in diameter and often contain ingested red cells. Cytoplasm is amphophilic and finely granular (varies with staining and fixation) with the nucleus blue. The nucleus is smaller (the size of a red cell) and more regular than that of a macrophage (*Plate 6a*). A PAS stained section may identify the area of the section where they are present but will also stain macrophages.

- Diagnosis. Stool or body fluid smears for cysts and trophozoites, biopsy for trophozoites and demonstration of tissue invasion.

3.4.2 *Acanthomoeba* spp

Causes ocular keratitis in contact lens wearers and may cause necrotizing and granulomatous meningoencephalitis from a nasal sinus infection. Skin lesions of a similar type also occur. The trophozoites (22 μm.) are larger than *E. histolytica* and *Acanthomoeba* spp. cysts are usually seen in sections, in contrast to *E. histolytica*.

3.4.3 *Naeglaria fowleri*

May cause purulent meningoencephalitis. Trophozoites (12 μm) are smaller than *E. histolytica* with an apparently absent nuclear membrane, prominent nucleolus, and vacuolated cytoplasm.

Both the above usually need to be isolated and cultured (Chapter 6) for identification in a reference centre.

3.5 Ciliates

3.5.1 Balantidia (*Balantidium coli*)

Tropical or subtropical infection uncommon in the UK which may be symptomless or produce an acute dysenteric picture similar to amoebic dysentery. In acute disease the entire colon is affected usually with distal predominance and small to large crater-like ulcers, resembling amoebic ulcers, which may perforate. Trophozoites are found in the lumen, the gland crypts, and the base of ulcers. A chronic inflammatory infiltrate with polymorphs is usual. Dissemination may occur to other parts of the bowel and lymph nodes. It is the largest parasitic protozoan of the gut in man.

The trophozoite (50–200 μm) has a black nucleus and red cytoplasm when stained with H&E, often with a clear space in the posterior part which represents the contractile vacuole. Cilia are seen on the external surface.

Free-living ciliated protozoa contaminating the water used for staining can give a false positive.

- Diagnosis. Stool for cysts and trophozoites or biopsy.

4. Histopathology of infections caused by rhabditida

4.1 Strongyloides (*Strongyloides stercoralis*)

Although not transmitted in temperate zones infected persons can carry the worms for life due to a cycle of auto-infection. Some 30 years after incarceration 9% of Far East prisoners of war were found to have larvae in their stools. Any suppression of cell-mediated immunity may lead to rapid and life-threatening dissemination. An infective proctitis with eosinophils and granulomas is usual. Light infections are easily missed. The filariform larvae (average 15 μm) lie in the glands, crypts, and invade the mucosa. There is a differential diagnosis with *Capillaria philippinensis*.

- Diagnosis. Examination of faeces or duodenal contents, biopsy.

4.2 Spirurida

All of the major filariases are seen as imported infections.

4.2.1 Lymphatic filariasis (*Wucheria bancroftii* or *Brugia* spp.)

Lymphatic filariasis presents as a lymphadenitis due to the adult worms (responsible for most of the symptoms) in the lymph node sinuses. Lymphatics are thickened with a chronic inflammatory infiltrate adjacent to the worm and in the adjacent tissue. Granulomas develop in association with degenerating worms often with an acute necrotizing inflammatory focus.

Microfilaria may also be seen in lymphatics and can evoke an eosinophilic inflammatory reaction, when they degenerate, with formation of microabscesses. Invasion of the walls of small vessels can cause focal vasculitis with thrombus formation.

Adult worms: *Brugei* 80–170 μm, *Wucheria* 300 μm in diameter. Microfilaria have a 10 μm cross-section.

4.2.2 Loiasis (*Loa loa*)

Adult worms migrate through subcutaneous tissues to any part of the body. Diagnosis is often made as they pass across the conjunctiva or bridge of the nose. Calabar (fugitive) swellings occur most frequently on hand, forearm, ankles, and orbit and appear to be more common in expatriates than natives. The dying worms elicit suppurative inflammation with secondary granulomatous and fibrotic changes. Microfilaria may be found in the skin particularly in capillaries around the sweat glands. Adult worms are 300–500 μm, microfilaria 5 μm in diameter.

4.2.3 Onchocerciasis (*Onchocera volvulus*)

The most likely presentation in the UK is of a subcutaneous nodule. Deposition of larvae on the host skin is followed by infiltration and development of onchocercomas as the larvae mature to adult worms over a period of up to one year. Microfilariae invade adjacent tissue and become distributed systemically.

The subcutaneous nodule is fibrotic, usually easy to separate from surrounding tissue, and contains small (1 mm) cavities filled with worms, seen in multiple cross-section in fibrous tissue where microfilariae are also found. Viable worms excite little active inflammation but dead ones are associated with acute inflammation. Inflamed nodules show the characteristic features of an abscess. Other skin manifestations of chronic infection are inflammation with an eosinophilic and histiocytic response to dead microfilariae, hyperkeratosis and acanthosis, hyper- or hypopigmentation, or atrophic dermatitis with dermal fibrosis. Microfilaria are usually easily found in skin lesions. In the eye chronic inflammation with eosinophils is usual with disorganization of the pigment layers. Lymph nodes show fibrosis, scarring, and atrophy with microfilariae.

The worm has a diameter of 350 μm (female) and 125 μm (male). The cuticle appears two layered and has distinct transverse or spiral ridges. The inner cuticle layer has striae which stain red with Masson Trichrome stain. Microfilariae are up to 360 μm long and 6 μm wide, but are often not seen in total in tissue sections.

- Diagnosis. Skin snips examined under saline solution or a stained preparation. The site of choice for skin snips is the scapular region.

4.3 Ascaridia

4.3.1 Ascaris (*Ascaris lumbricoides*)

The rhabditdiform larvae (hatching from an ingested egg) penetrate the small intestine to lymphatics and venules, are passed to the portal circulation, and then to lung and heart. The larvae break through alveolar capillaries, migrate up the bronchi, and are swallowed into the oesophagus and small intestine where the adult and egg-producing worms reside. During the lung migratory phase an eosinophilic allergic-type hypersensitivity reaction is common. Haemorrhagic pneumomia due to large numbers of migrating larvae or secondary pneumonia may occur. In some cases larvae embolize from passage through the left side of the heart. Intestinal infection may be complicated by invasion of the biliary tree, pancreatitis, perforation, peritonitis, and fistula formation to the skin or secondary bacterial infection may lead to an abscess. High worm loads can cause obstruction, intussusception, and volvulus.

Adult worms are 10–35 cm long and eggs 45–70 × 50 μm; larvae 0.02–1.5 μm depending on stage of development.

- Diagnosis. Eggs or worms in stool or biopsies, larvae in lungs.

4.3.2 Toxocariasis (*Toxocara canis, T. catis*)

Humans are an accidental host of these parasites of unwormed or young cats and dogs. Ingestion of embryonated eggs leads to penetration of the intestinal mucosa and carriage to the liver, lungs, and other organs. In the process they cause inflammation with eosinophilic granulomas. The characteristic lesions in the liver, 4 mm in diameter, are epithelioid granulomas with giant cells around larvae and frequently Charcot–Leyden crystals. Extensive hepatic parenchymal necrosis may occur and eosinophilic granulomas without larvae are frequently seen at the sites of dead or degenerate larvae. Lesions may occur at any site but particularly in the eye, which may lead to macular inflammation.

- Diagnosis. Demonstration of larvae (14–20 μm diameter, 290–350 μm long) is definitive together with serology.

4.3.3 Anisakiasis (*Anisakis* spp. and *Pseudoterranova* spp.)

Infection from eating raw or partly cooked fish is reported, uncommonly, in the UK and USA. Larvae burrow into the gastric or small intestinal mucosa usually with a florid eosinophilic reaction, which may perforate, cause peritonitis, or a granulomatous reaction. The nematode is 1 mm diameter and 3 cm long.

- Diagnosis. Endoscopic biopsy.

4.4 Oxyurida

4.4.1 Enterobiasis (*Enterobius vermicularis*)

The pinworm has the widest geographical distribution of any helminth and is common in children presenting with perianal and perineal itching, due to migration of the adult worms. The causal relationship of pinworm infection and other gastro-intestinal complaints is uncertain but they are found in resected appendices, both inflamed and non-inflamed, when the adult worm is seen in cross-section (150–350 μm diameter with lateral alae).

- Diagnosis. Perianal swab to identify eggs or adult worms.

4.5 Strongylida

4.5.1 Ankylostomiasis (*Ankylostoma duodenale, Necator americanus*)

Infection by these hookworms usually presents as skin itching at the site of penetration, followed by a pneumonitis with eosinophilia (Loefflers syndrome), and intestinal symptoms. The latter may occur without preceding lung symptoms if larvae are directly ingested. Histological descriptions are scanty and they are rarely found in tissue sections. Mucosal and submucosal nodules and abscess containing adult worms have been described.

4.6 Trichinelloidea

4.6.1 Trichuris (*Trichuris trichiura*)

Symptoms are related to the number of worms and duration of infection. In heavy infections proctocolitis and mucosal prolapse is common with diarrhoea/blood and in severe cases anaemia. The colon is congested, bleeds readily on contact, and frequently has small ulcers. Large numbers of worms are found attached to prolapsed mucosa. The worms are seen within a mucosal tunnel, with a roof of epithelial cells and the posterior end of the worm protruding into the gut lumen.

Worm diameter is 100–150 μm with 8 μm cuticle, the bacillary band in the inner layer of the cuticle is related to the oesophagus of the worm and consists of cuticular pores. This portion is seen in the parts of the worm embedded in the mucosa. Sections of the worm in the colonic lumen usually show the posterior part (up to 0.5 mm diameter) which contains the central genital tube.

4.6.2 Trichinella (*Trichinella spiralis*)

This infection is indigenous to temperate zones and usually contracted from the consumption of undercooked pork or wild animal meat. Adult worms infect the gut and larvae infect striated muscle. The small intestinal lesions show variable chronic inflammation, occasional small haemorrhages, and worms within crypts in a tunnel similar to those of trichuris infection. Muscular lesions are first degenerative with the gradual development, over about five weeks, of the encapsulated larva within the muscle fibre. The capsule is bland hyaline material and during encapsulation a myositis of single fibres occurs. The fate of the larva is death with calcification. Myocardial involvement differs in that larvae are rarely encapsulated. There is an eosinophilic myositis and secondary endocardial damage with mural thrombi.

Unencapsulated larvae are 13–15 μm in diameter, encapsulated 35 μm diameter and tightly coiled (*Plate 5f*). The pseudocyst is up to 350 μm with a capsule of about 15 μm.

- Diagnosis. Fresh muscle biopsy, small portion (approx. 5 cubic centimetres) squashed between slides and examined unstained for larvae. In sections eosinophilic myositis is suggestive and larvae identified by size and morphology. The differential diagnosis is with hookworm larvae.

4.6.3 Capillaria (*Capillaria hepatica, C. philippinensis*)

Rare in the UK. *C. hepatica* causes an acute or subacute hepatitis with peripheral eosinophilia. The liver shows focal liver cell destruction with mononuclear and eosinophilic inflammation and immature worms. Perioval granulomas develop later. Multinucleated giant cells form with phagocytosis of eggs and fibrosis and focal calcification develops.

Eggs are 48–62 μm × 28–37 μm. Females worms are 130 μm and males 80 μm in diameter. The intestine of the worm stains dark blue with H&E.

In intestinal capillariasis (*C. philippinensis*) numerous adult worms are found in the mucosa usually with marked inflammation. Small intestine may show flattened villi and dilated crypts and epithelial cells metaplastic changes. Sections show worms deep in mucosal crypts (female 47 μm, male 28 μm diameter).

5. Histopathology of infections caused by trematodes

5.1 Schistosomiasis (*Schistosoma mansoni, S. haematobium, S. japonicum*)

Schistosomiasis is contracted by paddling or bathing in water where the necessary intermediate snail hosts are found, which are infected by ova passed in urine or faeces. Free-swimming cercariae released from the snail enter the skin and via dermal venules are passed to the lungs where many are destroyed. Survivors pass to the systemic circulation and mature into adult worms in the portal venous system. After copulation the eggs deposit in fine venous radicals of the bladder, intestines, and occasionally other sites. *S. mansoni* and *S. intercalatum* commonly cause hepatic and gastro-intestinal lesions, *S. haematobium* genito-urinary, and *S. japonicum* gastro-intestinal lesions.

In any infection the worm and egg load determines the extent of organ and tissue damage. Many infections are light with minimal symptoms and little inflammation. In all species the lesions are due to the host reaction, usually consisting of eosinophils with granulomas of epithelioid macrophages and lymphocytes. The adult worms appear to acquire an outer layer which is probably of host origin and become resistant to the host immune response. Ova are highly immunogenic and the response may destroy tissue 100 times the volume of the egg. The bladder shows chronic inflammation and fibrosis with dead eggs becoming calcified. Pseudo-epitheliomatous hyperplasia, squamous metaplasia, and squamous carcinoma may develop. In the gut granulomas are found around viable or dead eggs with fibrosis and diffuse inflammation which may result in the development of inflammatory polyps. In the liver hepatic granulomas may be encountered which in severe cases may lead to pipe-stem fibrosis of portal tracts. Haemozoin pigment, produced by the adult worms, is usually seen in Kupffer cells. In the lung granulomas, vasculitis, and intestitial fibrosis with pulmonary hypertension may all occur. Dead ova are eventually digested and in long-standing cases a diagnosis may be difficult to make. In any site it is not unusual to find dead or calcified ova with no active inflammation around them.

Dead ova usually retain a brown refractility to the shell even when the internal miracidia have been phagocytosed. PAS staining may help to find eggs. The spines on the ova may be visible, apical in *S. haematobium*, lateral subapical in *S. mansoni*. Adult worms may also be seen (*Plate 6f*). The differential diagnosis of eggs producing granulomas includes: *Enterobius vermicularis, Ascaris lumbricoides, Capillaria hepatica* and *Paragonimus* spp.

- Diagnosis. Stool or urine examination and rectal snips with a squash preparation are best, biopsy is less sensitive.

5.2 *Clonorchis* spp. and *Opisthorcis* spp.

These are rare in the UK but have been reported in Europeans. Both produce infection of the hepatic and biliary systems resulting in biliary obstruction, jaundice, dilatation, and thickening of small and medium sized ducts due to fibrosis and adenomatous epithelial proliferation. There is usually slight inflammation and little damage to parenchyma. Viable dead or degenerating adult parasites are found in the duct lumen and eggs are often found in collections of inspissated bile. Both infections are associated with the development of cholangiocarcinoma.

- Diagnosis. Stool sample for eggs. Biopsy and resection specimens for eggs and adult worms. If eggs are recovered from a specimen they should be stained and examined directly, not put through histological processing. Worms found in tissue sections have the features of trematodes.

5.3 *Fasciola hepatica*

The liver is the primary site of infection where the adult worms usually produce abscesses and the eggs granulomas. The multiple small pale areas may resemble metastatic tumour. Adult flukes may be seen in the bile ducts. The abscesses may be related to bile ducts and partially lined by epithelium. Lesions are often track-like. Early lesions usually contain polymorphs and eosinophils. Older lesions undergo fibrosis and calcification. Ectopic lesions may occur almost anywhere, usually present as an abscess and parasites or eggs are usually found in the tissue.

Eggs are 130–190 μm × 63–90 μm, and the adult worm has the features of a trematode with an outer tegument and internal organs, including a characteristically highly branched intestine.

6. Cestodes

6.1 Hydatid disease (*Echinococus granulosus, E. multilocularis*)

This parasite has a wide geographical distribution including the UK, and human infections occur in nearly all these areas as a result of ingesting the eggs. The embryo liberated from the egg rapidly enters the tissues and via lymphatic or venous channels to other sites where differentiation and growth lead to development of hydatid cysts. They are commonest in the liver (but other sites may be involved), slow growing reaching up to 20 cm diameter, and have a characteristic appearance, being filled with clear fluid, are partly loculated or several cysts may coalesce and are composed of three layers. The outer layer is fibrous, the middle layer is white and laminated and separates easily from the fibrous layer, and the inner germinal layer is semi-transparent yellowish-white and contains numerous brood capsules. Daughter cysts may be present within the main cyst which together with the brood capsules form the hydatid sand if the cyst fluid is allowed to stand. Inflammatory response to the cysts is usually minimal unless there is rupture or secondary infection.

The laminated membrane is PAS positive, the protoscolices may be recognized by their hooklets. Dead cysts are often necrotic or calcified but should be carefully examined for areas of viability and daughter cysts.

E. mutilocularis is more often fatal and produces ectopic lesions more commonly although the liver is still the commonest site. The cysts are smaller and less well organized than in the case of *E. granulosus* infection. There is usually a marked granulomatous inflammatory response and the PAS stain may help to recognize fragments of the laminated membrane.

6.2 Intestinal tapeworms (*Taenia solium, Taenia saginata, Diphyllobothrium latum*)

Most infections are diagnosed on clinical grounds and stool examination. Occasionally a worm may be found in a resected appendix but larval infection may present a histological problem. Cystercicosis due to *T. solium* commonly produces intramuscular and subcutaneous lesions, and more importantly produces central nervous system and ophthalmic lesions (cystercerci). Death of the cysticercus in the tissues results in an inflammatory response which is more marked in tissues where a fibrous capsule is not well formed (e.g. brain and eye). Calcification occurs in relation to dead cysticerci. In removed tissue, elements of the cestode structure are recognizable both in dead and viable cysticerci.

References

1. Bancroft, J. D. and Stevens, A. (ed.) (1991). *Theory and practice of histological techniques*. Churchill Livingstone, Edinburgh.
2. Loose, J. H., Sedegran, D. J., and Cooper, H. S. (1989). *Am. J. Clin. Pathol.*, **91**, 206.
3. Curry, A., Turner, A. J., and Lucas, S. (1991). *J. Clin. Pathol.*, **44**, 182.
4. Orenstein, J. M., Chiang, J., Steinberg, W., Smith, P. D., Rotterdam, H., and Kotler, A. P. (1990). *Hum. Pathol.*, **21**, 475.

5. Bryceson, A. D. M. (1987). In *Oxford textbook of medicine* (ed. D. J. Weatherall), 2nd edn, pp. 5.524–5.532. Oxford University Press, Oxford.
6. Lynch, N. R., Malave, C., Infante, R. B., Modlin, R. L., and Convit, J. (1986). *Trans. R. Soc. Trop. Med. Hyg.*, **80**, 6.
7. Sells, P. G. and Burton, M. (1981). *Trans. R. Soc. Trop. Med. Hyg.*, **75**, 461.
8. Sargeaunt, P. G., Jackson, T. F. H. G., and Simjee, A. (1982). *Lancet*, (**i**), 1386.

Further reading

1. Gutierrez, Y. (1990). *Diagnostic pathology of parasitic infections with clinical correlations*. Lea and Febiger, Philadelphia.
2. Beaver, P. C., Jung, R. C., and Cupp, W. C. (1984). *Clinical parasitology*. Lea and Febiger, Philadelphia.
3. Coleman, D. V. and Chapman, P. A. (1989). *Clinical cytotechnology*. Butterworths, London.

A1

Suppliers of specialist items

Alpha Laboratories Ltd, 169 Oldfield Lane, Greenford, UB6 8PW, UK.
American Hospital Supplies, Station Road, Didcot, Oxfordshire OX11 7NP, UK.
American Type Culture, Collection, 12301 Parklawn Drive, Rockville, Maryland 20852, USA.
Amicon, Upper Mill, Stonehouse, Gloucester GL10 2BJ, UK.
Ames Division Miles Laboratories Ltd, P.O. Box 37, Stoke Court, Stoke Poges, Slough, Bucks SL2 4LY, UK.
Anderman & Co Ltd, 145 London Road, Kingston-upon-Thames, Surrey KT2 6NH, UK.
Bayer plc Pharmaceutical Division, Bayer House, Strawberry Hill, Newbury, Berks RG13 1JA, UK.
BDH Laboratory Suppliers (Now Merck Ltd), Hunter Boulevard, Magna Park, Lutterworth, Leicestershire LE17 4XN, UK.
BDH Chemicals Ltd, Poole BH12 4NN, UK.
Becton-Dickinson UK Ltd, Between Towns Road, Cowley, Oxford IX4 3LY, UK.
Bibby Sterilin Ltd, Tilling Drive, Stone, Staffordshire ST15 0SA, UK.
Biokit SA, 08186 Llissa d'Amunt, Barcelona, Spain.
API-bioMérieux (UK) Ltd, Grafton Way, Basingstoke, Hants RG22 6HY, UK.
API-bioMérieux, Marcy-l'Etoile, 69752 Charbonnieres-les-Bains, Cedex, France.
Bioquote Ltd, 3 Mount Pleasant Court, Ilkley, W. Yorkshire LS29 8IW, UK.
Bio-Rad Laboratories Ltd, Bio-Rad House, Maylands Avenue, Hemel Hempstead, Herfordshire HP2 7TD, UK.
Boehringer Mannheim GmbH, D-6800 Mannheim 31, Germany.
Boehringer Mannheim Bioquimica, Rua Nair 170, Olaria, CEP 21021 Rio de Janeiro, RJ, Brazil.
Boehringer Mannheim Corp., 9115 Hague Road, Indianapolis, Indiana, 46250, USA.
Boehringer Mannheim UK, (Diagnostic & Biochemicals) Ltd, Bell Lane, Lewes, East Sussex BN7 1LG, UK.
Camlab Ltd Nuffield Road, Cambridge, Cambridgeshire CB4 1TH, UK
Cellabs Diagnostics Pty Ltd, P.O. Box 421, Brookvale, NSW 2100, Australia.

Cetus Corporation, Emeryville, California, 94608, USA
Citifluor Ltd, Connaught Building (Room 303), Northampton Square, London ECN 0HB, UK.
Dako Ltd, 16 Manor Courtyard, Hughenden Avenue, High Wycombe, Bucks HP13 5RE, UK.
Dako Corporation, 6392, Via Real, Carpinteria, CA 93013, USA.
Difco Laboratories, P.O. Box 1058A, Detroit, MI 48232, USA.
Du Pont (UK) Ltd, Biotechnology Systems Division, Wedgwood way, Stevenage, Herfordshire SG1 4QN, UK.
Du Pont de Nemours Inc, Clinical Systems Division, Wilmington, DE 19898, USA.
Du Pont NEN Research Products, Schleicher & Schnell, VKR, P.O. Box 4, D-33 54 Dassel, Germany.
Dynatech Laboratories, Daux Road, Billingshurst, Sussex RH14 9SJ, UK.
Eiken Chemical Company Ltd, 33-8 Hongo 1-Chome, Tokyo, Japan.
Endecott's Ltd, 9 Lombard Road, London SW19 3UP, UK.
Fisions Scientific Equipment Bishop Meadow Road, Loughborough, Leicestershire LE11 0RG, UK.
Flow Laboratories, ICN Biomedicals USA, P.O. Box 5023, Costa Mesa, CA 92626, USA.
Flow Laboratories, ICN Biomedicals, Eagle house, Peregrine Business Park, Gomm Road, High Wycombe, Bucks HP13 7DL, UK.
Fluka Chemicals, Peadkale Road, Glossop, Derbyshire, UK.
FPC, Evergreen Scientific, UK Suppliers: Lab M, 52 Wash Lane, Topley House, Bury BL9 6AU, UK.
Ernest F Fullam 900 Albany-Shaker Road, Latham, New York, 12110, USA.
Gallenkamp, Fisons plc, Scientific Equipment Division, Belton Road West, Loughborough, Leicestershire LE11 0TR, UK.
Gelman Sciences Ltd, Brackmills Business Park, Casewell Road, Northampton NN4 DE2, UK.
General Diagnostics, Division of Warner-Lambert Company, Morris Plains, New Jersey, 07950, USA.
Gibco Biocult Ltd (Life Technologies Ltd), Trident house, Renfrew Road, Paisley PA3 4EP, UK.
Hawksley and Sons Ltd, 12 Peter Road, Lancing, West Sussex BN15 8TH, UK.
C A Hendley Ltd, Oakwood Hill Industrial Estate, Loughton, Essex, UK.
Arnold R Horwell Ltd, 73 Maygrove Road, W. Hempstead NW6 2PB, UK.
Integrated Diagnostics Inc, Berkeley, California, USA.
Institut Pasteur, 3bd Raymond Poincaré, BP 3-92430, Marnes-la-Coquette, France.
Jencos (Scientific) Ltd, Cherrycourt Way Industrial Estate, Stanbridge Road, Leighton Buzzard, Bedfordshire LU7 8UA, UK.
Kirkgaard-Perry, Gaitherburg, Maryland, MD 20879, USA.

Laboratory Diagnostics Company Ltd, Morganville, NJ 7751, USA.

Launch Diagnostics Ltd, 16 Upper Street South, New Ash Green, Longfeld, Kent DA3 8JJ, UK.

LIP (Equipment and services) Ltd, 111 Rockfield Road, Shipley, West Yorkshire BF17 7AS, UK.

Luckham Ltd, Labro Works, Victoria Gardens, Burgess hill, Sussex RH15 9QN, UK.

Marathon Lab Supplies, Unit 6, 55-57 Park Royal Road NW10 7JJ, UK.

Mercia Diagnostics, Mercia House, Broadford Park, Shalford, Guildford, Surrey GU4 8EW, UK.

Millipore (UK) Ltd, The Boulevard, Ascot Road, Coxley Green, Watford, Hertfordshire WD1 8YW, UK.

Millipore Intertech Inc, Ashby Road, P.O. Box 255, Bedford, Massachusetts, 31730, USA.

National Collection of Type Cultures, Central Public Health Laboratory, Colindale Avenue, London NW9 5HT, UK.

NBL Gene Sciences Ltd, South Nelson Industrial Estate, Cramlington, Northumberland NE23 9HL, UK.

Northumbria Biologicals Ltd, Cramlington, Northumberland NE23 9BL, UK.

Nucleopore Corporation, 7035 Commerce Circle, Pleasanton, California, 94566, USA.

Nunc—from Gibco BRL Ltd, Unit 4, Cowley Mill Trading Estate, Longbridge Way, Uxbridge, Middlesex UB8 2YG, UK.

Nycomed (UK) Ltd, Nycomed House, 2111 Coventry Road, Sheldon, Birmingham B26 3EA, UK.

Oxoid Ltd, Wade Road, Basingstoke, Hampshire RG24 0PH, UK.

Paramount Reagents Ltd, Mast House, Derby Road, Bootle, Merseyside L20 1EA, UK.

Path/Pact, 4 Nickerson Street, Seattle, Washington 98109-1699, USA.

Peteric Ltd, Unit C, 120 Oyster Lane, Byfleet, Surrey KT14 7LE, UK.

Pharmacia Ltd, Pharmacia House, Midsomer Boulevard, Milton Keynes MK9 3HP, UK.

Pharmacia Ltd, AB Fortia, Box 604, S-75125, Uppsala, Sweden.

Promega, Delta House, Enterprise Road, Chilworth Research Centre, Southampton SO1 7NS, UK.

Rocialle Medical Ltd, Dales Manor, Business Park, Swaston, Cambridge CB2 4TJ, UK.

Shandon Southern Products Ltd, Chadwick Road, Astmoor, Runcorn, Cheshire WA7 1PR, UK.

Sigma Chemical Co Ltd, Fancy Road, Poole, Dorset BH17 7NH, UK.

Sigma Chemicals, P.O. Box 14508, St Louis, MO 63178, USA.

SWS Filtration Ltd, Great Chesterford, Saffron Walden, Essex CB10 1PL, UK.

Tri-Continent Scientific Inc, 12555 Loma Rica Drive, Grass Valley, CA 95945, USA.

Tropical Health Technology, 14 Bevills Close, Doddington, March, Cambridgeshire PE15 0TT, UK.

Wellcome Diagnostics, Temple Hill, Dartford, Kent DA1 5AH, UK.

Wellcome Diagnostics USA, Boroughs-Wellcome Company Division, North Building, 3030, Cornwallis Road, Research Triangle Park, NC27709, USA.

Whatman International Ltd, St Leonard's Road, 20/20 Maidstone, Kent ME16 0LS, UK.

Index

Index

Index